PRAISE FOR *THE NEW FEMININE BRAIN*

"The brain of today's average woman is a lot different from that of her grand-mother. The modern brain has evolved to meet the demands of a much more complex world. But if we want to be healthier and happier, it also pays to listen to old-fashioned women's intuition. Dr. Mona Lisa Schulz unlocks the mysteries of the mind in her book *The New Feminine Brain*."

—from CBS's *The Early Show*

"Schulz draws on the body's emotional centers and the body's memories to assist her work, to which she brings acute observation, remarkable experience and memory, and deep empathy."

—*Booklist*

"Recommended."

—*Library Journal*

"If you're fortunate, you'll cross the path of an authentic teacher once or twice in a lifetime. If you're wise, you'll jump at the opportunity to learn with him or her. Mona Lisa Schulz is that kind of teacher. And she's exactly what she writes about: a woman who has found her unique genius and intuition. Furthermore, she's hilariously funny, with the rare ability to take complex material and make it seem perfectly simple. Her insights on the brain are brilliant. Her insights on life are remarkable. This is a book that every woman should read—a must for our times."

—Joan Borysenko, Ph.D., author of the *New York Times* bestseller *Minding the Body, Mending the Mind* and *Inner Peace for Busy Women*

"Mona Lisa Schulz applies her unique, intuitive genius to bring us the science underpinning the Feminine. This is a must-read for anyone who seeks balance or hopes to guide others to discover it."

—Michael J. Gelb, author of the *New York Times* bestseller *How to Think Like Leonardo da Vinci* and *Discover Your Genius*

"By the end of Dr. Schulz's remarkable book, women will understand why their unique female perceptions of the world give them a rich experience of life but also leave them vulnerable to stress and illness. With its optimistic, empowering message, women will be referring to *The New Feminine Brain* for years to come."

—David Edelberg, M.D., author of *The Triple Whammy Cure*

"At last, someone with medical expertise and wisdom has laid down the genius of feminine power. This book has bridged the body and mind with such exquisite clarity that it reads ~~~~ ry. This is the first to give a medical explanation for the special power of women's minds . . . that has been seen as inferior and shameful because women do not think like men. Most important, women can understand how to enlist their full capacities and unique contributions. The feminine brain, whether it be in a male or female body, offers healing for our bodies, minds, and spirits."

—Frank Lawlis, Ph.D., *New York Times* bestselling author of *The ADD Answer*

"*The New Feminine Brain* should be in every family's medicine chest. It offers both a new model and new tools for healing and empowerment. In this era where every difference is a disability, Dr. Schulz offers us a perspective that helps us inhabit and master the universe that exists within our own brain. This book will change the way you live your life!"

—Laura Day, author of *Practical Intuition* and *The Circle*

"Dr. Mona Lisa Schulz has written a wise guidebook for women on how to thrive in a complex world filled with bewildering challenges and multiple roles. Women who do not understand the information in this book will be severely disadvantaged. Men, listen up. You need this wisdom, too."

—Larry Dossey, M.D., author of *The Extraordinary Healing Power of Ordinary Things, Reinventing Medicine,* and the *New York Times* bestseller *Healing Words*

"You don't have to be female to enjoy *The New Feminine Brain*. With her unique gift for blending rigorous knowledge and intuitive insight, hard medical facts and poignant storytelling, Mona Lisa Schulz has written a book certain to enchant everyone."

—Elkhonon Goldberg, Ph.D., author of *The Executive Brain* and *The Wisdom Paradox*

"Dr. Schulz explains why my husband needs my brain to find small objects for him and why only the left-brain, linear, step-by-step explanations of my intuitive leaps register with him! *The New Feminine Brain* will help you see why your and your mate's brains are different and how you can work better together."

—Carolyn Dean, M.D., N.D., author of *Hormone Balance*

"Prepare to discover your uniqueness, your story, and your gift in this fascinating read. A brilliant expert on the brain and a medical intuitive, Dr. Schulz is one of the most interesting healers I've ever met. As a baby boomer, I'm also now using her medical advice on keeping brain cells activated to retain memory, stimulate brain flexibility, and stabilize good moods. This is an authoritative guide on my favorite subject—the human (female) brain."

—Naomi Judd, author of *Naomi's Breakthrough Guide*

"When Mona Lisa Schulz became my doctor back in 2000, I had no idea what a profound effect she would have on my life. She is one of the most gifted women I have ever met and had the great fortune of working with."

—Wynonna Judd

f**P**

Also by Mona Lisa Schulz, M.D., Ph.D.

Awakening Intuition: Using Your Mind-Body Network for Insight and Healing

THE NEW
FEMININE BRAIN

*Developing Your
Intuitive Genius*

MONA LISA SCHULZ, M.D., PH.D.
Foreword by Christiane Northrup, M.D.

FREE PRESS
NEW YORK LONDON TORONTO SYDNEY

*f*P

FREE PRESS
A Division of Simon & Schuster, Inc.
1230 Avenue of the Americas
New York, NY 10020

First Free Press trade paperback edition 2006

FREE PRESS and colophon are trademarks of Simon & Schuster, Inc.

For information about special discounts for bulk purchases,
please contact Simon & Schuster Special Sales:
1-800-456-6798 or business@simonandschuster.com

Designed by Davina Mock

Manufactured in the United States of America

10 9 8 7 6 5 4 3 2 1

The Library of Congress has catalogued the hardcover edition as follows:
Schulz, Mona Lisa.
The new feminine brain: how women can develop their inner strengths, genius, and intuition / Mona Lisa Schulz; foreword by Christiane Northrup.
p. cm.
Includes bibliographical references and index.
1. Women—Psychology. 2. Women—Mental health. 3. Intuition. 4. Mind and body.
5. Self-help techniques. I. Title
HQ1206.S4429   2005
155.3'33—dc22   2005040149

ISBN-13: 978-0-7432-4306-3
ISBN-10:   0-7432-4306-4
ISBN-13: 978-0-7432-4307-0 (Pbk)
ISBN-10:   0-7432-4307-2 (Pbk)

NOTE TO THE READER

The information in this book is not meant to be a substitute for medical care. If you have a medical or emotional problem, see your physician or other licensed practitioner in your area. Medical intuition does not diagnose illness nor does it prescribe specific medical treatment. You should only make medical decisions in a trusting relationship with your doctor.

Human vulnerability to disease cannot be reduced to a single physical or emotional cause. Many genetic, nutritional, environmental, emotional, and other unknown factors contribute to the development of illness and disease. Although many scientific and medical studies will be cited in this book, no study is perfect. There are limitations to any scientific inquiry. Patients should work with their health care practitioners to examine for themselves what problems, relationships, habits, and situations in their lives contribute to disease and what medical, herbal and nutritional solutions are available to create health.

The client studies and medical intuitive readings presented in this book are composites of several similar cases. None represents a single identifiable individual. Sexes of partners and children have been switched frequently; occupations, names, and locations have been changed. Any similarity to any real person's name or identity is coincidental.

CONTENTS

FOREWORD
Christiane Northrup, M.D.

Mona Lisa Schulz is as close to a modern day shaman as anyone I've ever met. She moves between the worlds of the seen and unseen, the intellectual and intuitive, the conscious and the unconscious, shedding considerable light and knowledge on the areas of our lives that have remained in darkness—and have unwittingly affected both our brains and our bodies. Once she illuminates these areas and points out how and why they are affecting our life and health, she then applies her considerable clinical knowledge and expertise to assist us in healing both our bodies and our lives. I have directly benefited from this both personally and professionally.

I first met Mona Lisa in 1992, when she was in her final year of medical school and also putting the finishing touches on her Ph.D. thesis in behavioral neuroscience. She wanted to do an ob/gyn elective with me, but I declined. I was in the midst of writing *Women's Bodies, Women's Wisdom,* had two young children, and had my hands full with a large clinical practice. Though I didn't have the time to take on another student, I was fascinated by her alleged intuitive ability. So we made an agreement. She would come and spend a day seeing patients with me if she would do intuitive readings on all of them beforehand. I wanted to know how accurate she was. The answer to that was and is, "Very accurate." More important, she was able to name the emotional patterns that were often driving a patient's state of health in the first place—something that I had long suspected. Having her—a newly minted M.D./Ph.D. in my office who was also extremely intuitive—helped to validate my medical approach. Adding her intuitive data to the objective findings on physical exams and medical test data helped me care for my patients (and myself) more thoroughly and effectively. I soon changed my mind about teaching this particular student. Thus was born a long, fruitful collaboration and friendship.

In the early days of our collaboration, I often called Mona Lisa into the operating room so that she could see physically what she had "seen" intuitively. This turned out to be a perfect way for me to develop trust in my own intuition and the role of clinical intuition in medicine. Intuition doesn't take the place of intellectual and technical skills. It simply adds a much needed dimension. Quite frankly, doctors who trust their gut instinct (intuition) are better doctors.

The other invaluable credential that Mona Lisa brought to the table came from the school of life—where no formal grades are given, but which can provide the most rigorous testing program known to humanity. She earned this credential through facing life-threatening illnesses and using them as an opportunity to heal her life. Having traveled the dark territory of a twisted spine, severe dyslexia, ADD, epilepsy, narcolepsy, several massive spine operations, and a run-in with a panel truck that collapsed a lung and shattered her pelvis, she has learned a lot about what it takes to be healthy. In the process of healing from all of this, Mona Lisa developed a brain, a body, and an attitude that are very unusual. And the compensatory strategies she has come up with to work around her challenges are both practical and teachable. *The New Feminine Brain* is the result. Mona Lisa often says, "I study the most wild and woolly abnormalities there are so that I can titrate back to normal." Indeed, the patients she sees with head injury, stroke, dementia, and developmental disorders are often on the very fringes of mental health and ability. They are challenging to every branch of medicine. And she helps them and their families because she grasps the nuances of neuroscience, psychiatry, and intuition. Mona Lisa says, "I find out what's intact and pump it up—maximizing the areas of my patients' brains and lives that are sound or preserved." Having done precisely that in her own life, she knows exactly what she's talking about.

Mona Lisa's unique approach has also been hard-won because of the rather striking cultural divide between intellectual and intuitive knowledge—particularly in medicine. For years, she had to keep her identity as a medical intuitive completely separate from that of medical doctor—

despite the fact that each enhanced and strengthened the other. (She has always had to keep two completely different résumés.) In fact, she had to hide her intuitive abilities during her training. I'll never forget the time that one of her professors at the hospital told her that she had to stop her intuitive practice (something that she kept completely separate from her medical duties) or the powers-that-be would not allow her to complete her residency training. These authorities didn't believe that intuition existed or that she could "see" what she said she could see. As has happened throughout history, they were threatened by a phenomenon that they didn't understand. When she wrote *Awakening Intuition,* she "came out" as a medical intuitive but downplayed her medical knowledge.

Finally, after years of working with a "split" in her own life—trying to keep medical information and intuitive information separate, Mona Lisa has found the courage and skill to bring these two worlds together where they belong. The result is this brilliant book, *The New Feminine Brain.* It contains exactly the kind of unique information that women everywhere need to validate their own unique ways of thinking, feeling, and being in the world. And it will give them the practical tools they need to deal effectively with the challenges of mood, anxiety, attention, and memory that so many are facing today. It has been a pleasure and an honor to have witnessed and midwifed Mona Lisa during the years that it has taken to articulate the information you are about to read in the following pages. And as you will soon see, all the work and time have paid off very well indeed.

CHRISTIANE NORTHRUP, M.D., author of *Mother-Daughter Wisdom: Creating a Legacy of Emotional and Physical Health* and *Women's Bodies, Women's Wisdom*

PART ONE

This Is Your Brain

Introduction

Women have a unique feminine brain. It is different from a man's brain. And it has its own styles of thought. Yet for the last fifty years women have had to fit their brains into a "male" world. We have had to learn how to, as the song says, "walk like a man," and "talk like a man," but stay a woman inside. To accommodate these two divergent roles, our brains have had to rewire themselves.

It's a biological fact that the process of learning any new skill creates physical, structural changes in the brain. Much research has demonstrated learning-induced changes in the brain. A recent study showed that even learning to juggle objects caused physical changes in brain anatomy. When a woman learns to juggle the traditional feminine role with newer, once typically male responsibilities, her brain changes physically and functionally. And as our world has gotten more technologically complex, the task of assuming roles common to both sexes has taken its toll on women's emotional and physical health.

So just being a woman today gives you some inborn mental and emotional challenges. However, the unique wiring of your brain and body also gives you some unique gifts and abilities.

In this book, I'll tell you how, as a woman, you can keep your brain tuned in to your natural mood cycles and thought patterns, but also be able to tune in to the new challenges that you face as you go to work in the boardroom, the home, the hospital, or the office—without compromising your health.

I can help you do this because I have done it myself.

The New Feminine Brain

After four years of medical school and three years of a Ph.D. program in neuroanatomy and behavioral neuroscience, I knew how traditional science viewed the female brain. I had studied it and compared it to the male brain. I had researched how emotions are wired in the brain; how memory and attention are wired; how morality, movement, desire, and passion are wired; and how the brain and body are interconnected. But fourteen years ago, when I walked onto the medical floor at Boston City Hospital as a medical student doing a clerkship, I looked around at the other doctors and realized that a lot of women working there didn't have the traditional feminine brain I'd learned about. Sure, there were the empathetic, motherly types who went into pediatrics or family practice and in their spare time ran recycling drives and worked for the homeless. But one woman we all had pegged for pediatrics shocked us by going into surgery—the most macho of all medical specialties.

In short, my understanding of how a woman's brain is wired was turned on its head. And what I had learned in seven years of training didn't amount to a row of pins when it came to making clinical decisions about my patients. At no time was this more obvious than my first day in the hospital, when I was sent to the emergency room to examine my first patient. I looked the part of a traditional doctor in my brand-new white 100-per-cent-cotton doctor's jacket, carrying my brand-new black doctor's bag. But it soon became apparent that despite two advanced degrees and $275,000 in tuition (and student loans), the traditional—read, masculine—approach to medicine wasn't going to work for me.

All I was told about the patient was her name and age. But as soon as I heard her name, information about her started coming to me intuitively. I could see in my mind's eye where her body was affected, and at the same time, I could sense her emotional state and how that might have predisposed her to illness. With these clues, I quickly checked the reference books in the on-call room for background in illnesses and conditions associated with her symptoms and made a note of tests I might need to do to make a diagnosis. It was the intuitive information, combined with all the knowledge packed in the traditional doctor's bag of my brain, that helped me approach that first patient with some degree of skill, if not poise. Even so, using my ophthalmoscope that first time, I shone the light into my own eye, not the patient's, to her great amusement.

Though I quickly realized I wasn't going to be a traditional doctor, it seemed that I wasn't going to be like some of my female colleagues either. I still couldn't get my hair and wardrobe organized like many other women, and I didn't go for the bib jumpers and clogs of some of the female doctors headed for family practice. I knew I had to figure out how *my* brain worked so that I could fit into this system and be successful.

Today, I know that's what we all do when thrust into a new situation or encountering a problem: We learn where our strengths lie, where our areas of genius are, where our flaws and "loose screws" are, so we can cultivate the areas in which we excel, and work around our shortcomings. Back then, I figured it out by trial and error. I learned, for example, that I was really good at finding a vein and drawing blood, but I was terrible at figuring out blood gas—checking the oxygen level of the blood leaving the heart, a delicate procedure that involves inserting a needle into an artery. We medical students learned each other's strengths and weaknesses, so that together, as a team, we could combine our skills and create one big brain. Some drew blood; others took blood gas readings.

This book will show you how you have done much the same thing in your life—compensated for your weaknesses by developing your strengths. When you were born, you had a traditional female brain that combined the genetic heritage of your parents and the in utero environment in which your mother developed you until you were born. Then, as you grew up in the incubator of your childhood, that genetic heritage was molded and acculturated to life in this society.

At the same time, you discovered the ways in which you weren't Everywoman. You found unique parts of yourself that were decidedly your genius, and other parts that tripped you up. You learned very quickly what your flaws are, and chose whether or not to show that vulnerability in relationships, in vocational settings, or even in your family. You learned very quickly whether you had the attention span of a gnat or you could stare for hours at a flower or a puzzle, trying to figure it out. Your mother and father learned whether they had to give you a list and copy it in triplicate because your memory was like a sieve and you lost everything. And your friends learned very quickly whether you had a memory like the Encyclopaedia Britannica and recorded anything they said or did.

Perhaps your personality, your temperament, was your foible but also your genius. Maybe everyone thought of you as a Mother Teresa, always ready to help with a kind and caring smile. Perhaps when you became a teen, you hit a dark, rainy week and cloistered yourself until your mood lifted. Maybe you were habitually irritable, but were also capable of focusing that edginess into creating an amazing short story or a play that kept your entire class riveted. Perhaps you jumped a mile when someone sneaked up behind you; anxiety and nervousness were your challenges, but also kept you alert to what others wanted or needed. Maybe you put your obsessiveness and compulsivity to good use in a detail-oriented after-school job such as shelving books at the library or canned goods at the grocery. As you were thrust out into the adult world, you learned to identify your particular struggles with attention, memory, personality, and mood.

We all have challenges in every one of those four areas. We are not Everywoman; each of us is unique. Contrary to what I learned in my medical and scientific training, *there is no longer a traditional female brain.* This is confirmed over and over in my clinical work as a neuropsychiatrist and as a medical intuitive. The complex world we now live in—like the complex hospital world into which I was thrust in 1991—has molded, remolded, and rebuilt our brains. This capacity of the brain to remold itself is what science calls "plasticity." Women's brains today physically reflect our responses to the unique challenges that confront us. And our brains continue to change as we struggle with our list of expectations: to be mothers, to hold down full-time jobs, to come home and run households, to be attentive to our mates or partners, to be active in the community.

While juggling all these roles, we are further challenged by all the ways in which information comes to us today. Centuries ago, we got our information by talking to friends and neighbors over the back fence, and from letters, telegrams, books, and newspapers. Then came the telephone, radio, and TV. Now we have satellite radio and cable TV, email, pagers, cell phones, the personal digital assistant, the Web. We have to perceive and pay attention to all this information, sort through it for what's important, and try to remember that. Even if you choose only one television information channel, such as CNN or ESPN, you're really getting several: The newscaster is speaking on the main audio/visual track while running text across the bottom of the screen feeds you updates; and then there are the commercials.

All of this input affects your perception, attention, and memory circuits. A recent study showed that children who watch too much television too early in their lives have an increased risk of developing attention deficit disorder (ADD). Cartoons in particular feature frequent changes of scenes with manic activity that can "prime" a child's brain to shift quickly from one topic to another instead of learning to focus and maintain attention in the way needed to learn and stay on task in a classroom.

Your temperament, too, affects your capacity to perceive, pay attention, and remember. If you are moody, irritable, or nervous, or if you're even a bit obsessive or compulsive, your ability to perceive, process, attend to, and remember information will be challenged by today's information environment. And finally, even though the brain's capacity for adaptation is immense, your unique genetic predisposition for handling information will place certain limits on your brain's ability to change. All these factors will remold the brain you were born with so that it can be as efficient as possible. But still your brain can get tripped up by the main demands it faces.

This book will teach you how to appreciate, care for, and cultivate your unique genius, your brain's special power. You'll come to understand *how your brain works, how it is wired*—both your traditional brain and your *New* Feminine Brain. You will learn how your particular challenges are also wired into your brain. For instance, perhaps you have problems paying attention to a lecture or to directions your boss gives you for finishing a task or you have trouble remembering names and dates. Perhaps you have a winning personality that can get you in any door, but you also have problems with temperament and mood, with irritability or anxiety, any of which can affect how you fit in, as well as how you follow rules. Or, perhaps your challenges affect your ability to cultivate your own creative impulses in your vocation, to express your purpose in life.

Are you able to use your brain's power for building a sense of security and self-esteem, for feeling rewarded in life, and for avoiding addictive behavior? How do you use your brain's unique gifts in relationships? Are you able to feel a healthy empathy or do you love and feel so much that it hurts? Can you bond with children, your own and other people's? Do you have a capacity to love others? To love yourself? How do you express your uniqueness or eccentricities? Can you appreciate them? Can you learn to love the eccentricities of others? We'll deal with all these questions and how the New Feminine Brain's makeup affects your answers.

When I speak of the *New* Feminine Brain, I don't mean to imply that the brain of our female ancestors was not as good as ours today. Newer is not better, just different. Calling it the New Feminine Brain simply acknowledges the huge impact of all the different challenges women face today. As a result of the many competing pressures we have to deal with, we also have an increase in chronic fatigue syndrome, fibromyalgia, environmental illness, multiple sclerosis, alcoholism, eating addiction, compulsive gambling, eBay addiction, ADHD (attention deficit and hyperactivity disorder), and obsessive-compulsive and attachment disorders. Many of these illnesses of body and brain that women struggle with now simply were not as prevalent in the ancestral brain—even a couple of generations ago.

Intuition

As we talk about all of these psychological and biological challenges, we will also talk about the importance of intuition—the ability to make good, beneficial, or correct decisions with insufficient information. Normally, we make decisions based on concrete information that we can see or hear. However, when we can't get enough facts from the outside world—or we are overwhelmed by too much information—we can function effectively by using our intuition. Despite what you've been led to believe, intuition doesn't come to you through tea leaves, tarot cards, a Ouija board, or from another world. *Intuition is a natural product of your brain and body.*

In all my university studies in neuroscience there was never any discussion of intuition. Yet we cannot talk about the New Feminine Brain *without* talking about intuition. Our lives as women today are bombarded with greater and greater complexity, so the New Feminine Brain has to exaggerate—to overdevelop—its intuition. We women today need to appreciate our intuition, which has sometimes been denigrated by our culture. We need to understand how it's wired into our brain and body and develop it further. Intuition helps us learn to adapt to what the world demands of us.

Many people try a variety of routes to gain access to their intuition and improve it. There's a lot of New Age nonsense about how to increase intuition, from burning incense to help pump up your intuitive circuits to wearing crystals to sitting under a pyramid. But intuition isn't enhanced by New Age paraphernalia. You don't need external devices to be intuitive.

If you have a brain and a body and you sleep at night, by definition, you have all the equipment you need to be intuitive. By managing problems with mood (Chapters 4 and 5), anxiety (Chapters 6 and 7), attention (Chapter 9), and memory (Chapter 10), you can clear out and open up brain pathways for intuition on your own. Learning your unique left brain/right brain style (Chapter 1), and learning your body's tendencies toward illness, also helps you find and use your intuition. In fact, the areas of your feminine brain and body that make you unique—whether you have an exceptional talent or are challenged by depression, anxiety, or other health problems—are exactly where to look to find your intuition.

I depend a lot on my own intuition and started to learn to do so almost as soon as I joined the working world of the hospital. During one of my first days on the medical floor at Boston City Hospital, I wrote an order on a patient's chart but forgot to put up the little red flag that alerts the nurses to check for a new order. I was standing near the nursing station in my white doctor's coat, when an immense presence started moving toward me from the other end of the hallway. Dressed all in white, from the old-fashioned nurse's cap to the white stockings and lace-up shoes, this wasn't just any nurse: It was the head nurse. Boom, boom, boom, boom, she marched up the hallway, barking "Doctor! Doctor!" I was looking all around to see who she was talking to, until I realized she was talking to me. "Did you put this chart on the order stand?" she demanded. I could only stammer, "Ah, ah, ah." "You didn't put the flag up," she continued. "This isn't going to happen again, is it, Doctor?" she said pointedly. All I could squeak out was a meek, "N-n-no." After that, I realized that the nurses are the ones really in charge.

During those first weeks on the medical floor I realized very quickly which female doctors would survive this hazing and which ones would not. If you tried to be Marcus Welby—to issue orders like one of the male doctors—the nurses would run you into the ground. If, on the other hand, you tried to be empathetic or overly familiar—to bond as one of the girls—they would also cut you down. They could detect a brown-noser a floor away. Yet, in spite of the nurses' toughness, they were also the most tuned in to their patients—the most intuitive—of all the health professionals. I had to learn very quickly how to utilize both my brain and my intuition to master the subtleties of the situation.

Different Women, Different New Feminine Brains

You can see how differently New Feminine Brains are wired by looking at how you and your friends act in different situations. Let's take three women, Norma, Mildred, and Mandy, each of whom decided to redecorate her living room. On Saturday mornings Mandy would phone Norma and suggest that they go pick out a fabric for Norma's couch. Norma would put her off by saying, "I've got to pay my bills," but Mandy would arrive at her door anyway, honking the horn and waving a cup of coffee. Off they'd go to the store, and Norma would pick out swatches and bring them home. For three solid years, they looked at fabrics. Norma would come home, drape the swatches over her couch, and never choose one, because nothing seemed quite right. "Quite right" and "just so" behavior is the sine qua non of an obsessive-compulsive, anxiety-ridden kind of wiring in the brain. Suddenly, one Saturday, Norma found a new couch in a fabric she loved, bought it, and paid in cash. Everyone, including Norma, thinks the couch is perfectly divine.

Mandy, too, had been thinking about decorating for a long time. Then one Saturday night, while she was watching television with her best friend, Liz, she suddenly announced, "Come on, we're going to buy a couch." Off they drove to L.L. Home—a subsidiary of L.L. Bean that is open twenty-four hours—where Mandy ordered an entire living room set in leather. She had never visited the store before or picked out a swatch. Yet at 10:45 p.m. on a Saturday night, she slapped down her credit card and bought an entire suite. Liz thought Mandy was having a psychotic episode, but Mandy loves her furniture, and her cats love it, too—something she had failed to consider in her enthusiasm. And then there's the impulsively incurred credit-card debt that she's still paying off. (Unlike Mandy, Norma not only plans her purchases carefully but never incurs any debt.)

Norma and Mandy represent two extremes. On one end is Norma with her swatches, an example of compulsivity and perfectionism—organizing and planning. These functions occur in one area of the brain and usually lead to the area that governs movement. But Norma takes a long time to get out of one brain area and to the next for movement and execution. Mandy is the other extreme—impulsive. Her brain areas for imagination and perception are very active, but then she skips organization and planning almost completely and goes right to movement—often without thinking through the consequences.

Their friend Mildred is the head researcher in the medical firm for which they all work. She falls somewhere between Norma and Mandy. When Mildred decided to buy a couch, she looked through catalogues for a week or so, then drove calmly (and always within the speed limit) to the furniture store. She had a relaxed, twenty-minute discussion with the salesperson, then wrote out a check and arranged for delivery, after checking her appointment book to make sure she could be at home. Mildred's brain in this circumstance progresses in an orderly way from the area for perception and attention to organization and planning, and then to movement and execution.

Yet, for all her balance, Mildred often has to rely on her friends. Norma, as Mildred's business administrator, lends Mildred her perfectionism and supreme organizational skills. Mandy, Mildred's research partner, has tremendous creativity and isn't held back by convention; she lends Mildred her spontaneity. Together, the three friends have one complete brain.

In this simple example of buying furniture, you can see clearly how three different feminine brains, each with its own unique genetic heritage, approach a task and execute it according to their unique styles of attention, memory, personality, temperament, mood, and anxiety. But while the brain is highly adaptable, the body is less so. One of the important lessons you'll learn in this book is what happens to your body when you ignore or override your brain's unique gifts and challenges.

Keeping Brain and Body Together

I learned this the hard way. After I completed my M.D./Ph.D. program in Boston, I was all set to go south for a residency in neurology. Several days before I was supposed to begin, I blew out two vertebral discs in my neck, which paralyzed my left hand, so I had to postpone the residency. In the interim, I took a job working with Christiane Northrup, M.D., an expert on women's health, well known for her innovative work as an obstetrician-gynecologist at her clinic on the Maine coast. Still, the last place I ever expected to find myself was working with another doctor, especially one like Chris, who had an angel mobile flying over her desk, and ate roasted tofu instead of prime rib. I'm sure people who knew me thought I'd gone soft in my head, because from that moment on, half of my career turned to intuition. I had learned in medical school that I had a talent for medical intuition, but even more important, it seemed that whenever I *didn't* use my intuition, my own body got sick. So while I took advanced training in psychiatry, I began to do phone consultations as a medical intuitive.

How this works is that a person calls and gives me his name and age, and I describe a specific emotional situation in his life that might predispose him to illness. Then I scan his body intuitively to see where he might be prone to physical challenges. Our relationship isn't that of doctor and patient; my clients are required to sign a consent form before our session acknowledging that. But in our sessions, people learn how their body and brain are uniquely wired for intuition, and how, if they don't listen to their *brain* intuition about what they need to do with their life, their *body* intuition will let them know through symptoms of illness.

For a while, I was leading a double life. I was either in the hospital being a medical doctor or I was on the phone being a medical intuitive. I even wrote a book, *Awakening Intuition,* to teach people how to use their mind-body connections for insight and healing. Then I blew out eight more discs in my spine and had to have surgery implanting a series of steel rods from my neck to lower back. (On an X-ray, my spine now looks like the Brooklyn Bridge standing on end.) Shortly after I recovered, I was at a bookstore signing copies of my book, when an ethereal-looking woman planted herself in front of me and asked, "Do you think that your health problems in your spine are because you're living a split life? They say that if people have two divergent personalities, they snap. Do you think having two separate careers is bad for your body?"

At that moment I had my Sharpie pen poised to write an inscription, and a long line of people waiting to have their books signed. I was in no mood to have some stranger named Ariel telling me about my health or my career. But weeks later, when I went to my doctor after rupturing yet another disc in my neck, he said, "You know, you can't keep doing this. You have to find out why you're blowing all these discs."

I walked out of his office feeling really shaken, because I finally realized that my body couldn't take it anymore. I hated to concede that Ariel was right, but I had to admit, *I'm a doctor and I'm a medical intuitive, and separating those two identities in practice, legally, is important. But trying to separate them in my psyche—in my understanding of who I am—could kill me.*

Mine is an extreme case—in line with my extremely intuitive and impulsive temperament—but you can see that, if you don't perceive, accept, and appreciate your own unique genius, and adapt your life to it, your body will snap. Maybe it already has snapped to some degree or other. You will learn where your body's vulnerable spots are when you take the body questionnaire later in the book.

Another good way to see how the different parts of the brain express themselves is for me to take you on a brief visit to my neuropsychiatry clinic. My patients are unique among the medical population. They have disorders that most doctors in my part of Maine don't treat, such as autism, mental retardation, Asperger's syndrome, brain injuries, stroke, dementia, epilepsy, and multiple sclerosis. All of these disorders exaggerate one or more of the brain networks you'll be learning about in this book. In medical school, we were told that cases could be divided into two groups: "horses," or common disorders, and "zebras," out-of-the-ordinary complaints. I had trouble paying attention to ordinary cases. Zebras, on the other hand, sparked my interest. I don't treat horses. I treat zebras.

My clinic is a symphony of eccentricity and uniqueness. At one moment, we might have someone locked in the bathroom, while outside the door, a very normal, horse-like caretaker is saying, "Mary, Mary. Unlock the door. Come out of the bathroom, now!" Inside, Mary is carefully tearing apart the toilet paper and making a neat pile of the individual sheets. At the same time, in the waiting room someone is changing the dial of the radio from easy listening to a rock station that's playing the Rolling Stones' "Nineteenth Nervous Breakdown." In the far corner, a man with fifteen TV remotes stuffed in his pockets is saying to no one in particular, "Honest, I wasn't there when they stole the TVs. I was just watching."

All of these people have wonderful hearts, and I find something to love in every one. Each one has an area of uniqueness—and though it's clearly extreme, it's only an exaggerated form of a behavior that we all have to a degree. Like Mary in the bathroom, we all have an area of compulsivity—something we pay extremely close attention to and want to dissect to pieces. We all have an area of sociopathy, like the guy with the remotes—the small white lies we tell in daily life that help us fit into society. And all of us have our unique music in the brain. In the following chapters, we will explore the symphony of sound in the New Feminine Brain. You'll discover the songs all women share, the unique sounds that are your genius, and the discordant notes that have kept you from fully utilizing your brain's power to adapt to life's changing demands.

COMING TO TERMS WITH THE UNIQUE FEMININE BRAIN

I first faced my own feminine brain's *emotional style* around puberty. On the first day of school in the eighth grade, I was fidgeting at my desk. The teacher looked at me and snapped, "Stop fiddling around with things on your desk . . . you're driving me crazy." I started crying, which really drove her crazy, and she sent me to the guidance office.

I told the guidance counselor why I was crying and he told me, "You're never going to be able to go anywhere in life if you cry like that in public. You've got to be more thick-skinned." (Not all girls and women are like this, of course, but some of us are.) I figured I'd make up for my emotional thin skin by building up my intellect and getting "brain-tough." From the age of seven, I had known I wanted to be a doctor and a scientist. I worked hard and got into Brown University.

During my sophomore year at Brown as a premed student, I was failing organic chemistry, which is known as a course that derails many wannabe doctors. The harder I studied, the lower my test scores were. Those scores went from 60 percent to a 26 percent to an all-time low of 6 percent (yes, out of 100 percent).

To continue in premed, I had to pass organic chemistry. So, I hired a tutor to study for the final exam, which counted toward half of the final grade. My average grade going into the final was so low, I overheard one of the teaching assistants say, "The Mona Lisa is going to smile again in this same class next year." After hours of tutoring, though, the information all magically came together in my mind at the testing, and I got 105 percent on the final. That did make me smile.

This embarrassing situation had actually turned into a learning experience for me. I had noticed that many other people were also failing and the majority of them were women. Then, as now, women tend to approach the learning process in classes differently. No matter how hard I work to learn something, I never learn well "in captivity," that is, in the situation where the teacher lectures and the student listens, takes notes, learns the information, and finally takes the test. As a result, I never did well in any of those large college lecture lab classes. But I learned what I needed to do to master the material.

When I was graduated from Brown, I got a job in a research lab. To my amazement, I found that I excelled at learning in the more "hands-on," practical, learning environment. Working as a scientist, I was able to pay my way through medical school. I created an artificial gonorrhea cell that did nearly everything a real cell does. I was able to publish several papers because I was well suited to designing experiments and learning the scientific principles as they applied to a project as I went along.

My success at research, not my premed grades, probably got me into an M.D./Ph.D. program at Boston University. Unfortunately for me, medical school classes are frequently taught in the same didactic style as premedical education. So once again I sat for six to eight hours a day listening to teachers lecture. I took notes, studied hard, and failed. Once again, I wasn't alone. By the end of the first year of med school, twelve people were failing at least one class and nine of them were women. Since our medical school class was almost exactly 50 percent women and 50 percent men, I couldn't figure out why a disproportionate number of women was failing. This time, the class I was having problems with was gross anatomy. Since I wanted to do my Ph.D. in neuroanatomy, I was scared and embarrassed.

I went to the head of the anatomy department to get a tutor. I showed Dr. Brown (not his real name) all my diagrams, charts, and notes, and asked him to please tell me what I was doing wrong, why I had failed the exam. I looked at him, he looked at me, and I started to cry, just like when I was back in the eighth grade. I felt like an absolute failure. First, I was an emotional failure, because I couldn't *not* cry when I was very upset. Secondly, I was an intellectual failure. I was starting to think I was stupid and didn't belong anywhere near a graduate school or a medical school, let alone a patient. As I stood there marinating in self-pity and despair, Dr. Brown said, "I can tell by your notes and charts that you have a different way of learning. You have to see the whole picture before you can understand and demonstrate your knowledge of the details on the exam. Don't worry. This will all come together on the makeup exam."

I thought he was just being nice because I was an "emotional woman" crying in his office. Having nothing left to lose, I said, "You're just being nice because I'm crying." He disagreed, saying he had already told a few students not to bother taking the retest but to instead come back and repeat the whole first year of medical school.

Using Woman's Intuition in a Field Dominated by Men

For the entire next few months, I studied with another failing female medical student, Lynn. We devoted ourselves to the material day and night. Yet we couldn't possibly memorize everything in the textbooks. We simply didn't have enough time. Intuitively, I got a strong sense that we should, however, learn in detail the anatomy of the male and female reproductive systems, especially its "lymphatic drainage."

Both Lynn and I passed the makeup final exam. I got 103 percent. We both nailed the essay, which was worth 30 percent of our score: "Please describe the lymphatic drainage of the uterus, ovaries, penis, and testicles."

Who knew? We had followed our intuition, we were prepared, and we succeeded. This was the first time I successfully used intuition in medicine. And it became clear to me that it was important to use that part of my brain along with the studying and hard work.

The best part of this difficult experience was not successfully passing gross anatomy in the first year of medical school and staying on the path to becoming a doctor. The best, most healing aspect was finding out that *intuition matters* and having the professor, Dr. Brown, validate that *there is merit in my unique style of learning*. That's why I know that I can help you learn about your intuition and your own brain's style of dealing with information—and with life!

Two Brains in One: Using Two Brain Styles to Succeed

I eventually figured out that the traditional "mind-set" with which other people approach class material and learn is typical of male brains. I'd listen to the teacher with my native feminine brain style, but learn the information in the male brain style. By also using my intuition, eventually I passed every test and was graduated. It was a lot of work, but it was worth it. I learned to see, think, and act like a man *and* a woman. But over time, that sort of overwork and overcompensation will wear you down and take its toll on your brain and body. It did for me—and it does for most women.

The world's changing demands on women force us to sprout dual brain types to adapt and accomplish all of our tasks. On top of our inborn feminine wiring, we must develop or sprout new pathways in the brain—new responses, actions, and behaviors, too—to survive in jobs and careers that require a more male, compartmentalized brain style. We have to develop more compartmentalized brain pathways for separating emotion and empathy so that we can make key business decisions. We have to develop a way of walking and talking in the business world that masks our moods and fears. We have to develop attentional pathways and memory pathways that accommodate the huge amounts of information that come at us from the media. And we have to figure out how to gain access to our intuition and use it to survive and thrive.

Developing more masculine brain pathways on top of her inborn feminine brain style comes at a cost to a woman's emotional, intellectual, and physical health. Her brain, the New Feminine Brain, doesn't have all the bugs worked out of it. Women may develop moodiness, depression, nervousness, anxiety, inattention, and problems with learning and memory. If you are emotionally porous, whatever you attempt to compartmentalize or shut down may actually get overloaded and increase your risk for developing certain health problems. The New Feminine Brain's recently acquired brain pathways can create tension with the old brain and body, leaving a woman stuck in the middle, unable to make key decisions about her life, including vocational goals, relationships, or her place in society.

"What should I do with my life?"

"Should I take this job or go back to college?"

"Should I stay in this relationship or get a divorce?"

"Should I have a baby right away, or should I wait?"

We are bombarded every day with too many choices and too many decisions to make.

Making balanced decisions every day requires a healthy brain. By that, I mean a brain that can learn and remember and has the capacity for stable emotions. If you have problems with depression, excessive anxiety and panic, attention deficit disorder, or problems with memory, you can get stuck when you try to make decisions. How do you live your life to its fullest and maximize your potential when emotional stress, information overload, or inertia overwhelms you? You learn to keep your brain-body pathways open and healthy.

Women's and men's brains are wired differently for mood, anxiety, attention, and memory. And women's and men's bodies are vulnerable to illness in different ways. How a woman's brain and body have been shaped by emotion, learning, health, and illness determines how her body receives intuitive information. Learning your body's tendency toward symptoms of illness also helps you get in touch with your intuition and use it.

In Chapter 1, you learn how your feminine brain may be wired between its left and right hemispheres. In Chapters 3–8, you learn how your feminine brain circuits are shaped for experiencing *feelings* that can predispose you to mood problems and anxiety. In Chapters 9, 10, and 11, you learn how your brain is uniquely wired for thought, which may cause you to pay attention, learn, and remember differently. *These feminine brain circuits that give you the most difficulty are the very areas of your brain through which intuition can come to you.* To put this in a more positive way: What makes you different—your tendency toward moodiness, depression, anxiety, panic, dyslexia, attention deficit disorder, or memory problems—can actually provide you with a unique capacity for intuition. You can learn to appreciate and maintain these natural mood cycles and thought patterns. And learning your personal language of intuition will ultimately help you have a healthier mood and lower, healthier levels of anxiety. It will also help you pay attention, have a sharper mind, and better memory.

This is not a passive book. Don't think you can just sit down and read it. You're going to need a pencil and some paper. You're going to be drawing. You're going to be filling out questionnaires. One questionnaire will walk you through a series of situations from daily life. Your responses will show you how your unique feminine brain works. You can also get your loved ones to answer the questionnaire and see how their unique brains are wired. Then, by filling out another questionnaire, you'll find out how your body speaks to you through symptoms, so that you learn to cultivate your brain's unique genius.

I'll also be telling you about typical cases from my neuropsychiatry clinic, and stories of some of my clients from my practice as a medical intuitive. From the stories of my patients and clients, you will see how various people have learned to cultivate the unique genius of their New Feminine Brains by understanding how their brains are wired and then rewiring those parts that made it harder to handle their lives. And you will learn how to rewire your own brain by learning new behaviors with the help of exercises, nutritional supplements, and—under your doctor's supervision—the latest medications.

In my first book, *Awakening Intuition,* I wrote about the science that supports intuition and the fact that emotions have very definite physical effects on the body. *The New Feminine Brain* focuses on how our femaleness is naturally wired into our brain and how to develop and use our feminine intuition in order to understand our brains, bodies, and emotions. We'll start with a look at how our brains work compared to men's.

All of this will help you see how to keep yourself well, prevent illness, and improve your health—because a lot of your health depends on what you do for yourself.

Most of psychiatry—including talk therapy—doesn't work much of the time or for very long. In comparison, in internal medicine, most patients readily respond to treatment because the diseases are much easier to diagnose and treat. If someone has a bladder infection, you can see evidence of disease by reading the patient's vitals and looking at the bacteria in the urine under a microscope. After the patient gets antibiotics, her vitals return to normal, the bacteria disappear, and the patient rapidly gets better.

Treating the psyche is not nearly so straightforward. The most common forms of depression and anxiety cannot be accurately diagnosed with a scan or blood test and the treatments that are available, medicine and psychotherapy, do not have lasting, permanent, dramatic effects that can readily be measured. It's common for many women and men to be in "talk therapy" for years, even decades, without measurable change or improvement other than a sense of "social support." Millions of people take Prozac, Zoloft, Valium, Xanax, or go from medicine to medicine looking for relief and, although they may experience a year or two of improvement, eventually their symptoms return, limiting their relationships, careers, and finances.

What's worse, problems with the psyche don't stay in the psyche. Eventually, chronic depression and anxiety increase your chances of having debilitating health problems including obesity, heart disease, pain disorders, Alzheimer's disease, dementia, and cancer.

This book is going to show you how to get your life on the right track and on the track you want to be. It's going to let you pull together your hopes and your reality. You'll see why you keep going after the wrong goals and the wrong guys. You're going to introduce your right brain to your left brain so you can live in harmony with your body, capture your intuitive genius, and live out your dreams and potential.

Let's start with a look at how our feminine brains work compared to men's.

ONE

It Takes Two:
Right Brain, Left Brain,
Women's Brain, Men's Brain

Much of nature is organized in twos: male–female, yang–yin, right–left, rational–intuitive. We each have a unique blend of these opposites, a combination of male and female traits and right-brain/left-brain tendencies that we use every day of our lives. To have truly balanced emotional, mental, and physical health, we need to use both sides of our brain. Although it is possible to accomplish almost any feat alone if we apply ourselves, the process almost always goes more smoothly if we have support from someone or something. Sure, you can open a small jar with one hand tied behind your back, but it's easier to use both hands or a tool. Similarly, as you work and play, it will always be easier and better for you to use both sides of your brain.

If you've been in an airport recently, you've undoubtedly heard this announcement: "Before you leave the baggage claim area, check to make sure you have your own bags. Many bags look alike." The same can be said for the female and male brains, which are more alike than they are different. Yet the differences are crucial to understanding ourselves and each other. There is an obvious difference, for instance, in how men and women feel emotions and think about things: Women tend to pay attention to the world differently than men do and have different styles of remembering things. Women also have greater problems with depression, mood, and anxiety.

Why are women more prone to depression and anxiety? What makes women more likely to suffer from attention problems (ADD or ADHD), although they are underdiagnosed, and memory problems (including Alzheimer's disease)? Hormones determine how your brain is organized and the degree to which your brain is more feminized or more masculinized. The "sex" of your brain—its hormonally associated tinge—affects how much you use your right or left brain to think, feel, listen, and use language. It also affects how you see the world, what you pay attention to and ultimately remember, and how you attend to your inner experiences. Whether your brain is more hormonally masculine or feminine also affects the likelihood of your developing ADHD/ADD, memory problems like Alzheimer's disease, or mood disorders, like depression and anxiety. The sex of your brain will ultimately determine how you want to maximize your brain's potential, that is, what kinds of treatments or efforts will work and which will fail. Finally, how your brain has been organized by hormones and whether you depend more on your right or left brain also determine how your mind and body are wired for intuition.

The Traditional Female Brain Versus the Traditional Male Brain

Women's brains are changing as a result of internal and external opportunities and pressures that are unique to our time and culture. But to understand the New Feminine Brain, we first need to know how the traditional female brain functions.

THE TRADITIONAL FEMALE BRAIN HAS MORE CONNECTIONS BETWEEN BRAIN AREAS

Male and Female Brain Traits

Traditional Female Brain Traits	Traditional Male Brain Traits
More connections between brain areas	Fewer connections between brain areas
More connectivity	More compartmentalization
More likely to think about multiple things at a time	More likely to think about one thing at a time
Greater capacity for growth and change over time (plasticity)	Less capacity for growth and change, more anatomic stability

The traditional male brain is 10 percent larger than the traditional female brain but has *fewer connections* between the cells. The traditional female brain may be smaller but it has more connections between brain cells. The corpus callosum, which connects the two hemispheres, is bigger in women. These basic structural differences may explain some of the differences between men and women in how they see the world, what they pay attention to, how they remember events, and how they get in touch with their intuition. These differences also help explain the unique challenges that the New Feminine Brain has with attention, memory, mood, and anxiety—the Big Four challenges that we'll be dealing with in the next chapters. They also provide insight into how women and girls approach relationships, eat and sleep, and deal with weight and pain.

Although it is larger, the traditional male brain, with more nerve cells and fewer connections, is like a house with a lot of incoming phone lines but no extensions: You can only talk to one person at a time. The traditional female brain, on the other hand, is like a house with only one incoming line but multiple extensions: Several people can talk on the line at the same time, so there are more connections among all the parties. It's more integrated and integrative. The male brain functions more like a cell phone—only one party or part of the brain can talk at a time. Like a two-way radio, on a cell phone, when one person talks, the other person's speaker automatically shuts off, so the receiver can only listen. This is not a normal way to converse, as far as I'm concerned. It reminds me of a dinner party at a friend's house where I practically had to take a number if I wanted to speak. One person would say something, then there would be a long pause. Finally, someone else would say, "Are you finished? Can I say something?" and the first person would say, "Yes, I'd really like to hear what you have to say." Silence. "Well, in response to what you said, I was thinking . . ." It made me want to shriek. Where I grew up, everyone talked at the same time, so you could listen to what others were saying and also interject. We didn't consider it rude; it seemed natural.

With fewer connections, the traditional male brain has more precision in its focus and differentiation (or specialization) between its various parts. When one area of the brain is functioning, the other areas are relatively silent; you get one clear signal, while the others are relatively muted. So in the traditional male brain, one issue appears on the neural screen at a time. As a result, it may be easier for the individual with such a brain to block out intuitive information while going about daily tasks. That's not true of the traditional female brain: When more areas "talk" at once, there won't be one clear signal, but the various signals will be closely integrated—including intuition. So, in the traditional female brain, many issues appear on your mental screen simultaneously. The kids, the pets, the job, the taxes, the upcoming payroll, the lawn, a possible war, the abducted teenager in the news, all of it. The traditional male brain may seem to process things more tidily: It opens a single file at a time, deals with it, and closes it. But it can't always compare information between files, understand them as a whole, or make associations and inferences—which is part of intuition's genius.

On the other hand, because the feminine brain has so many issues actively processing simultaneously, this can take a toll on attention and memory. Juggling all those files at once can affect organization and "neatness." For some genetically susceptible individuals, the feminine brain can be predisposed to depression and mood disorders and anxiety. In others, it may increase the risk for obesity and eating disorders, hormonal and reproductive problems, and immune system disorders.

One type of brain isn't superior to the other—they're just different. From an evolutionary standpoint, the way the traditional male and female brains are organized makes sense. Hundreds of thousands of years ago, the specialized male brain adapted to perform highly focused tasks, such as hunting and protecting the tribe, while the traditional female brain with its greater connectivity was well suited to the more diversified simultaneous tasks of child rearing, gathering diverse food substances close to home, and maintaining cohesiveness of the family unit and connections among the tribal families.

THE TRADITIONAL FEMALE BRAIN HAS A GREATER CAPACITY TO SPROUT CONNECTIONS, OR CHANGE "SHAPE" OVER TIME

Not only are there more connections in the female brain, those connections can proliferate and change over time in response to stimulation and new, more challenging environments. This capacity for plasticity—sprouting new connections and changing over time—is influenced by hormones, among other factors, which shape, and turn on and off, the brain's development. With the onset of puberty, hormones catalyze a wave of remodeling of brain cell connections (synapses). How fast a girl matures depends on the balance between the gas pedal of growth (estrogen) and the brake pedal (progesterone). Hormones even govern our brains' responsiveness to injury: It is well known that women have a greater capacity for recovery from brain injury and stroke, which seems to be mediated by hormones.

Repeated changes in hormone levels through the menstrual cycle, pregnancy, childbirth, and menopause may help the female brain develop its characteristic extensive pathways between cells. Additional pathways in the brain can also sprout as a result of medical treatment with hormone replacement therapy and birth control pills, and treatments for infertility and cancer (particularly with tamoxifen). All these additional pathways may help your feminine brain adapt better than the male brain to changes and challenges in your internal and external environments.

The "Sex" of Your Brain

I don't mean to imply that differences between male and female brains are clear-cut. The degree of feminization or masculinization—the "gender" of the brain—varies widely from woman to woman and from man to man. At one extreme of the spectrum is the traditional male brain; at the other, the traditional female brain. Yet the masculinization or feminization of brain regions may vary from one area to another *even within one brain.* So, it's possible that you could have both the mood circuits of a traditional female brain and the visuospatial, map-reading capabilities of the traditional male brain. You might "throw like a boy," for instance, but "talk like a girl."

Language and the Female Brain

I heard about a fascinating case study at a neurology lecture. An expert Braille instructor, a woman who had been born blind, had a stroke in her fifties. The stroke knocked out the visual area in both the right and left hemispheres of her brain. When the neurologist first visited her in the hospital, he said, "Mrs. Jones, I have bad news and good news. The bad news is you have had a stroke in both sides of your brain in both the occipital lobe areas that are critical for vision. The good news is that since you're blind, you won't even miss these areas." Mrs. Jones was encouraged and reassured, and said, "Please hand me my address book so I can call and tell my friends." But when the doctor handed her the Braille address book, Mrs. Jones was horrified to find that she could no longer read it. When she placed her fingers on the elevated dots on the pages, they meant nothing to her.

When women have a left hemisphere stroke, they initially lose language but almost always have a nearly complete recovery. Why? Women's language is more likely than men's to be organized bilaterally, that is, in both the right brain and the left brain. In addition to having a sex-based advantage for plasticity and sprouting new pathways around the injury, a woman is more likely to be able to use her "spare" right hemisphere to pick up the slack in language function.

Unfortunately, Mrs. Jones had stroked out both hemispheres' "visual" areas, which had adapted to allow her to "read" Braille with her hands. Since both sides of her brain were affected by the stroke, she didn't have a "spare" brain area with which to recover that reading function. Any remaining plasticity wasn't likely to help her recover from such a devastating stroke. She also had such severe underlying cerebrovascular disease—heart and blood vessel disease—that she was at high risk to suffer subsequent strokes. If her underlying disease hadn't been quite so advanced, I would have encouraged her to follow some of the recommendations in Chapter 10 of this book in order to try to promote healing in the brain and the growth of pathways that would compensate for those the stroke had destroyed. Mrs. Jones's body obviously had trouble handling cholesterol, which promotes narrowing of the arteries, and had what's called an inflammatory response. If caught earlier, she could have taken massive amounts of antioxidants under her physician's supervision and gotten acupuncture to treat her cerebrovascular disease. Traditional Chinese Medicine and Chinese herbs are also sometimes helpful in opening the energy flow between brain and heart and in blood vessels.

Mrs. Jones's tragic experience, like many severe brain injuries, helps us understand how the brain works. The occipital lobe, or visual area, of the brain of a blind person doesn't receive visual input from the outside world. This area of the brain normally takes images and translates them into electrical signals that the brain can process for emotions, behavior, learning, and memory. But the brain is resourceful and a congenitally blind person's occipital lobe can be trained to "bring sight" to his fingertips. The previously unused visual area in the brain learns how to process sensation and movement in the fingers and its cells "morph," changing their electrical properties, so that they acquire the properties of another sense—the sense of movement.

Women Use Their Right and Left Brains Differently Than Men

Because the left and right hemispheres of the brain differ anatomically in the functions they perform, we say that the brain is asymmetrical. The right brain usually controls movement of the left side of the body and the left brain usually controls the right side of the body.

Both men and women need to use both sides of their brains to be healthy. We all need to see the world accurately, pay attention when we need to, remember things, make decisions, and use our intuition. However, women and men use their right brain and left brain differently. Traditionally, men have ways of distributing "brain function" between both hemispheres that are different from women's. Of course, individuals may deviate from this typical organization, but generally a man uses his head differently than a woman to:

1. Write or perform *skilled movement* like painting, hitting a baseball, etc. (called *handedness*)
2. Use *language*: talk about feelings; take a gut feeling, a hunch, and translate it into words
3. Experience *emotions* and communicate those feelings via facial expression, voice tone, and gesture
4. *See in three dimensions* (called visuospatial perception)
5. Pay *attention* and *remember* things
6. *Feel pain* and have awareness of the state of health in one's body
7. Be in contact with one's *intuition*

Since women's and men's brains are wired differently, they have differing susceptibilities to emotional and physical health problems, too. For example, women are more likely to *recover movement* after suffering a stroke. Men are more likely to be born with *dyslexia* (or a language problem), but women who are dyslexic are more likely to recover and compensate. Yet women are twice as likely to suffer from *depression, anxiety,* and other *mood disorders.*

Of course, all women aren't the same in how they feel emotions, put ideas together when they think and learn, or use their intuition. Many individuals deviate from the general, typical points we can make about the specific ways the brain is organized.

I am a tireless people-watcher wherever I am—in a restaurant, airport, or on the street. You can tell an awful lot about a person by watching him in his everyday world. By observing how a woman approaches any task— and how *you* approach any task!—whether it's writing, drawing, flipping through a magazine, or reading a book, you can tell how her brain is organized. You can also predict with some degree of accuracy any tendencies toward mood and anxiety problems, attention and memory problems, and a host of other physical health disorders.

Let's look at each of your brain function areas to see if you have:

a. A traditional feminine brain style
b. Nontraditional feminine brain style
c. Traditional masculine brain style
d. Nontraditional masculine brain style

Skilled Movement

If you are left-handed or ambidextrous, you are more likely to have either a *nontraditional feminine* or *nontraditional masculine* brain style. Your speech and mannerisms may appear more emotional. You may pay attention and learn differently than your friends. This may increase your chances of being labeled ADD or LD (learning disorder). Being a "southpaw" or an ambipaw helps you blend traditional right-brain emotionality and "three-dimensional" spatial capability in almost everything you see, do, or say. Traditionally, studies on left-handed people have shown them to be more emotional and creative, but being left-handed is also associated with some health challenges, including hormonal and immune problems.

Usually, we are more skilled with one hand, one side of our body more than the other, and handedness is the most obvious way of figuring out how a person's brain is wired for skilled movement. Ninety percent of people prefer to use the right hand more than their left for a variety of tasks, so their left brain is dominant for hand control. *Handedness,* however, is a measure of degree. Most people think if you write with your right hand, you are by definition right-handed. However, some people write with their right hand, but do a lot of other things (bowl or bat) with their left hand, so these people are either left-handed or ambidextrous.

Handedness is in part genetic, and left-handedness is more frequent in men than in women. The left brain usually dominates control of skilled movement, which makes most people right-handed. However, trauma or stress in utero or around birth can increase a female baby's chances of being born left-handed. One theory suggests that if a developing brain gets higher levels of testosterone in the fetal environment, the right hemisphere develops more than the left. The right hemisphere then takes over the job of creating skilled movement, which makes the girl left-handed or ambidextrous. Since men and male fetuses have more testosterone, they would ultimately have a greater tendency to be left-handed, but some female fetuses in a high-stress, testosterone-laden prenatal environment may also become left-handed.

Elevated testosterone somehow also aggravates the development of the immune system. There is an association between left-handedness and immune system disorders like asthma, allergies, rheumatoid arthritis, and lupus. There is even an association between left-handedness and premature grayness, among other conditions. Left-handers (or more appropriately, non-right-handers) are also more likely to die sooner than right-handers.

So, if you are left-handed, if you use both hands for skilled movement, and if you have had a lot of immune system problems or infertility, you may have been born with a brain that has nontraditional organization for language, perception, attention, memory, emotion, and intellectual capacities. You may have more spatial and creative talents, and also be highly intuitive. Being left-handed or ambidextrous may exaggerate your intuition because the right brain has more input into everything you see, do, and say. So, right-brain intuition, body intuition, and dream intuition are more likely to be infused into everything you experience. Yet because your left-handedness is often associated with an unusual brain wiring for language (see below), you may not be able to easily articulate your hunches or gut sense.

Language: Dyslexia and Being Able to Talk About Your Feelings

In most men, the left brain controls the capacity to speak, read, and write. It takes sounds (called phonemes) and translates them into words (called graphemes). This hemisphere governs grammar and stores vocabulary words (called syntax and semantics). The man's right brain adds emotional tone, inflection, metaphor, and humor. Since the traditional man's brain is more compartmentalized, language is created mostly by the left brain.

In contrast, the traditional woman's right brain has a greater role in language and communication. Having language in both hemispheres gives the traditional feminine brain distinct advantages, for instance, in recovering from a stroke, as we've discussed. It does not necessarily give women better speaking skills than men. Yet, when women speak, they use both their analytical left brain and their emotional right brain simultaneously. Therefore, women may be anatomically encouraged to talk about how they feel about anything and everything. They are also more likely to discuss their hunches and gut sense.

Traditionally, when men speak, they use mostly their left analytic rational brain and are anatomically more likely to segregate their right-brain emotions. So men are ultimately biologically primed to talk more about *things* than *feelings* and are less likely to talk aloud about their intuition.

The differences between the sexes in the wiring of language in the brain also have enormous implications when it comes to treating depression, anxiety, and other mood problems. Traditionally, it may be easier for a woman to talk about her feelings, and individual talk therapy can be helpful. However, if a woman feels her husband doesn't talk about his feelings with her, asking him to share his feelings with a therapist is unlikely to help either spouse. Since the man is likely to have fewer connections between right-brain emotions and left-brain language, talking about what he feels in the "captivity" of marriage therapy or even during moonlit walks may feel akin to eating ground glass. If a woman measures the level of her husband's love and devotion by how much he puts his feelings into words, she is setting herself up for repeated disappointment and frustration. Her husband's right-brain emotions of love and passion are more likely to be communicated through *behavior* (buying flowers or wanting to do things together).

At family events when I was growing up, when people first arrived, the women usually were very talkative. Most of my uncles and male cousins just stood around, looking uncomfortable. Over time, people would begin to clump together as they started to relax. The men would watch the ball-game or go outside and talk about how long it took to get to the party, what routes were best, what the traffic was like. The men usually did the driving in those days, and their "car talk" showed that traditional men's brains are more skilled at processing visuospatial information and maps. The women usually gathered in the kitchen to talk about babies and family matters. No matter their sex, though, people tend to talk a lot when they're interested in the topic.

Experience changes the brain and its anatomy. Connections for language, perception, and attention are remodeled throughout your life, and help you learn and adapt to new situations. The degree to which experience can change your innate brain style is not yet well understood, and it's not clear whether a male language style can change to become more feminine. Typically, men don't want to talk about their feelings—even mood problems that hurt their health, such as depression. A great book about depression in men, entitled *I Don't Want to Talk About It,* agrees that the male brain structure keeps men from discussing feelings, and points out that society creates pressure on men to adhere to sexual identity roles. Yet this pressure can shape a man's brain so that he learns to stuff his feelings. This same culture encourages a woman to talk (and even complain) about her feelings. This social pressure may also affect women's memory. Women's brains generally have a better capacity to hear and remember what is said, an advantage that occurs in all age levels, regardless of the content and meaning of what is said.

Not all women and men fit into these typical brain sex types for language. One way to figure out your own brain style is to ask yourself the following questions: Do you read slowly? Have trouble with writing? Did you do much better in math in school than English or history? If you answered yes to all of these questions, your brain may have unusual language circuits and a nontraditional, masculinized brain structure. In other words, you have a certain kind of New Feminine Brain.

Dyslexia is a developmental brain disorder in which the wiring for language is not normal. An individual with dyslexia not only has a reading disorder, he or she also has problems with writing. Dyslexics may have difficulty with "left-brain" reading because small lesions occurred in the left brain while they were growing in the womb. They are more likely to be left-handed, ambidextrous, and have an increased risk for immune system problems.

Dyslexia can take a different form in women than in men. Since the female brain has more plasticity and is generally more adaptive, the lesions tend to have less effect on language development. Women also seem more successful at developing ways to compensate for their reading problems. As a result, a woman with a traditional feminine brain can more easily hide or overcome dyslexia than a man. When a dyslexic person reads, he or she uses the right brain to guess or intuit the text. Women may do this better because they have more connections between the two hemispheres. As a result of this compensatory strategy, an adult woman's dyslexia may only show up in her writing and not in her reading. Most dyslexic adults have more difficulty with writing than reading, since they've had more practice reading and have devised more intuitive ways to compensate for their reading problems.

A woman's inborn capacity to compensate for a developmental problem like dyslexia can give her a wonderful ability to adapt in different educational and vocational environments. Yet her ability to "hide" a developmental disability may prevent her from getting appropriate help, remedial education, or support. Generally speaking, a man's developmental disorder would be more obvious to teachers and he would ultimately get more help sooner.

Trying to Fit a Round Peg into a Square Hole

Ann, age twenty, called me because she was concerned about her grades in college. Although she always had trouble focusing in class, she had managed to dig in and get straight A's in high school, enough to get into an Ivy League college. Her family was filled with overachievers. Her father was a lawyer and her mother a psychiatrist. Her oldest brother was a heart transplant surgeon, a sister was a neurosurgeon, and a younger brother was studying astrophysics. Although Ann was trying to follow in her family's footsteps by being premed, she was doing poorly in nearly all of her freshman courses. She couldn't finish the reading on time and was having a hard time keeping up with all the papers. The only class in which she excelled was an elective in clothing design. Ann had always been very artistic and creative with sewing and needlework as a child, and had dreamed of designing a line of clothing and couture. Knowing that this plan would be criticized by her family, Ann ignored her creative bent for the more practical career of being a physician, which would also please her family.

After getting a 2.0 grade point average in her freshman year, Ann had a neuropsychological evaluation to see if she had any learning disabilities, and was given a diagnosis of ADD and dyslexia. Ann's neuropsych test scores do not come close to describing her gifts, talents, and weaknesses. All of the individual subtests for attention and language were terribly low, while the right hemisphere visuospatial "artistic" skills were off the board high. Given that Ann was left-handed, it makes sense that most of her genius was in her right hemisphere, and why she was attracted to a creative pursuit. As fate would have it, her "learning disabilities," dyslexia and ADD, would make it hard for her to enter into a medical career especially if she were doing so for parental approval and social status.

I helped Ann look at her neuropsych test scores and learning disabilities in a different light so that she could appreciate how her brain was wired for skilled movement and language. Her ADD and dyslexia may be the downside of a brain model whose genius is in creative and artistic design, but Ann saw that she could use her mind to excel in a field for which her brain was uniquely wired.

EMOTION: DEPRESSION, MOODINESS, ANGER, AND ANXIETY

The right brain is dominant for expressing your feelings and picking up the emotions of others. You can in fact see how someone's brain is organized by looking at her mouth and face. When someone smiles or expresses an emotion, the two sides of the face rarely mirror one another. Typically, the left side (controlled mostly by the right brain) is more emotionally expressive, especially for right-handed people.

Recently, some friends and I visited a vitamin company (USANA) and met its president, Myron Wentz. He had just written a book and was proudly signing copies. The book jacket pictured a man on an ocean beach, facing to the right. I assumed it was the author, but it didn't *look* like the man in front of me signing the book. So I said, impulsively (a trait I have difficulty managing), "Excuse me, Dr. Wentz, who is the man on the cover of your book?" (As soon as I said it I knew I was knee-deep in trouble!) Dr. Wentz looked up and said, "That's me!" I then tried to explain to him that since the picture only revealed the right side of his face (reflecting his left hemisphere), I simply didn't recognize him. The speed with which my friends ushered me out of the room and back to our car led me to believe this hadn't gone over well, but I couldn't really tell for sure since I was seated in the car on the far right and could see only the right sides of their faces.

If you were to look at photographs of well-known personalities like Elvis, Muhammad Ali, and Marilyn Monroe, the left side of the person's face has more emotional expression. Some notable exceptions would be Rock Hudson and Leonardo Da Vinci's painting of the "Mona Lisa" (which many believe is a self-portrait). Their facial expressions of emotions are much more obvious on the right than the left. We'll find out why that is later.

Left-brain language in isolation, without the right brain's influence, tone, and prosody, is like the voice on computer software that reads aloud typed words. It feels and sounds mechanical and nonhuman. We've all had teachers who bored us silly. Ben Stein's portrayal of a teacher in the movie *Ferris Bueller's Day Off* is a perfect illustration of left-brain information without the right-brain warmth that makes language come alive with meaning.

The right brain controls our capacity to be in touch with intuition and emotions in general, but the left brain does have a role in the experience of positive moods like love and happiness. In both the traditional male and traditional female brains, the left brain is more important for positive words such as "joy," "happiness," "love," and "cheer," while the right hemisphere is more important for negative words like "fear," "anger," and "sadness."

Women's moods change with the menstrual cycle. Before ovulation, your left brain is more active, so you're better able to hear positive words, and more likely to be rational, analytical, and focused. After ovulation, the right brain dominates, and you're more likely to be intuitive and hear negatively charged words. Women in general are more likely to hear and talk about negative emotions, due to their cyclic hormonal changes and the increased connectivity between their two brains. At certain times in the monthly cycle, you may experience what I call the "pool-backwash system," which cleans out painful emotions—like the filtration system in a pool—and helps you get in touch with your intuition.

From an evolutionary standpoint, these cyclical mood swings may have a purpose. Depending on which part of the menstrual cycle you're in, your brain organization changes, bringing different skills to the fore. The traditional male brain has more compartmentalization and as a result men are more able to censor right-hemisphere emotion and intuition when they are trying to perform a left-brain, rational task. But a traditional woman's brain has more communication between the two hemispheres, so the right brain's emotions and intuition are more likely to have constant input into every task. Being less able to censor her emotion and intuition makes a woman more likely to be consciously aware of the health and happiness of her children, spouse, friends, and others around her. This constant awareness has many advantages, but also makes us easily distractible in the classroom or boardroom. For instance, I am basically a right brain on a stick and I have ADHD. Ritalin helped me focus. When you're supposed to be paying attention to the chemistry lecture but you are keyed in to how distressed the professor looks, you're going to miss some important information you might need for the exam.

A woman's menstrual cycle gives her two mind-sets with which to approach the world. For two weeks before ovulation, we're more likely to be in our left brain, with its better mood and more analytical, rational, focused frame of mind. At that time, we are more closed to our intuition. After ovulation, we are more intuitively open and emotionally porous to what's going on in our life and the lives of loved ones because high levels of estrogen flow to the left brain. Once we get our period, estrogen levels wane and the relative level of testosterone increases. The right brain takes over.

With the onset of menopause, this cycling between the left and right hemispheres stops, and the brain can constantly be in this intuitive, porous state. Across your lifespan, your brain's masculinized or feminized style may vary from month to month (due to your menstrual cycle) and from era to era (due to pregnancy or menopause). It may also vary due to weight, percentage of body fat, or medicinal treatments for breast cancer, infertility, or other hormonally mediated illnesses. Some women may more easily adapt to this "rubber-band" brain—these cyclic changes in brain style. Other women's brains may be innately more sensitive to the fluctuating levels of estrogen, progesterone, testosterone, and other hormones, and also be more susceptible to acquiring problems in attention, memory, mood, anxiety, panic, addiction, pain, sleep, or eating disorders. Some women who early in life had only a few days of PMS with moodiness can suffer at midlife for weeks of mood disorders. PMS can turn into years of perimenopausal symptoms, and can even make a woman wonder if she's drifting into early-onset Alzheimer's disease or late-onset mental retardation.

Obviously, you need adequate right-brain skills to function emotionally and socially, but environmental pressures on the New Feminine Brain may require that you force yourself to stay in your left brain—to create more separation from your feelings at home and work. And you may have to do this in spite of the changing phases of your menstrual cycle. Over time, constantly censoring your feelings is going to cause problems, however. Your body will eventually acquire what I call the "stigmata" of trying to push your brain beyond what your body will accept. You may start to develop health problems such as chronic fatigue syndrome, fibromyalgia, environmental illness, obesity, and other disorders that are showing up with increasing frequency as the New Feminine Brain is stressed.

The Dangers of Getting Stuck in Left-Brain Emotions

Some people's emotions come from one hemisphere more than the other. Those who are "stuck" in a left-brain, positive perception of life develop anosognosia, or denial of problems in their life in general. Refusing to accept the bad, they see only the good in others and turn a blind eye to difficulties. If you look only on the bright side, however, you basically have to put a tourniquet on your corpus callosum and force yourself to stay in your left brain.

Yet even as you try to stay in a left-brain frame of mind, your right-brain/body connections and intuition won't let you get away with the sham, and your body will rebel. People who smooth over major issues and traumas in their life, or rationalize their problems, eventually suffer physical disorders. Emotions that you deny and refuse to admit into your conscious brain go into your body and lead to illness.

Women tend to have a keener sense than men of whether someone is hostile, friendly, sincere, or in distress. Women may have developed this greater "social perception" early in our evolutionary history in order to pick up emotions in others, to detect fear or illness in an infant's facial expression, or read someone's body language especially at a distance, to help protect their children.

Achievement, social standing, and power leave their mark on the body and the brain. Studies of male monkeys show that social status can alter hormone levels. As the monkeys achieve more dominance and social status, their testosterone levels go up. But as their power and status in the community decline and their submissive behavior increases, their testosterone levels go down. In the fish species *Haplochromis burtoni,* the more territory an individual commands, the more the brain cells in its hypothalamus puff up with testosterone. When your place in society changes, so does your brain.

Testosterone causes differences in the brain at many stages of development, not just in utero, but across the whole lifespan. Testosterone secreted by a woman's ovaries and adrenal glands can cause reversible but real activation of specific brain circuits. Female rhesus monkeys who have been exposed to testosterone during late fetal life later develop "rough-and-tumble play," that is, more aggressive, less sedate play that is thus labeled "masculinized." Women who are born with excess testosterone and androgen levels (a condition called congenital adrenal hyperplasia or CAH) exhibit what is called "masculinized behavior," that is, higher levels of aggression and more rough-and-tumble play. These women have masculinized brain styles as well, with better spatial ability. In addition, their interests are also what society would call masculinized—they have less interest in infants, marriage, and motherhood and a higher incidence of homosexuality and bisexuality.

Excessive testosterone levels have been associated with people who are aggressive, hostile, and usually unfriendly and with the frustration and excessive assertiveness of competitive environments. People with these characteristics can be found in all walks of life—from prison to a crowded city, to being stuck in traffic in the suburbs. Five studies of older individuals and male prisoners have found evidence between aggression and testosterone levels. Women convicted of violent crimes also have higher testosterone levels compared to women convicted of nonviolent crimes. And higher levels of testosterone aren't found just in prisoners. In the general population, aggressive people usually have higher testosterone levels. No one knows if the testosterone (or other androgens) causes the aggressive behavior (angry outbursts, competitiveness, road rage, etc.) or whether the aggressive behavior itself drives up the testosterone levels.

Changes in estrogen, progesterone, and testosterone may not just rewire the New Feminine Brain's capacity for attention, learning and memory, mood, anger, anxiety, behavior, and relationships. They also affect the function of a woman's immune system. Testosterone and progesterone lower the immune system's ability to defend the body against infection and cancer. Estrogen induces white cell maturation and encourages the production of immunoglobulin protein products, which fight infection. Testosterone, in contrast, inhibits immunoglobulin production, thus inhibiting the immune system. Women with excessively high estrogen and lower testosterone levels also have a higher incidence of autoimmune illnesses like allergies, rheumatoid arthritis, and thyroid disease. When androgen (testosterone) concentrations were higher than normal in utero, they were associated with left-handedness (decreased left hemisphere function), impaired immune function, increased susceptibility to autoimmune problems, and dyslexia.

In the twenty-first century women (and men) are living in a more populated, technologically sophisticated, competitive, "rough-and-tumble" world. The resultant changes in estrogen, progesterone, and testosterone that influence the female brain and immune system may predispose women to immune system dysfunction, changes in hormones that increase her chances of getting cancer of all types (especially breast, ovarian, and colon cancers, which are hormonally sensitive) and immune disorders (including chronic fatigue, fibromyalgia, environmental illness, and others).

An Emotional Mother Teresa: Feeling Emotions for Someone Else Who Can't

Annabelle, forty-six years old, called me for an intuitive reading.

The reading: Annabelle's brain and body seemed to be a sort of "satellite dish" for picking up emotional distress in loved ones. I saw her as nearly continuously tuned in to a relative who was emotionally handicapped, someone who had overly compulsive left-brain functioning and an inadequate level of right-brain social and emotional functioning. Annabelle's body seemed to suffer from carrying the weight of someone else's emotional pain. I saw lifelong problems with attention and memory, which were aggravated by anxiety and depression. In addition to a hyperactive immune system prone to allergy and infection, Annabelle's body seemed to struggle with cravings that affected her weight and digestive tract.

The facts: Annabelle had a daughter, Bethany, with Asperger's syndrome, a right-hemisphere developmental disorder that is similar to autism. Bethany's emotional and social handicap made it difficult for her to make friends because she seemed blind to others' feelings and social cues. Bethany was a left-brain savant, with an amazing ability to learn languages, but her right brain's disability made her clueless about why she couldn't get along with others, despite repeated, obvious rejections. Time after time, classmates turned down Bethany's invitations to go to movies or other after-school activities.

Bethany's handicap placed a burden on her immediate caregiver, Annabelle, who had to become a "right-brain donor" to her daughter. Over time, this was causing emotional and physical health problems for both of them. As Annabelle served as her daughter's right brain, she had nightmares about her daughter's problems and suffered from repeated colds, flus, and frequent allergies. Annabelle could always intuitively tell when her daughter was having a bad day at school. She would feel panic, anxiety, and worry, and had food cravings for chips, popcorn, Coke. She also admitted that she would chain smoke. Eating and smoking would dull the panic and anxiety, and numb a sense of impending trouble. Invariably, Annabelle's right brain and body intuition would be confirmed once she arrived at the school to pick up her daughter. Bethany would have an emotional meltdown once she got into the car, telling the usual story of rejection.

Annabelle's right brain was functioning overtime, doing double duty picking up emotions in her own life as well as the emotional problems of her daughter. Although Annabelle's intuition and great empathic abilities could make her a successful, gifted psychotherapist, the continual over-working of her right brain had a painful detrimental effect on her emotional and physical health. She suffered from chronic anxiety, panic attacks, depression, was forty pounds overweight and a two-pack-a-day smoker. Her doctor had prescribed Zoloft for her mood, Buspar for chronic anxiety and insomnia, and Ritalin for attention deficit disorder. Taking the Zoloft had caused her to put on fifteen pounds and the Buspar was upsetting her stomach.

I taught Annabelle how her unique feminine brain was wired for mood (Chapter 4), anxiety (Chapter 6), attention (Chapter 9), and intuition (Chapters 8 and 11). She learned that she was self-medicating her panic, depression, and distractibility by eating and smoking and in order to turn off the distressing intuitive signals she was getting about her daughter's life. I recommended that she learn about the herbal, nutritional, and medical solutions that you'll read about later in the book that can ease melancholy and panic and focus attention. Annabelle eventually mastered the intuitive language that was imbedded in her mood, anxiety, and attention disorders and learned how to stay healthy and help her daughter realize her potential.

SEEING IN THREE DIMENSIONS: MAP READING, GETTING LOST, AND FINDING YOUR WAY

The right hemisphere is typically dominant in drawing three-dimensional shapes and other so-called visuospatial tasks. Drawing accurate shapes, angles, length, distance, width, and three-dimensionality shows that your right brain is on task. The left hemisphere will add specific details, but overall appreciation of space and dimension comes from the right brain.

By examining your visuospatial capabilities (for instance, are you good at reading maps; do you have a good sense of direction; can you rotate an object in your mind's eye and visualize it from different angles and dimensions?), you can figure out whether your brain is traditionally feminine or masculine.

Sex hormones in the womb affect the development of spatial areas in the brain. So do later experiences in life. Interestingly, women evolved unique spatial abilities—quite different from men's—and we are much more skilled at fine motor tasks. As our species evolved, many scientists believe, women developed survival skills that included detecting and gathering small foods (grains, berries, small game) in many different ecosystems during different seasons. This skill can be seen today in women's unique spatial abilities of identifying objects in smaller defined areas. In contrast, men are believed to have adapted to hunting over large territories and to making large tools, so this may have influenced their development of a generally superior capacity for aiming across long distances and their capacity to mentally rotate objects.

As Doreen Kimura, the queen of gender differences in the brain, writes, "the tasks that women were predominantly engaged in in preliterate societies . . . [were] . . . making pottery, weaving, manufacturing thread and cordage, and so on. The Purdue Pegboard, a standard test originally designed to select for factory jobs requiring manual skill, shows a consistent advantage for women. . . . Some have argued that women's advantage on such fine motor tasks is accounted for by their smaller fingers, but while this may contribute to the sex difference in some studies, we have not found this to be the case in ours."

Social pressures eventually led to women with these fine-motor talents being forced to do factory work, piecework, and other low-paid jobs, yet this same fine-motor aptitude would enable them to be superior brain surgeons, architects, and professional musicians.

By contrast, navigation and sense of direction are characteristic of a more masculinized brain style. Map reading, for instance, is easier to accomplish if you have a sense of direction, and a sense of direction combines both visuospatial and mental rotation skills. Map reading and navigating across roads involves developing the ability to recognize a scene from different viewpoints, mentally rotating surroundings in your mind. For example, when you are given directions to a party, to be able to go home afterward successfully without getting lost, you have to reverse the directions in your mind. And if you take a route that involves a lot of one-way roads, you need to be able not only to reverse directions but also reassemble parts of the route piecemeal by mentally rotating part of the scene. This skill seems to be better developed in the traditional male brain due to androgen or testosterone environmental stimulation in utero but also may be due to evolutionary influences millennia ago that supported the traditional male role of nomadic hunting across long distances.

Scientists have found that men and women use different strategies to find their ways when navigating. Women tend to use landmarks and objects en route to remember how to get somewhere: "The McDonald's will be on the right" or "The bridge is on the left." Traditionally, men tend to use visuospatial directions, like "go west" or "go five miles on route 295."

Men tend to learn the route in fewer trials than women, but women tend to recall more landmarks. When using maps, men tend to recall more details about directions and distances, while traditionally women recall more details about landmarks and street names. Perhaps traditional women's way of compensating for their traditionally less developed visuospatial abilities is to rotate the map, rather than mentally rotate landmarks in their mind.

But traditional women's brains are better adapted to find objects in small spaces. Today, for instance, if you can't find the ketchup in the refrigerator or the heirloom in the attic, who are you generally going to call? Your mother. And how many times do you have to tell your husband what drawer the spatula goes in? Many scientists believe that women originally developed this ability so that they could detect small changes in their surroundings, such as noticing whether a stranger or animal had entered their environment, so that they could protect the tribe, or find lifesaving foods in difficult terrains and ecosystems. This talent for distinguishing objects makes women particularly skilled at jobs such as private investigation, detective and police work, scientific research, dentistry, ob/gyn, and nursing in intensive care units, to name just a few.

Again, not all women and men are the same. Increasing numbers of women with New Feminine Brains have developed more typical traditional masculine visuospatial skills due to either environmental demands or hormone stimulation of their brains. (Think of Venus Williams and her 120-mile-an-hour serve, or the Olympic gold medalists on the U.S. women's soccer team.)

I actually have both the masculine and feminine visuospatial direction senses, and I have a great ability to find lost objects. I regularly find money on the ground and four-leaf clovers. In every lab in which I've worked, my colleagues have called me the Patron Saint of Lost Objects. In addition, I have the direction sense and map-reading ability of what would traditionally be found in a man's brain. Whenever I travel to a new city, I quickly figure out what direction is north, south, east, and west, buy a map, and memorize the general grid or orientation of major roads. With this in mind, I usually make my way around like a native.

A woman's capacity to perform spatial tasks in a masculine or feminine style varies with her hormonal levels. During the menstrual phase of her period, when estrogen is at its lowest, she acquires a more masculine, increased visuospatial skill. In contrast, premenstrually (during the luteal phase after ovulation, in the second half of her cycle), when estrogen is at its highest, she demonstrates a more feminized style of visuospatial capacity (less skill). A little advice: If you have a traditionally feminine brain, restrict your map usage to the two weeks prior to ovulation. Between ovulation and menstruation, you'll want to rely on someone else's left brain.

Changes in estrogen, progesterone, and testosterone due to environmental changes, social status, infertility treatments, or treatment for breast and other hormonally responsive cancers can also affect the New Feminine Brain's perception and visuospatial abilities. As more women enter very competitive traditional male fields such as law enforcement, firefighting, and the military services, stress causes testosterone levels to rise. As a result, women are helped hormonally to acquire new visuospatial skills, such as the ability to use weapons and tools and read a map, whether of a war zone or Greater Los Angeles. In fact, women are helped hormonally to adapt to virtually any career and pursuit in a man's world that they want.

ATTENTION AND MEMORY

Traditionally, women and men have different ways of paying attention to the world around them, which may explain the different ways that the sexes demonstrate problems in distractibility or "attention deficit disorder." Both have to focus on a variety of settings on the job, at home, or in school. Both are constantly bombarded by honking cars, blaring radios, and ringing phones. Yet, men's and women's brains differ in being able to shift attention moment by moment *to* what needs to be in the center of their awareness and *away* from what seems to have lower priority.

Many brain areas link together to help us pay attention (more on this in Chapter 9). However, the right brain is the "dominant" hemisphere for attention and more critical for intuition. Traditionally, men and women have different innate abilities in dividing their attention between rational and intuitive senses, and also to "disconnect" from their intuition when necessary.

Since women's brains traditionally have more connectivity and less segregation of function between the two sides of the brain, it makes sense that our attentional style would be different from a man's. Since hormone levels influence the function of the right and left hemispheres, the menstrual cycle's changes in hormones and moods can also create changes in attention. During the first half of the menstrual cycle, when estrogen levels are lowest, attention to rational, left-brain information may be at its peak. In contrast, during the two premenstrual weeks, as estrogen levels increase, we can become more easily distracted by intuitive input, to which we tune in more. In women with attention deficit disorder, symptoms of inattentiveness worsen premenstrually and during menopause. At these times, we're less able to divide attention between rational left brain and intuitive right brain pools of information. Altering the dose of Ritalin or other medications according to the phase of the menstrual cycle is said to help some women with ADHD function better. For some ADHD women at menopause, hormone replacement therapy may alter the Ritalin dose they need. In fact, many more ADHD women than men *do not* improve with Ritalin treatment.

Testosterone levels influence attention and definitely are associated with impulsivity. Men traditionally have higher testosterone levels and are more impulsive. Women traditionally have lower testosterone levels and are less impulsive. This difference in testosterone and impulsivity may explain why men and boys are more likely to have ADHD (attention deficit disorder with hyperactivity and impulsivity) whereas girls and women are more likely to have a more "dreamlike" or "spacey" type of ADD.

At menopause, however, the brain's attention circuits change. With a decrease in estrogen and an increase in testosterone, women are more impulsive, more hyperactive, and less attentive. These changes make some women feel as if their brain is turning into a "fuzzball." Menopausal women with ADD may become even more inattentive, impulsive, and hyperactive. Many women also become more emotionally porous—they hear their intuitions more than ever and may be distracted by the pain in others' lives at this time. Men, who go through a "testepause," have decreasing testosterone levels and a relative increase in estrogen, so their attention may actually become more acute.

But in the New Feminine Brain, a woman's attention may be more similar to the typical masculine pattern, as a result of the life pressures and hormonal changes rewiring her circuits. More women may be diagnosed with ADD and ADHD, and not just because more doctors are aware of this diagnostic category, but because of the increase in women's social status and the increase in testosterone levels that goes along with that.

PAIN AND BODY AWARENESS

Men and women experience pain differently. There are at least three reasons why women's brains may be more finely tuned to register pain than men's:

1. The pain areas in a woman's brain have more cellular receivers to detect pain.
2. Women's brain cells are more sensitive to pain.

3. Men's brains are more compartmentalized and therefore more anatomically capable of shutting out pain.

Women also have a more sensitive sense of touch, so we have a lower threshold for pain, especially in our joints and lower digestive tract. The right brain has more connections to the body and intuition comes more readily to us through our right brain–body connections. People rely on this brain–body intuition every day when trying to make decisions even if they are not consciously aware that they are doing so. Pain and any other uncomfortable body feeling can be a signal from the brain–body intuition letting us know that we need to pay attention to and change something in our life. Someone might say, "I could feel in my heart it was the right thing to do," or "I got a bad feeling in my gut about it." If your two brains are more segregated from one another, as in the traditional man's brain, you may be more able to shut out pain and the intuition associated with it by distracting yourself and escaping into left-brain activity, like reading a book or performing some soothing, skilled task. A typical woman's right and left brains are more intertwined, however, so even when she is using her left brain—reading, speaking, or writing—she is still tuned in to a channel of body awareness from her right brain.

Women are anatomically less capable of escaping pain. Yet the more masculinized your brain is, the more likely you will be to escape, neglect, or deny pain and illness in your body. Men's brains may have evolved the ability to escape or be numb to pain in order to survive while hunting or fighting over territory. Traditionally, a woman may have had to have more body awareness than a man. She had to know what was going on inside her body in order to ensure her and her children's survival. However, for a woman to survive as a pseudo-hunter or warrior in the working world of the twenty-first century, her brain has adapted so she can compartmentalize, dissociate, or deny a certain amount of body pain.

Women today have a more masculinized brain style superimposed over their traditional feminine brain circuits. We have sprouted brain pathways that mute the right hemisphere's lifesaving body awareness and intuition, and segregate away parts of reality in order to adapt to modern life. As a result, many women may be losing touch with their bodies in order to manage their work in the outer world and at home. By dissociating pain so that she can compete, survive, and thrive in the outer world, a woman may achieve short-term success but increase her chances of having health problems later in life.

There are ways to balance the need to masculinize your behavior, keep in touch with your intuition, and still maintain your health, which we'll discuss later in the book.

INTUITION: GAINING ACCESS TO INFORMATION

The six brain functions that we have discussed—*movement, language, emotions, attention, memory,* and the capacity to *feel pain*—are all involved with creating and perceiving intuition. Since traditional women's and men's brains are wired differently for these functions, it's safe to say that women and men also gain access to their intuition differently. Yet both sexes get intuition through these six brain-body pathways.

It was long thought that women had cornered the market on intuition. A woman is likely to say she made a decision based on "women's intuition," while a man is unlikely to admit to using intuition at all. Yet women and men have the same basic components in their *intuition network*. These include:

a.   The right brain
b.   The left brain
c.   The body
d.   The dreaming or sleep mechanism

Compared to men, we women have more pathways between our right and left brains *and* between our right brain and body. This hyperconnectivity between the sides of the brain makes us more likely to make right-brain emotional hunches and to talk about them with left-brain language. Similarly, a woman has an exaggerated capacity to sense stimuli, pain, and health changes in her body. Because she is in touch with these right brain–body information nerve highways, she may be more likely to talk about intuition that she gets from her body. She may say that she "feels it in her bones," or "has a gut sense," or "has to go by what her heart tells her."

She is also more likely to notice her right-brain dreams and use left-brain language to talk about them with friends or a therapist, or to write about them in a journal.

Let's be clear: Traditional men *do* get intuitive information. They may not talk about it; their right-brain or body intuition may simply be shunted directly into making choices or taking action with little discussion. Of course, some nontraditional men's brains are wired for the hyperconnected, verbally fluent, intuitive style. And there are nontraditional women who act intuitively from their gut and have little recognition of where their decision-making capability comes from.

Ultimately, you want as many windows open as possible into your intuition. But if you have problems with mood, or attention, if you've been labeled ADHD, or have chronic pain and health problems, some of the portals into your intuition may be clogged. By learning how your own feminine brain works and by creating healthier circuits for mood, anxiety, attention, and memory, you can gain greater access to intuition and make better decisions.

Let's start with learning more about how you can integrate your right and left brain and become even more aware of the masculine or feminine nature of your mind.

TWO

Someday, We'll Be Together: Embracing Your Rational and Intuitive, Masculine and Feminine

The 1972 movie *What's Up, Doc?* reminds me of the differences among brain styles. It opens with the main character, a charming ditz played by Barbra Streisand, walking into a San Francisco hotel carrying a red plaid bag. In the lobby, there are three other red plaid bags identical to hers. One contains secret documents belonging to a government whistleblower. Another is packed with a wealthy woman's jewels. The third is filled with ancient rocks that belong to a musicologist played by Ryan O'Neal. It's a screwball comedy, so naturally, the suitcases get mixed up, and for the rest of the movie, the characters chase each another all over San Francisco in pursuit of their bags.

Like those red plaid bags, our brains look pretty much alike from the outside. But functionally—the way they work—they vary a lot, depending on their sexual identity and hormonal influences.

Help! I've Been Taken Prisoner by My Left Brain!

The intuition we get frequently points to the need for us to change something about a job, a goal, or a relationship. Unfortunately, change frequently means we have to give up something we think we need, so we try to avoid it. But, like a trapeze artist, you need to let go of one swing in order to grab onto a new one. Flying between them is scary because you're not sure that you'll arrive safely at the next point. Being "up in the air" in your life, being in transition, too, is frightening. Not knowing where you're going to land if you leave a bad job, relationship, or social circle is enough to make you cling to what you know—even when it's bad for you—rather than let it go so that you can follow your intuition to a better life and better health.

Our left brain's frontal lobe is a censor and can dim or block our intuition. The left brain is good at dulling pain, including painful insights that ask us to change our goals, career, or relationships. Here's what can happen if you ignore your intuition and allow your left brain to overrule intuitive insights.

Arguing with Intuition: Explaining Away Possible Solutions to Your Problems

Betty, age forty-one, called me for a reading.

The reading: I saw that Betty was not doing the work of her heart. Her daily job wasn't using all of her gifts, talents, and skills, but it made her feel safe and secure, and provided some financial stability.

Betty had received intuitive messages from several sources in her feminine brain that she needed a greater sense of purpose. For instance, Betty's lifelong tendency toward sadness and fearfulness seemed to be deepening. Her brain's fear and sadness emotional circuits, part of her intuitive network, were signaling that something was out of balance. I saw that Betty's *body* was her greatest source of intuition, screaming at her through symptoms of illness. Illness has multiple contributors—including diet, pressures in work and home environment, and emotional and behavioral patterns. Emotions trigger the release of chemicals in the body that increase an individual's risk of getting ill. (We'll talk more about this in Chapters 3, 4, and 5.) In Betty's case, I felt as if her escalating sadness and anxiety were targeting her immune system and colon.

The facts: Betty had been in school studying to be a psychologist when she met her husband, Carl. She was inwardly relieved when she got pregnant so she could opt out of the competitive process of applying to graduate programs. When her two children went to school, Betty joined a local hospital system as a crisis worker. After working in the system for twelve years, she began to get bored with her job. The state regulations had gotten tighter and Betty had lost quite a bit of freedom. She now had less patient contact and more paper-pushing duties.

Betty grew depressed and anxious in her dead-end job. She knew it was unhealthy for her, but she found reasons to reject any and all solutions to breath new life into her career identity.

1. *Long-term goals:* Betty believed that she couldn't go back to school because she had "lost her intellectual edge" and couldn't possibly get back into a graduate program in psychology.

2. *Relationships:* Betty had a "second family" with some of her friends at work and couldn't imagine separating from them.

3. *Organizations, family, and society:* Betty had "put" twelve years into her employer's retirement system. If she could find another position at the hospital in which she could feel fulfilled, she could kill two birds with one stone: get a job that was more interesting to her *and* keep her retirement funds. However, the only positions that piqued her interest were nursing or social work, both of which required her to go back to college, which terrified her.

So Betty stayed stuck in her job, and suffered in silence. Soon after we spoke she was diagnosed with an attack of shingles, and a routine blood test found her to be anemic. After an exhaustive battery of tests, doctors found a tumor in her large intestine.

Each time Betty had considered changing her job, her mind gave her so many excuses not to change that she got stuck. While her intuition was screaming for her to *move,* her left brain's frontal lobe was rationalizing that she *stay.* As a result, Betty was *stuck* in her vocational rut. The stress of unresolved anxiety and depression filtered down into her body, increasing her chances of getting an illness to which she was genetically predisposed. Her body was insisting that she reconsider her vocational future before she didn't have one. Thankfully, Betty's diagnosis of colon cancer made her stand up and take notice that her retirement benefits weren't worth dying for.

The Brain Censors Intuition and Facts

Like Betty, we all have had times when we have become unhappy with our job, dissatisfied with a relationship, or discouraged with our life in general. The right side of our feminine brain may warn us that our life is out of control: We feel afraid, angry, or sad. If it's inopportune to think about how much you might want to change a relationship or a career, however, your left brain may "reason" away your feelings. The left brain may then dominate, causing you to

1. *Judge* your fear, anger, or sadness as foolish, ridiculous, or unwarranted;

2. *Ruminate and obsess* about various details of the situation, and so prevent you from ever seeing the whole picture and creating change;

3. *Feel shame* about your emotions and coerce you into doing what others think you *should* do; or

4. *Feel artificially happy and joyful* to distract you or neutralize your distress.

Ultimately, your left brain is important in helping you control your emotions, fit into society, and function in relationships and a career. However, if your left brain dominates and overwhelms your right brain—and drowns out your intuition—you will end up with an imbalanced brain and an imbalanced life. Most of us are born with a tendency to be more in the left or the right brain. You can find out on what side of the feminine brain you *tend* to reside at the end of this chapter. Some of us, however, are born to spend time in both sides of the brain equally. Remember, though, your tendency can change due to your hormonal status, what part of your menstrual cycle you are in, whether you're peri- or postmenopausal, or if you have experienced significant trauma or challenge. Your job may also encourage you to try to live in your left brain and turn off the right brain's emotional and intuitive circuitry.

Neither man nor woman can live by one brain alone. You don't want to trap yourself in the comfort of your left brain's more tidy, pleasant, socially ordered environment. If your right brain's emotions and intuition don't have equal input into decisions and actions, they initiate biochemical and hormonal events that trigger physical and emotional problems: Chronic depression, anxiety, panic, dementia, heart disease, immune system dysfunction, and cancer are the products of an overly dominant left brain, a silenced right brain, and censored intuition.

On the other hand, excessive intuition can also set the scene for painful consequences.

Help! I've Been Taken Prisoner by My Right Brain!

Making decisions purely on the basis of hunches or intuition is as unbalanced as ignoring intuition entirely and basing your life purely on facts and rationalizations. Going with your gut without considering the practical aspects of career and finances, relationships with friends and family, or your place in a larger community can get you into trouble, as you will see in the following story.

Talisman (or Tali for short), forty-one years old, called me because she, like Betty, felt "stuck." Tali had chosen her name after leaving home and going to college. Born with a normal name to a normal family, Tali had never felt normal and didn't think she could function normally in the world.

Always called "space cadet" by her friends, Tali seemed to spend more time in the ether than on earth. From an early age, Tali had trouble paying attention in school and always seemed to be daydreaming. She never approached the assignments in a way that the teacher expected. Even though Tali got a few points for being "unique," "creative," or "original," she lost many more points for being disorganized and handing in work that was incomplete or late. She had a hard time remembering deadlines and taking standardized multiple choice tests like the SATs. Evaluated and found to have ADD—attention deficit disorder, "inattentive type"—she nonetheless had an amazing capacity to zero in on the distress of a family member or loved one. Tali's intuition was razor-sharp. She always knew when a loved one had died because she'd get a hint of it in a dream.

Tali's biggest problem when she called me was finding the right kind of job. She just couldn't figure out where she fit in because she always felt that she was operating on a different wavelength. Even so, Tali had completed a master's degree in counseling psychology. Her first job was in the teaching hospital of a medical school. Soon, however, Tali felt at odds with the administration and other personnel in her department. Proper billing procedures for her department required Tali to diagnose her patients by listing the symptoms that fit criteria in a diagnostic manual. Tali's brain just wasn't able to dissect someone's psyche into seemingly artificial "left-brain" analytical categories, even if it meant her job was on the line. Her overly right-brain "global" approach to her patients got her bad job performance evaluations.

Tali was great at intuitively understanding was what going on with staff members and patients alike, however. In seconds, she could use her right-brain talents to assess why staff members weren't getting along or which patient was in danger of committing suicide. But she had difficulty communicating this intuitive information in a left-brain analytical style that was acceptable in the academic environment of the psych unit. In contrast to Tali's emotional, blunt, direct style, other staff members used only clinically "appropriate" terms during their long, detailed "team" meetings.

Discouraged, Tali grew tired of all the dos, don'ts, and shoulds involved in academia and left to work in a private practice. Soon, she attracted various corporate clients who wanted the benefit of her unique insights to solve their staff disputes. Tali's career took off. Her "no-nonsense," practical approach helped her mediate even the most difficult situations. Yet Tali's intuitive insights were taking over her life. During her nonbusiness hours, at home, various scenarios would "play in her mind" about her clients' conflicts and she couldn't seem to turn them off. When she exercised, took a shower, or did everyday tasks, clients' faces would flash through her mind.

Tali's intuition was both a gift and a curse in her private life. Although her closest friends appreciated her emotionally blunt, direct style, they frequently had difficulty with her tendency to be overly involved in their lives. Whether she liked it or not, Tali's intuitive mind wandered into the lives of those she loved. She would always know when someone was in pain or likely to be harmed and felt compelled to do something to try to help or stop the suffering, but many of her friends and loved ones didn't want to be rescued. On more than one occasion, Tali had become involved in a family dispute, or tried to save someone from "making a terrible mistake," only to be scapegoated or labeled a busybody. Even when Tali practiced self-restraint and avoided getting involved, her mind would be consumed with the pain of her family.

Soon, both Tali's emotional and physical health were affected. Her lifelong tendency toward anxiety became panic attacks in her twenties. She became depressed and had chronic insomnia that she was able to hide, but other medical problems cropped up, including hypothyroidism, irritable bowel syndrome, food allergies, and lower back pain.

Tali had to learn to direct and contain her hyperactive right-brain intuition circuits. She needed to pump up her left-brain censors so she could gain some mental buffers between herself and others' emotional reactions (you'll see how to do this in Chapters 8 and 11).

Insufficient access to intuition as well as excessive intuition increase your tendency to develop emotional and physical problems. Yet more than anything, not having a handle on your intuition makes your feminine brain circuits go haywire, and leads to problems with mood, anxiety, attention, and memory.

The Difficulties with Unbridled Intuition

Our Western society favors "left brain-centric" thinking, since it is tidier, more easily controlled by rules and regulations, and generally more pleasant. Ultimately, it's less common to have a dominant right brain, because anyone with that mind-set will have a difficult time surviving and thriving. Individuals who think and feel in a more right-sided way most likely train themselves to pass as "normal."

By virtue of our genetic and hormonal makeup, women generally have more contributions from our right brains in almost every area of our life. Right-brain dominant thinking results in a number of characteristic tendencies:

1. *We become overwhelmed by emotion* to such a degree that it's often difficult to fit easily into the demands of a social group, career, family, or relationship.
2. *We become overly global* in our thinking. We tend to make generalizations, focusing on the whole picture and neglecting the details.
3. *We take shortcuts through someone's psyche during conversations.* Relying on emotional expression, a gesture, and other forms of nonverbal communication, we may have a hard time actually focusing on the words a person is saying.
4. *We focus our attention* so much on others' feelings that we may not know what we ourselves feel and want.
5. We experience *mixed negative emotional states* of fear, anger, and sadness that make it hard to see the world optimistically.

Ultimately, for a healthy mind, body, and intuitive capacity, we need to use both sides of our feminine brain.

Sex Hormones and the Brain

Hormones and life experiences mold how our right and left brains process feelings and thoughts and lead to a feminized or masculinized brain style. Most people's brains fall somewhere between these two extremes, but I have to repeat here that neither left nor right is superior, more intelligent, more intuitive, or more creative than the other.

Hormonal changes help explain why women have more fluid brain styles throughout their lives—and why we may try out different identities at different times. Several studies have shown that changing hormonal levels affect the brain's degree of masculinization and feminization, and consequently affect how a woman uses her left brain and right brain. Waning levels of estrogen and rising levels of testosterone actually rewire the female brain. During the childbearing years, as estrogen levels rise and fall within each menstrual cycle, the brain regularly cycles between the left and right hemispheres. When a woman's social status rises, her testosterone levels rise, further rewiring her brain.

But if her brain is subjected to additional hormonal fluctuations—which can be caused by factors from fertility drugs to professional success—the cycling between right and left hemispheres will be affected even further. A female brain that has been masculinized by testosterone in the womb is more likely to have unusual intellectual gifts in right-hemisphere areas, like map reading, mathematics, mechanical technology, and athletics. Of course, development doesn't stop in the womb. It continues to be shaped throughout life by education, parenting, mentoring, nutrition, social status, and trauma. The "raw material" of the exceptionally feminized or masculinized brain that begins to develop in a mother's body can either be "normalized" postnatally or become even further polarized. If a girl is born with a strongly masculinized, right-hemisphere brain, with gifts in mathematics and science, but is labeled a "geek," she may "deep-six" her gifts, and choose to stuff her nontraditional brain into a more traditional mold. Lack of appreciation and acceptance of the skills, talents, and gifts that are wired in her brain may lead to low self-esteem, depression, eating disorders, addiction, and other problems with relationships, fertility, and parenting.

Testosterone Isn't Just for Men, Estrogen Isn't Just for Women

Hormones help shape our minds in utero, but they are also critical for brain function throughout our lifespan. When an egg unites with a sperm, if the baby is going to be a girl, genetically it will have two X chromosomes, and if it's to be a boy, it will have an X and a Y chromosome. The male Y chromosome is responsible for testosterone production in a boy. Since the X chromosome controls the brain's and body's sensitivity to testosterone and other androgens, and a woman has twice as many X chromosomes as a man, a girl is doubly sensitive to even small amounts of testosterone during development. If the mother is stressed, her adrenal glands pump out testosterone-like molecules called androgens that masculanize the developing baby girl's brain, or feminize a developing baby boy's brain, increasing his susceptibility to depression, anxiety, language disorders like dyslexia, and certain health problems later in life.

What sort of stressors might influence a mother's hormones and increase the level of androgenic "male" hormones in her body? Perhaps she is struggling to hold down two jobs while raising two children. Maybe she's supporting her husband, who is in school or out of a job. Maybe she's part of the "sandwich generation," who take care of both children and aging parents. All these pressures increase the stress androgen hormones in the mother's body, reshaping and masculinizing *her* brain as they masculinize her unborn baby girl's brain.

Sandra Bern, a psychologist at Stanford University, has shown that cultural changes have shaped a woman's personality more than a man's. From the 1970s to the '90s, women's degree of masculinization increased even though their "femininity quotient" stayed the same! In contrast, men's degree of masculinity stayed the same. When social learning changes behavior, it shapes brain pathways and changes a woman's tendency toward problems with mood, anxiety, attention, and memory.

Prenatal stress feminizes a male brain and masculinizes the female brain. Some people erroneously generalize this finding to say that maternal stress in pregnancy causes homosexuality. This is simply wrong and this assumption has been shown to be incorrect by many studies. All left-handed men who are poor at map reading are not gay nor are all left-handed women who are good at target shooting lesbians. Some but not all women whose brains were masculinized by a prenatal adrenal gland problem have the male-oriented visuospatial ability. Scientists have shown that our femininity and masculinity—our gender traits and role behaviors (toy choices, rough-and-tumble play, cognitive style, and personality characteristics such as aggression and nurturance)—are housed in multiple areas of the brain, and lie in networks that are different from those for sexual preference.

But hormones do shape our brains from the moment we are conceived to the time we die. Estrogen, testosterone, progesterone, and others help determine how we think and how we emotionally experience the world.

Of course, "masculinization" or "feminization" is a matter of degree, so the girl will still become a woman and the boy will still become a man. However, each will have subtle emotional characteristics and some of the thought styles associated with the opposite sex, since their brains are tinged by hormones usually associated with the opposite sex. A woman whose brain has been prenatally altered by testosterone may be more likely to be left-handed or ambidextrous, and have specific talents usually seen in men, for example, map reading. However, she will still have to deal with the feminine brain's increased risk for moodiness, depression, anxiety or nervousness, addiction, pain, sleep, or immune system disorders. In addition to brain changes, she may also have physical changes in her body that cause problems in her female reproductive system and immune system dysfunction.

A Female Baby's Brain May Become Nontraditional If Her Mother Takes Hormones

Gerry was fifty-one years old and very concerned about her physical and mental health. When she came to see me, she had been suffering for ten years from SLE (lupus), infertility, premature menopause, and depression. After years of illness and remissions, and steroid treatment, her depression deepened and she was diagnosed with osteoporosis.

Gerry had recently found out that during her pregnancy her mother had taken DES (diethylstilbestrol), a synthetic estrogen that was believed to help prevent miscarriages. Gerry wondered if that had anything to do with her lifelong history of mental and physical challenges. DES masculinizes the brain of the female baby. "DES daughters" have higher rates of menstrual, infertility, and pregnancy problems. Like the female babies who developed in utero in stressed mothers with excess androgens, DES daughters have an increased frequency of being left-handed, having ADD/ADHD, learning disabilities, and high spatial abilities.

To assess Gerry's feminine brain's mind-body challenges, I looked further into her areas of talent and strengths. Gerry's brain had many specific characteristics that are more frequently seen in a man's brain.

She was *ambidextrous:* Gerry wrote with her left hand but was ambidextrous in softball and when doing manicures. She was the only one of her girlfriends who could skillfully apply nail polish with either her left or right hand.

She had *majored in traditionally male-dominated subjects in college:* Gerry had been in premed and was at the top of her class in physics and chemistry.

She *designed and built the addition to her house:* Gerry had a flair for building projects. Her favorite show was *This Old House* on PBS.

Having the masculinizing effect of DES on her developing brain may have also greatly increased her chances to experience certain emotional and mental health problems including:

- *Depression:* Gerry also suffered from PMS, but her irritability and depression got out of control during infertility hormone treatments and during steroid treatment for lupus.

- *Immune system dysfunction:* Gerry developed lupus and infertility, two conditions thought to be autoimmune in nature.

I helped Gerry to understand that she had a unique brain organization, a model much different from the traditional feminine brain. Many of the prototypical left-brain functions were Gerry's weaknesses. Rather than focus on how she was different from other women, I helped Gerry open her right-brain areas of genius: her capacity for math, science, and three-dimensional design. However, Gerry would have to accept that her immune system and mood were both her weakness and her source for intuition. By learning how her feminine brain was wired for mood, learning, memory, and intuition, she could learn how to utilize her genius and maximize her emotional and physical health.

Your Developmental Stage Shapes Your Moods and Intellectual Capabilities

Just as sex hormones administered to a pregnant woman will shape her developing daughter's brain later in life, different estrogen, progesterone, and testosterone levels during certain stages of the menstrual cycle, pregnancy, postpartum, and peri- and postmenopause can facilitate emotional and intellectual abilities.

Mary, a forty-eight-year-old, was obsessing about her work. She said, "I can't stand it; the same worry repeats over and over in my head like a skip on a CD." Mary was a medical research technician and had made a minor mistake, contaminating a small batch of samples. Despite the trivial nature of the error, the thought of it went around and around and around in her head. In her twenties, after her husband left her, Mary had had a "nervous breakdown," but since then she had done well. She suddenly went into menopause after a total abdominal hysterectomy for a fibroid (the doctor removed her uterus and her ovaries). Following the surgery, her doctor told her she needed only estrogen, mistakenly thinking she no longer needed progesterone, too, since he had been taught its only purpose was to prevent uterine lining buildup.

Mary reported, "After that surgery, my mind went down the hopper. I can't think straight, I make mistakes, and I'm really blue."

All the so-called reproductive hormones have profound effects on the feminine brain throughout our lifespan. Estrogen is an antidepressant hormone and critical for bonding in relationships. It is also critical for good memory function and paying attention. Progesterone is a mood stabilizer that not only quells anger and irritability, but lowers anxiety. Testosterone helps promote initiative and motivation for many kinds of goals in the outer world, not just sex.

Mary needed progesterone as both a mood stabilizer and antianxiety agent. She needed all the emotional stabilization she could get, since she had had a nervous breakdown earlier in her life. When the doctor removed Mary's ovaries, Mary suddenly lost an important source of progesterone and estrogen, her own body's way of balancing mood and anxiety states. By replacing estrogen but not progesterone, Mary became anxious and moody, increasing her chances of having another depression.

Mary learned an array of solutions for her depression (Chapters 4 and 5) and anxiety (Chapters 6 and 7), and also figured out that her intuition was telling her that she needed to reexamine the intimate relationships in her life.

CHEMICALS IN THE ENVIRONMENT SHAPE THE NEW FEMININE BRAIN

A woman's brain in the twenty-first century faces a lot of new environmental challenges that it has not evolved protection against. Hormone-like molecules that show up in our food, "xenoestrogens," affect our brains' emotional and cognitive abilities. Herbal compounds (phytoestrogens like the isoflavone genistein from soy) may enlarge specific areas of the hypothalamus and hormonally alter it. Some widely used insecticides have an estrogenic effect on the developing prenatal brain, altering it in a way that causes problems with the menstrual cycle later in life. DDT, PCBs, methoxychlor, and other insecticides are either masculinizing or feminizing to brains and bodies of other animals and may also present a challenge to the New Feminine Brain. They have been shown to feminize seagulls, alligators, and rats. PCBs bind to estrogen receptors on turtle eggs, and the young produced are only female. These environmental xenoestrogens may also affect the way the feminine brain learns, remembers, and creates moods. Environmental xenoestrogens may also increase the incidence of breast cancer, fertility, and gynecological tumors.

Androgens (like tamoxifen and other related medicines) are currently used to control certain types of cancer. Some scientists believe caution is warranted with these medicines because they change the shape of certain nuclei in the brain cells that are responsible for sexual behavior. Alcohol, cocaine, and monosodium glutamate (MSG) can also change the shape and size of certain fetal brain areas if taken by a pregnant woman.

Here are three different women with three kinds of conflicts and health challenges.

Pressures to Maintain Roles Rewire the Brain

Chloe was a high-powered, successful writer before her marriage to Don. At thirty-nine, Chloe knew her biological clock was ticking so she had two children quickly. Having done a lot of reading on parenting while pregnant, she decided to be a stay-at-home mother. At first, Chloe basked in the warmth of the home fires. She kept the house clean and took care of the children while her husband ran a local real estate firm.

By the time her first child was seven and the younger one was five, Chloe began to experience physical and emotional problems. After the second child, she had suffered some fatigue and depression, but no matter what medicine she took or how much she rested, her symptoms didn't improve. Chloe developed a goiter and hypothyroidism, but taking thyroid replacement didn't improve her mood, her fatigue, or help her lose the forty pounds she had gained. Chloe became so depressed, she was suicidal.

Chloe's husband was desperate to have her feel better. He got her someone to help with the kids and help keep the house clean, to open up space in the day so she could return to writing. They built a home office for Chloe complete with computer and stereo system. Despite her husband's loving efforts, Chloe couldn't get any serious work done on her writing. She had trouble "disconnecting" from the role of being a mother and homemaker enough to "connect" with her writer's identity. When Chloe was in her office, her mind wandered toward how her children were doing or what needed to be done in the house. When she was being a mother and homemaker, she was beating herself up for not being more organized and productive in her writing.

Chloe's feminine brain had been rewired, before she was married, by the immense success and social perks that came from being a famous writer. Higher social status increases testosterone, which increased her drive in the competitive business world.

When a woman suddenly interrupts a "high-voltage" career, she is at greater risk for depression and other mood disorders. If she trades in that high-testosterone career for the estrogen-soaked vocation of motherhood, her brain will be two brains in one. Like Chloe, she has both the traditional feminine circuits for nurturance and bonding and the more masculinized testosterone brain pathways of her career. Chloe's twice-rewired brain was trying to find a balance.

Neither Chloe's mother nor any of her aunts had had her medical problems so early in life. Chloe's New Feminine Brain had some glitches to work out—an increased risk for depression and thyroid disease.

Trying to Make a Square Peg Fit in a Round Hole

If you have a nontraditional feminine brain, it's critical for your emotional and physical health that you do what Dolly Parton suggests, "Find out who you are and do it on purpose." Don't try to fit your unique brain style into a career and lifestyle that makes other people accept you but makes you miserable. Excessive exercise, anorexia nervosa, and excessive dieting can alter estrogen and progesterone levels and affect the female brain.

Debra was always the apple of her father's eye. In a Christian family of seven (two girls, three boys), she was the free-spirited tomboy. She rode four-wheelers with her father through the backwoods, bought her first motorcycle at age sixteen, and excelled in math and science, especially chemistry. While her sister was cooking for church picnics, Debra was riding her motorcycle with the boys behind the church. This all worked until she was to go off to college.

Debra had wanted to be a doctor, but her parents wanted her to go to a Christian college to become a teacher. Debra had to choose between her father's love and acceptance and her future. She ran away from home and used her savings to become a nurse. Although Debra reveled in working in the medical environment that she had always craved to be in, she also felt somewhat unsatisfied. Back at home, her sister, "the normal daughter," got married and had several children.

The rift between Debra and her family healed over the years, but an inner core in Debra did not. She became depressed, gained a lot of weight, and grew unsightly body hair. At the age of forty-two, Debra became conflicted over whether or not to have kids. Even though being around kids had always irritated her and she had never really wanted children, society and her family had programmed her to believe that she wouldn't be a real woman until she became a mother. So Debra tried to have children anyway, couldn't get pregnant due to irregular periods, and finally was given a diagnosis of polycystic ovary disease. Debra was trying to take her masculinized brain style and fit it into a traditional feminine life, and it was making her sick and miserable.

Polycystic ovary disease (PCO) is a complex disorder in which a woman's hormonal rhythms go haywire. Patients often become obese, depressed, and infertile; they grow unsightly hair and their menstrual cycles become wildly irregular as their levels of testosterone and other androgens go up. The prolonged, unstable elevated hormonal patterns increase the incidence of endometrial and breast cancer. Hyperinsulinism and obesity increase the chances of hypercholesterolemia, heart disease, stroke, and diabetes. Although physicians used to treat patients with PCO with a variety of hormonal treatments, including the Pill, we now realize that a food plan low in carbohydrates and fat with moderate levels of protein can reduce insulin resistance and normalize weight, hormones, and the menstrual cycle. No one really knows how many people have this disorder because many women may have some but not all of the symptoms. Now, many scientists believe that, with the epidemic of obesity in the United States, many women have elements of the insulin resistance that sets the scene for the hormonal problems characterizing PCO.

Traditional Desires

In the twenty-first century, society sometimes denigrates women with traditional female brains who want to focus a large portion of their adult life on nurturing and motherhood. If a woman believes she must tough it out and fit into the newer societally dictated role of "having it all," combining a career with motherhood, she may snap under the pressure emotionally and physically. The following story is a case in point.

Nadine, thirty-five, had gone to Columbia University in New York and majored in both English literature and political science. She also had been a fiercely competitive tennis player and an intensely perfectionist, serious student. Her father had a law firm in which she had always been slated to become a full partner. Once she finished law school, Nadine married a schoolmate and moved into one of the best corner offices. Everything was "on schedule." Nadine even passed her law bar exams on the first try.

Once Nadine began her first year of practice, however, a nameless discomfort and fatigue took over her. She began to think she was pushing herself too hard in her daily hourly workouts with her trainer, so she dropped them. She dropped her birth control for the first time in her life and tried to get pregnant. Months went by and the only thing that stayed on schedule was the growth of Nadine's law practice. She didn't get pregnant as she wanted, and her frustration and fatigue mounted.

Nadine went through three expensive rounds of IVF (in vitro fertilization) without success. Her fatigue got worse and Nadine became more obsessed with her weight. Some doctors were concerned that her teenage episode of anorexia had recurred.

When I talked to Nadine, she was miserable, exhausted, falling behind at work. She was obsessed by the idea that others in her father's law firm would perceive her as "slacking off." Nadine told me she secretly wanted to be a mother, stay at home with a baby, and even homeschool her kids.

She wanted five kids and didn't see herself as a lawyer for the rest of her life. Everything she had worked for, perfectly scheduled and executed, seemed hollow now. Once she actually felt what it was like to be a lawyer, she couldn't believe she had spent all that money for all those years of study.

Nadine was very concerned about her body. Her periods had stopped and she had severe constipation. She blamed these symptoms on residual hormonal imbalances from all the IVF treatments but it was obvious that at 5'7" and 110 pounds (having lost 30 pounds), Nadine was suffering from anorexia nervosa. In addition to having a distorted body image and episodes of overeating, vomiting, or overexercise, patients like Nadine with anorexia nervosa usually come from families where success, achievement, and appearance reign supreme. Nadine didn't want to even talk about the possibility of quitting law and leaving her father's law firm—it "just wasn't an option." Anorexia is said to develop when the "role of the perfect child" becomes too difficult. Ironically, it appeared that for Nadine to become pregnant and enter into the role of being a parent, she had to resign from being "The Perfect Child" with her family, and risk disappointing her father and other family members.

Some women so stress themselves that, in their quest for perfection and their attempts to fit into the competitive world, they tip the hormones in their body away from normal levels. For example, women who compulsively exercise their way into anorexia lower their body's estrogen levels; as a result, the androgen "male" hormonal level goes up. Nadine's straining to be a perfect daughter was ironically working against her ability to be a perfect wife and mother.

The Dangers of Low Estrogen and Rising Testosterone

Believe it or not, a lot of your brain is made of Fat! The neurons in the brain are coated with a protective, fatty coating called myelin that "shrinks" when you lose excessive amounts of weight. So it's not surprising that CT brain scans of patients with anorexia nervosa and bulimia show brain atrophy, which is reversible if the woman gains weight. PET studies of patients with bulimia show loss of normal, right-hemisphere activity. In our society, with its emphasis on thinness, competitiveness, and social status, women are unwittingly transforming themselves into hypertestosterone, hypoestrogenic beings. The pressure on women today to have the pseudoadolescent male body that is typical of today's runway model causes her brain to be more susceptible to moodiness and anxiety. Yet you can learn how to manage your desire for physical fitness and social acceptance, career and motherhood when you understand your New Feminine Brain's strengths and weaknesses.

What Kind of Brain Do You Have?

How can you tell what your brain style is? How do you know if you live in your right brain or left brain, or somewhere in between? Is your brain more feminized or masculinized? How has your brain been altered by diet, trauma, or other experience? Let's look at the various ways you can figure out what side of the brain you're on.

VISUOSPATIAL CAPABILITIES: SEEING IN 3-D, FINDING LOST OBJECTS, AND DRAWING

To find out what style of brain you have for perception, please look at Figures 1 and 2. Figure 1 shows two rotational tasks—the idea is to mentally rotate all the figures and decide which could be identical to the one on the left, rotated to a different orientation on the page (answers: B, D, and E). Traditional men are supposed to be better at this kind of mental rotation task. Ask a couple of men in your life to look at part B if you have trouble seeing which figures are identical. Figure 2 shows two groups of figures. You need to try to identify the items that have changed location from the top to the bottom groupings. Traditional women have been shown to be better at identifying locations of objects within a small area. Short-term practicing does not seem to reduce the differences between the sexes in performing visuospatial tasks. Some have suggested that differences between women and men in visuospatial skills has declined over the past few decades.

The long-term adaptation of a woman to perform dual roles in our so-

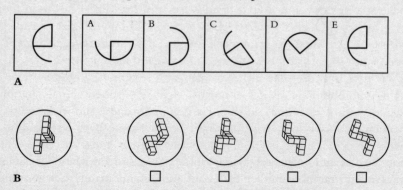

Figure 1. Mental Rotation: In an array of six boxes and five circles, which ones are duplicates?

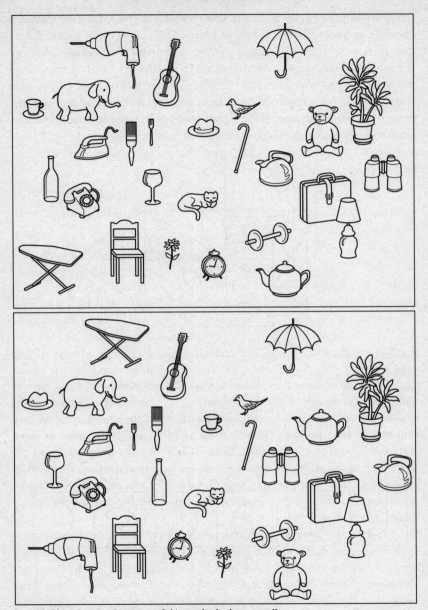

Figure 2. Object Location: In an array of objects, what has been moved?

ciety encourages hormonal changes in her body and a rewiring of path-ways in her brain, leaving her with new intellectual capabilities but emo-tional and mental challenges as well.

Now look at Figure 3. This is known as the Rey-Osterrieth Complex Figure. Get yourself three pieces of unlined 8½- by 11-inch paper. Take a few minutes to study and copy the figure on one piece of paper, then close the book and throw away the drawing. On another piece of paper, redraw the figure, as much as you can remember. When you've finished, set your drawing aside for a few minutes. Then, on the third sheet of blank paper, draw what you remember of the figure without looking at either your second drawing or Figure 3 in the book.

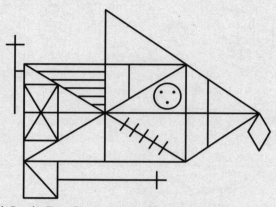

Figure 3. Rey-Osterrieth Complex Figure: Drawing to copy and by memory.

At the end of that time, look at what you've drawn and what you recalled. When you drew the first outline of the figure, how did you do it? Did you try to draw the overall configuration and then fill it in? If so, then you approached the task primarily from a right hemisphere point of view: You were looking at the gestalt, the whole. Did you start drawing in the figure piecemeal, filling in details as you moved across the page from left to right? If so, then you perceive and attend to the world from a left hemisphere perspective. Many people have a mix of both right and left hemisphere perspectives.

Most people approach this task by first drawing the outer configuration, then filling in the details. The right brain perceives the forest, then the left brain fills in the trees. This mirrors the order in which the brain develops—right frontal lobe first, followed by the left hemisphere. If you can remember the shape but you miss the details, you live in your right brain for perception, visuospatial skills, attention, and memory—and your left brain is a little on the loose side. On the other hand, if your paper is dotted with details—a cross here and a triangle there, and a circle with three dots over there—then you're likely to have a left brain that is highly functioning but a right hemisphere that has trouble seeing the overview—what the details add up to. This exercise gives you a good idea why we need both left and right brains to fully perceive the world.

LANGUAGE: THE HAIR WHORL EXAM AND OTHER TESTS

In the next test, you're going to check another sign of right-brain or left-brain dominance: hair whorls—the pattern your hair makes as it grows. Hair grows in a spiral, or whorl. As the brain develops, it pushes out the skull in a pattern that shows up on the scalp. Your hair whorls show how your brain is organized.

Stand or sit with your back to a large mirror, then hold up a hand mirror in front of you and angle it so you can see the crown of your head. Part your hair down the middle. Does your hair spiral to the left, in a counterclockwise pattern, or clockwise, to your right?

If your hair spirals in a counterclockwise direction over the left parietal area of the brain (roughly the crown of the left side of your head), chances are you process language mostly in the left hemisphere. This is the most common pattern. If your hair whorl is on the right side, you probably process language mostly in the right brain. You are also more likely to have learning challenges such as attention deficit disorder. If you have two hair whorls—one on the left parietal area and one on the right parietal area—your brain is most likely organized bilaterally for language. You may have more difficulty finding the ketchup in the refrigerator than someone with a traditional feminine brain, but you're probably better at visuospatial tasks such as throwing a ball, and right-brain skills such as geometry. If you can't figure out where your hair whorls are, ask your hairdresser. Sometimes only your hairdresser knows for sure.

When you've figured out your own hair whorls, you might want to take a look at your partner's hair and your children's.

Now, think about your occupation. Most people choose jobs that fit with how they think. There are exceptions, of course; I've known people who wanted to major in English in college, but when they found out they were dyslexic, selected another field. Generally speaking, someone majoring in a language-intensive subject like English would have more blood flow to the left brain, while someone in a visuospatial, "three-dimensional" discipline like radiology or architecture would have more flow to the right brain.

How Do You Speak and Converse?

Someone who processes language mostly in the right brain is likely to be blunter and use fewer words. She may lack the immense dictionary of the left brain. Her sentence structure tends to be less varied: She's likely to repeat the same word order, with the same cadence. If I ask someone, "Where's the newspaper?" and he responds, "It's in the car," I might ask, "Where in the car?" and he would probably simply repeat, "It's in the car." He may vary his tone, mannerisms, and facial expression, but he's basically just using his right brain. But if I ask someone else, who is more lateralized in the left brain, "Where's the newspaper?" that person's answer will be more precise and descriptive: "It's in the car, to the right of the gear shift, underneath the seat, beside the oil can." The person who speaks from the right brain will use broad, nonspecific phrases, such as "You know that thing we did that time down there with that thing?" She is more likely to speak in sentence fragments, with less attention to grammar and syntax. On the other hand, since the right brain is more directly connected to the body, she will likely use more gestures when speaking than someone who speaks more from the left brain.

Women are using more of their brains than ever before. On one level, nothing could be more exciting than to have increased brain capacity, including greater cognitive abilities. But the news is not all good, because, as we've seen, in changing the hormonal makeup of your brain, you may also increase your chances of getting various emotional and physical disorders.

Like a new car coming off the assembly line, the New Feminine Brain has an evolving style. The new model has a lot of options not available in earlier models, but it may take years—or decades—to iron out the way all the new features work together. The New Feminine Brain has some distinct advantages—it's fully loaded with increased connectivity, increased right-hemisphere use. But the female chassis or body struggles to keep up with its new brain style, its more complicated electronics and computer systems.

Throughout the rest of this book, we will explore how to help your New Feminine Brain approach any challenges you may have with mood, anxiety, attention, memory, and intuition. You will discover how your unique brain has developed and the best solutions to your problems and challenges.

PART TWO

The New Feminine Brain's Wiring for Emotions, Moods, and Anxiety

THREE

Emotional Feng Shui:
You Are What You Feel

**The only true currency in this bankrupt world is what you
share with someone else when you are uncool.**
From the movie Almost Famous

Emotions have always been an issue for women. Since the beginning of
recorded history, women have been described as the more emotional and
intuitive sex. In several scientific studies, the majority of women believed
that they were more likely than men to express positive emotions like joy,
love, affection, warmth, empathy, and sympathy clearly in relationships.
They also felt they were more likely to express "negative" emotions such
as distress, sadness, disgust, vulnerability, hurt, sadness, and shame.

I've never met a woman who didn't have a problem with one emotion
or another. Yet we have five basic emotions of fear, anger, sadness, joy, and
love. These can occur in a lot of permutations, however. For instance, we
can feel:

Attraction, adoration, and infatuation
Aggravation, agitation, and irritation
Humiliation, mortification, invalidation, dejection, rejection, and neglect
Ecstasy, gaiety, and joviality
Jumpiness, panic, and anxiety

It has been said that we are what we eat, but we are actually even more
what we feel. The emotions that your heart and mind contain—how you
feel—are the best predictors of your overall happiness, health, success at
long-term goals, and your place in society. Unresolved anger leads to in-

creased risk of sudden death from a heart attack. Optimism and love enhance the immune system and protect you from cancer and other illnesses.

Because the feminine brain is hyperconnected, women feel emotion in
almost everything they think, say, or do. With a brain suffused with emotions, it's no wonder that our feelings and emotional brain circuits are also
the foundation for our intuition. A capacity to be emotionally or intuitively "porous" to others' feelings is probably inborn, but is more frequently found in individuals, male or female, with the hyperconnected
feminine brain style.

Emotions Are Expressed Simultaneously in the Brain and Body

Negative emotions come from the right brain, which has millions of connections to the body. When we feel an emotion, especially anger or fear,
physiological changes take place simultaneously in all of the body's organs.
A physical symptom in our body can also evoke an emotion. For example,
when someone is nervous or anxious, he may experience shortness of
breath, and feeling short of breath can precipitate a feeling of panic or anxiety.

Each of the five basic emotions (see Emotional Feng Shui diagram,
p. 70) uses a distinct brain circuit. Each travels a specific highway, primarily from the right brain, through a section of the brain stem down to the
body, and then back to the brain again. These circuits in the brain and brain
stem help create internal emotions of fear, anger, sadness, joy, and love, as
well as typical patterns of physical reactions, like stomachaches, high blood
pressure, a lump in the throat, heart palpitations, and hot flashes.

Every illness has an emotional and behavioral component. Each of the
brain's emotional pathways for fear, anger, sadness, love, and joy also connects through the brain stem to specific organs of the body. For example,
if you are fried, steaming mad, or marinated in resentment, the anger circuit in your brain and brain stem areas increases your heart rate and body
temperature (thus the temperature metaphors). Your muscle tone changes
as well. Muscles tense in the mouth, face, jaw, vocal cords, hands, and fists,
which cause you to frown, grit your teeth, clench your jaw, talk in a louder
voice, clench your fists, or be more likely to pound or slam things or, in
some cases, drive fast. At times, we will suddenly feel "tense" or "shaky,"
"out of sorts," not knowing exactly what we are feeling. The unnamed
emotions in our brain and body fester, and if we don't get to the root of
what we are feeling and why, we tend to get sick. Learning "emotional
feng shui" can help you find out what you are feeling and why.

The five basic emotions parallel the five elements in traditional Chinese medicine. In fact, Traditional Chinese Medicine considers the illness/emotion, body/brain connection as a whole entity. Emotional disharmony can induce illness, and body organs in disharmony can induce painful emotional states. If fear, anger, sadness, love, and joy occur out of proportion to each other in the normal "even-tempered" emotional landscape, stress will result. One could say that an imbalance between the five basic emotions causes "bad emotional feng shui."

Emotional Feng Shui

To help you figure out your brain's emotional feng shui, I created a five-sided functional model of the feminine emotional brain (see Figure 4, "Emotional Feng Shui"). Each side represents a basic emotion: fear, anger, sadness, love, or joy. Each emotion is precipitated by specific events and is associated with typical thoughts and actions, and health reactions. Our mind-body circuits for *fear* start to fire away when we are in unfamiliar territory, or anticipate harm to ourselves or a loved one. When you are feeling fearful, for example, you are more likely to act nervous, talk quickly, cry, yell, run and hide, avoid what is terrifying you, or not move at all. When you are afraid, your heart races, you get sweaty, jittery, feel short of breath, tense your muscles, and your body temperature feels like ice. If you are genetically susceptible, sudden or prolonged fear can precipitate an asthma attack, cause immune system dysfunction (including allergies and colds), bowel problems (including irritable bowel syndrome and ulcerative colitis), skin problems, or thyroid disease. Sudden fear, if held long enough, turns to chronic worry and anxiety, and, in some genetically susceptible individuals, leads to ulcers, overeating, or obesity. Similarly, if a person has chronic ulcers or obesity for a long period of time, she is more likely to experience chronic anxiety.

In contrast to experiencing fear, *sadness* is more likely to be precipitated by loss of love and acceptance, having things turn out badly, or being with someone else who is sad. When you feel sad, you are more likely to walk, talk, and think slowly. Grief tends to make you tired and lethargic. Extreme sadness and depression can increase your risk of getting a virus or other infection, or even cancer.

You're more likely to feel *anger* after you've lost power, status, or respect, or things don't turn out the way you expected, or after feeling physical pain. Anger circuits tend to increase the heart rate, causing palpitations, and raising cholesterol, blood sugar, and blood pressure. Another physical by-product of anger is a change in hormone levels, which can lead to breast lumpiness, migraine headaches, and insomnia. If you are chronically angry, your simmering irritability or hostility increases your chance toward hypertension, cardiac arrhythmias, and other types of heart problems. And if you have hypertension, arrhythmias, or long-term heart problems, you are more likely to feel irritable, agitated, or on edge.

Being successful and getting what you want releases opiates in the body which relieve pain, enhance the immune system, and give you a sense of ecstasy, pride, and a feeling of well-being. *Joy* releases acetylcholine, serotonin, and norepinephrine in the brain, enhancing attention, learning, and memory. Joy subsequently increases the level of "energy" in the brain and body, making us feel excited, energetic, and talkative.

Similar to joy, you feel *love* when someone gives you what you want, makes you feel needed and secure. Like fear, love makes your heart beat faster, possibly because both emotional circuits travel through similar brain and brain stem areas that may prompt the sympathetic nervous system to make your heart go "pitter-patter." Love creates a mind-body biochemical environment that encourages bonding. It affects hormone levels in the body, especially oxytocin, which is critical for a mother to bond with her newborn baby and for falling in love. Serotonin as well as cholecystokinin (CCK) also signal feelings of love but are associated with food and appetite. You don't necessarily experience love only in a one-to-one relationship. Love circuits also fire when you feel kinship with other living beings (E.O. Wilson calls this "biophilia"). You can also feel love for a piece of land (for me, that would be the coast of Maine), or for your "calling" in life—which also causes the love circuits to fire. The neurochemical changes that love causes in the brain and body are very similar to the biological events of joy. Love also enhances (via oxytocin and opiates) the immune system and improves attention, learning, and memory.

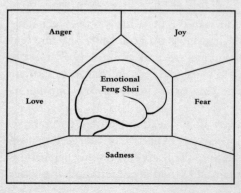

Figure 4. Emotional Feng Shui™. A balance of five basic emotions creates health.

EMOTIONAL FENG SHUI

Emotion	What the Emotion Is Signaling	Thought Pattern	Action	Health Reaction *if you are genetically susceptible*
Sadness	• Things turning out not the way you want or expect • Loss of love/acceptance or a significant relationship • Being in contact with someone who is sad	• Thinking that the pain from the loss will last forever • Thinking that things are hopeless, and that you can't do anything to improve the situation • Distractibility/problems paying attention • Forgetfulness, problems learning	• Face: Frowning/dull, droopy eyes • Body: droopy, slumped posture; slowed movements, slowed speech, slowed thoughts • Talking about things that are depressing • Criticizing, blaming, being "down" on things	• Fatigue/lethargy/apathy • Lack of initiative and motivation • Hollow feeling in chest, emptiness/chest pressure • Shortness of breath • Problems swallowing • Dizziness • Gaining or losing weight • Anorexia or obesity • Insomnia or excessive daytime sleepiness • Major depression • PMS depression • Menstrual and perimenopausal irregularities • Increase in cholesterol • Increased pain • Inflammation in body: increased risk of heart disease and dementia • Immune system dysfunction: increased susceptibility to infection, autoimmune illness, or cancer
Anger	• Things turning out not the way you want or expect • Losing authority, respect, or power • Having you or someone you love experience emotional and physical pain	• Thinking things are unfair, unjust • Thinking things should be different • Seeing only your point of view, thinking you are right and "they" are wrong	• Tight, red face: gritting teeth, clenched jaw • Tight, clenched hands, fists; rigid, tight neck and back • Surge of energy: loud voice, stomping feet, slamming things, crying	• Feeling hot, flushed face • Headache • Increased heart rate, blood pressure, elevated cholesterol • Depression • PMS irritability • Menstrual and perimenopausal irregularities • Estrogen dominance: breast lumpiness • Muscle tension/pain

Emotion	What the Emotion Is Signaling	Thought Pattern	Action	Health Reaction _if you are genetically susceptible_
Fear	• Entering into an unfamiliar situation • Being alone, or in the dark • Being threatened or hurt • Sensing someone you love is being threatened or hurt	• Awaiting rejection or criticism • Believing failure is imminent • Believing you are powerless • Losing control	• Frozen face • Nervous, shaky speech • Crying, yelling, running, hiding, fidgeting • Not moving • Avoiding what you fear	• Sweat, perspiring • Hot flash, cold chills • Shortness of breath, asthma • Palpitations, chest pressure • Lump in throat, difficulty swallowing • Nausea, abdominal pain, diarrhea, constipation • Hair loss • Thyroid dysfunction • Skin problems, rashes
Love	• Someone treating you favorably • Someone gives you what you want or need, or raises your status, your self-esteem • Wanting closeness • Sharing a special experience with a pet, animal, piece of land, or "great work"	• Someone makes you feel needed, gives you a sense of safety and security, or tells you that you are attractive • Wanting to do things for someone	• Face: bright eyes, smiling, increased eye contact • Acting "excited," giddy • Appearing calm and alert simultaneously	• Increased heart rate • Increased body temperature • Feeling strength in the body • A change in appetite • Improved immune response
Joy	• Getting what you want or have worked for • Being accepted by others • Achieving a goal	• Thinking that you are strong, powerful, capable, lovable, and successful	• Smiling, bright eyed • Talking freely and jubilantly • Moving with a light, carefree bounce in your step • Appearing energetic, charismatic, and enthusiastic	• Turning red, blushing • Enhanced immune system competency • Improved attention, learning, and memory

Sources: A Damasio (1999). _The Feeling of What Happens: Body and Emotion in the Making of Consciousness._ New York: Harcourt and Brace; J Panksepp (1998). _Affective Neuroscience: The Foundations of Human and Animal Emotions._ New York: Oxford University Press; M Lewis and JM Haviland-Jones (2000). _Handbook of Emotions,_ 2nd Edition. New York: Guilford Press, pp. 139–152. MM Linehan (1993). _Skills Training Manual for Treating Borderline Personality Disorder._ New York: Guilford Press, pp. 139–152.

What Are My Emotions?

We are all born with a temperament, a unique blend of emotions, thoughts, actions, and typical body health reactions or tendencies (see Figure 5). Our unique temperament makes us tend to travel in some of the basic emotional brain networks more than others. Some women are more fearful, some tend toward sadness, and others are more irritable or angry. Some lucky women are "even-tempered" and travel equally in all of the five basic brain highways.

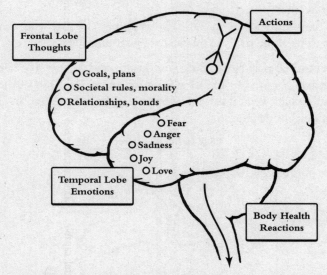

Figure 5. Feminine Personality Style: Emotions can be funneled into goals, relationships, or society.

Similarly, each of us has a unique personality style, a personal way that we tend to get our emotional needs met. Via frontal lobe "executive" pathways, we can funnel our passion into (1) work, (2) relationships, (3) society, and (4) physical activity. If we don't have a balanced way of getting our needs met, we can experience health problems. For example, if I have been born with an irritable, easily angered temperament and then suffered some type of abuse, I may take my anger and funnel it into a job as a lawyer fighting for social justice. Although this focus in life may benefit my clients and possibly my bank account, in the long run, living and breathing constantly in anger and fight mode is likely to cause me hypertension, high cholesterol, and heart disease. Your unique feminine brain is a product of your genes, temperament, personality, and later life experiences. Using some emotional pathways and frontal executive networks more than others, you can develop exceptional capabilities—your personal genius—but not without some cost.

How Your Emotions Affect Your Health

Do you:

- Shop compulsively when you are upset?
- Eat too much when you feel overwhelmed, rejected, or upset?
- Have trouble talking to a loved one or a boss when you are upset or hurt?
- Find yourself staying in a bad relationship because you don't want to be alone or feel you can't support yourself?

Your emotions may be affecting your health, and you need to become knowledgeable about your brain's wiring for emotions. Each of the five basic emotions has a typical pattern of feelings, thoughts, actions, and body health reactions (see Figure 6).

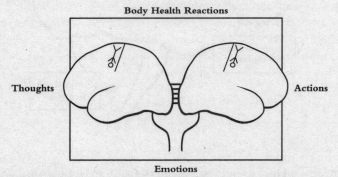

Figure 6. The New Feminine Emotional Brain: Emotions, thoughts, actions, and body health reactions.

In the four-sided box surrounding the brain, the bottom side represents the feeling associated with the emotion, and the left side stands for the thought patterns that tend to coincide with it. The right side of the square symbolizes how we act when we experience that specific emotion. Finally, the top of the square represents body health reactions that tend to occur. For health and consciousness, we need to be aware of all the typical patterns of feelings, thoughts, actions, and health reactions associated with fear, anger, sadness, love, and joy.

For example, suppose you feel chronically exhausted and stay up late into the night ruminating about all the things that are wrong in your life. You have an attack of the shingles, a very painful condition associated with immune system deficiency. You have the typical *actions, thoughts,* and *body health* reactions of *sadness.* Treating yourself for depression may stop the self-deprecating thoughts, improve your fatigue, and build up your immune system to make the painful shingles go away. It doesn't matter if you never felt sad, because you have three out of the four components of the sadness brain circuit, indicating that you have excessive activation of that brain-body network.

All of us have an inborn weakness in one or more of the five basic emotional circuits (see Figure 4, Emotional Feng Shui diagram) in the New Feminine Brain. For example, some women are predisposed to depression; others to panic and anxiety. The three columns of the Emotional Feng Shui chart will give you clues to whether or not your brain-body emotional circuits are firing in a healthy way. By examining your thought patterns, automatic actions, and health reactions in a specific emotional brain circuit (fear, anger, sadness, joy, or love) you can name the emotion, know what it's telling you, and learn what to do to soothe the feeling.

Every organ of the body has a connection to the emotional circuitry of the brain. If you can sense your emotions and how they affect your thoughts and behavior, you can tap into a treatment modality that could be cheap and free of side effects.

Let's see some ways this intertwining of brain and body works.

The Emotion-to-Disease Domino Effect

Mood problems over time eventually trigger the release of biochemicals that will unbalance your health. Vice versa, health problems over time set into motion a series of neurochemical imbalances that can cause depression, anxiety, and other emotional disorders. If you have had a back injury and suffer in pain for a prolonged period, you are more likely to develop a neurochemical imbalance of opiates and serotonin, which ultimately will increase your chance of getting depressed. Similarly, if you are chronically depressed, the consequent imbalance in opiates and serotonin increases your chances of developing chronic pain like lower back pain. Technically, it is inaccurate to say that pain causes depression or depression causes pain since the emotional brain is wired in such a way that both phenomena occur almost simultaneously.

What would cause some women to feel depression first and later experience its associated physical health problem? Some women have a higher threshold of physical pain—that is, our brains are constructed in such a way that they keep pain signals out of our awareness, leaving us a

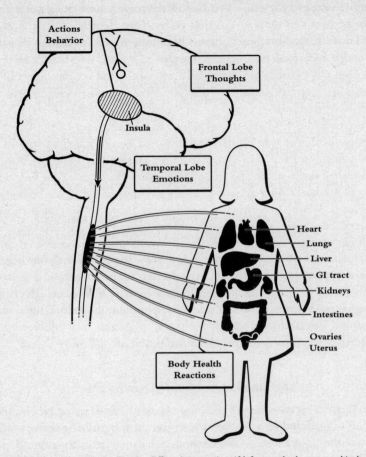

Figure 7. The Emotion-to-Disease Domino Effect: Any emotion, if left unresolved, sets up a biochemical chain reaction that influences the health of the body.

greater chance of experiencing emotional distress first. Others have a higher threshold for emotional pain. We may be less aware of our emotions, but are more conscious of thoughts, actions, and body health reactions. When each of the five basic emotional brain circuits fires, biochemical changes occur in the mind and body simultaneously. Depending on your wiring, you may be more susceptible to either the physical health reactions or the feeling state.

Ultimately, both your emotions and your body can be a source of intuition, specifically medical intuition about your health and life. Through sickness or health, your body will let you know how you *really* feel about how things are going in your life. Similarly, your feelings of fear, anger, sadness, love, and joy can let you know intuitively how good your health *really* is.

The feminine brain may have a higher incidence of depression, anxiety, and other mood disorders because:

- Women experience complicated mixtures of emotions that they have a hard time identifying (i.e., feeling "awful," "overwhelmed").
- Women attempt to numb their emotions to maintain the approval of others.
- Women who have a lower socioeconomic status find that communicating negative emotions can compromise their personal or financial safety.
- Women have complex hormonal cycles that may make their brain's emotional apparatus more susceptible to mood disorders.

If ignored, your emotional nature will take a toll on your physical health. Depression, irritability, anxiety, and panic increase a woman's chances of developing immune and autoimmune illnesses like lupus, rheumatoid arthritis, fibromyalgia, and other pain syndromes. Imbalanced emotions ultimately increase your chances of getting heart disease, stroke, cancer, and hormonal and reproductive problems.

Emotions, Stress, and Illness

Mary Kate is forty-six and is returning to work after having two children. She always wanted to have kids and create a family, having spent much of her childhood in and out of foster homes. However, due to cutbacks at her husband's job, she could no longer afford to stay at home, homeschool her children, and be the mother she always thought she'd be. So Mary Kate brushed up on her secretarial skills and got a job in a busy office.

Immediately, Mary Kate started having problems of fatigue, nausea, and stomach distress. She had such an upset stomach each morning that she couldn't get any breakfast down before leaving for work. Her doctor checked her hormones and found them normal, except for a slightly abnormal thyroid stimulating hormone (TSH) test, indicating mild hypothyroidism. Mary Kate's doctor put her on a low dose of Synthroid, but nearly a month later, she still wasn't right. She developed hot flashes and muscle tightness in her neck and jaw. Her blood pressure became elevated, her cholesterol skyrocketed, and at times she had heart palpitations. Feeling nervous and jittery, she went back to the doctor, who lowered her Synthroid. But then her fatigue and stomach distress, which had eased up when she started taking Synthroid, returned.

Mary Kate's brain and body were changing; her love and joy circuits were no longer firing as frequently. She had left a job she loved—being a stay-at-home mother—to become a secretary, a job she hated. The loss of satisfaction decreased her joy circuit's production of oxytocin and opiates, which made her anxious. The separation from her children also caused a precipitous decline in the levels of her love neurotransmitters, opiate, serotonin, and norepinephrine. Mary Kate's career change altered the emotional landscape of her brain and the neurochemistry of her love, anger, joy, sadness, and fear circuits, which led to depression, anxiety, and physical problems.

Mary Kate didn't understand why she couldn't get well. Her doctor asked her if she was having any stress in her life—if anything was making her anxious. Mary Kate had to think for a minute about what was stressing her out. If she could only get used to this new job, she was sure her "stress" would go away.

All of us, like Mary Kate, have found ourselves in situations where our body seems to be just out of control. At some crossroads in our life, our body will present us with one symptom after another. We may get lab tests, may even get a diagnosis and medical treatment. But our bodies will work around the medical or surgical treatment. The symptoms of illness will return or we'll have side effects from the medication. Sooner or later, someone will say, "Stress may be making your illness worse." Yet stress is a "wastebasket" term. By that I mean it tells us that we are feeling something that is causing us distress, but we don't know which emotion we are experiencing or what prompted it. Saying we're stressed doesn't tell us how we can respond to the emotion we are experiencing, or change our response, or make the appropriate life changes before we develop a chronic emotional and physical problem.

Even though Mary Kate felt that her mood was all right, her body's intuition was signaling that she had a problem she had to pay attention to. Mary Kate had never really felt depressed or anxious; she always considered herself pretty emotionally well-adjusted. From an early age, in and out of foster homes, Mary Kate had learned to "numb" herself to the ups and downs of life and focus on doing what she had to do in order to survive. Mary Kate knew that nothing would make her happier than to be a stay-at-home mother, but she felt she had to pull herself together and go out into the business world, even though it was obviously making her body uncomfortable.

Working with a psychotherapist, Mary Kate learned that an early traumatic history of abandonment is associated with having trouble with "emotional regulation." Many children with this background grow up to be adults who "numb" their feelings during stressful situations. Being "uprooted" from the safety of her home to work in a busy office reenacted the trauma of being continually uprooted and moved from foster home to foster home. Mary Kate came to realize that many of her body's symptoms of ill health were associated with fear, sadness, and anger. Unexpressed anger about having things turn out counter to what you want is associated with hypertension and hypercholesterolemia. Unresolved fear about being in a new, unfamiliar place is frequently associated with thyroid dysfunction and abdominal pain. Yet the only opportunity Mary Kate had to know any of this information was through the intuitive signals that her body was giving her, by developing hypothyroidism, hypercholesterolemia, high blood pressure, and stomach pain.

Mary Kate's primary care doctor and a psychotherapist helped her in several ways to establish a healthier brain and body. For six months, Mary Kate took a combination of antianxiety and antidepressant medicines and nutritional supplements to calm her fear and nervousness, elevate her mood, and lower her blood pressure and cholesterol. Mary Kate also learned which of her automatic thoughts censored both her emotions and intuition. These included:

> "A lot of people get what they want, but I can't get what will make me truly happy."
> "I blame myself for what goes wrong around me. When things go wrong, it's up to me to fix them."
> "Whatever I do, it will never been good enough."
> "I am not valuable unless I'm taking care of someone's needs."

Mary Kate learned that everyone has these kinds of rationalizing thoughts that keep feelings and intuition at bay during times of stress, but that eventually these emotions have to come out somewhere. In her case, they took the form of problems with her heart, thyroid, and digestion.

With the help of her loving husband, family, and medical team, Mary Kate began to rewire her thought patterns, challenging herself to grow beyond the survival patterns she had adopted as a child. She began to realize that she could get what she wanted and still contribute money to her family. Mary Kate kept her office job long enough to learn how to do basic bookkeeping tasks and run a computer, then quit and started a home-based business selling nutritional supplements. During the mornings, she home-schooled her children; in the afternoons, she ran her business. Mary Kate's business skyrocketed; she soon learned that the flexible nature and other social skills that she had adopted as a child, going from foster home to foster home, enabled her to relate to a variety of clients.

Eventually, Mary Kate weaned herself off all the medicines and said good-bye to her psychotherapist. Having learned about the emotional and intuitive wiring in her brain and body, she knew how it could alert her to when she was holding herself back or allowing herself to think she couldn't be happy. Mary Kate would be able in the future to tune in to her emotions in a way that could keep her healthy.

Making the Connection Between Emotion and Physical Illness and Healing

Connecting certain emotions and thoughts to the body symptoms to which they give rise doesn't seem to be enough to help you heal. What do you do with that information? Unless you learn how to rewire your emotional brain circuits, the intuitive signals behind your health problems will have to get louder and louder to get your attention, until you get sicker and sicker and *have* to change what's wrong in your life.

The following medical intuitive reading I did on Betty-Ann, age forty-six, illustrates the limitations of simply making the connection between stressful emotions, thoughts, and body symptoms.

The reading: When I looked intuitively at Betty-Ann, I could see that she worked like a dog. I saw her carrying the bulk of responsibility for money in a relationship. In contrast, I saw that her partner was very irresponsible with money and seemed to hate his job. Betty-Ann spent an awful lot of time walking on eggshells around her very discouraged partner. She seemed to pump up her partner's self-esteem by funneling her money into "his business," but at great emotional and physical cost to herself. When I looked at her body, I saw a tendency for her family to have an increased risk toward getting thyroid problems. She seemed to be at risk for having hormonally sensitive calcified "lumpiness" in both breasts, and she seemed to be about twenty to thirty pounds overweight.

The facts: Betty-Ann was very successful in her real estate career, but she frequently worked weekdays and weekends to make up for her husband's financial problems. After her husband, Norman, had lost his CEO position five years before, he had begun to spend a lot of time on the

Web "day trading" stocks. Unfortunately, he was bad at it, and his financial losses were taking a toll on his self-esteem. He had also lost $75,000 of their retirement savings and taken out a $25,000 line of credit on their house to fund new trading. Betty-Ann had not known about these losses until she tried to refinance their house. Norman was ashamed about losing his job and about losing their retirement savings, but when Betty-Ann tried to talk to him, his reaction was so angry and so filled with shame that she didn't feel she could bring it up with him again. It just seemed easier for her to improve their financial situation by selling more houses. Working longer hours also got her out of the house so she didn't have to see her husband glued to the computer screen. The sight of him "trying to make up all their losses" made her feel "crazy."

Working so many hours and being so busy helped Betty-Ann numb herself to the painful feelings between her and Norman. It also gave her a lot of joy, self-esteem, and social status in her community. Betty-Ann took Synthroid for hypothyroidism but was otherwise very healthy, except for a "few extra pounds" on her hips. She did have a tendency to get fibrocystic disease in her breasts, which scared her, since her mother had died of breast cancer. Betty-Ann's work addiction prevented her from being present to or "conscious" of the fear, anger, and sadness that could be intuitive warnings of impending health problems and financial danger.

Although Betty-Ann truly loved her husband, she was beginning to suspect he was jealous of her success. Yet he was the only partner she had ever had who made her feel needed, acknowledged her intellect and gifts, and with whom she also shared an excellent sex life, at least until recently. So, the love Betty-Ann felt for her husband together with the joy from her business success worked to neutralize the negative emotions that were her intuitive warning signals. Betty-Ann was feeling only a paralyzing numbness, because her positive emotions of joy and love were undercut by fear, anger, and sadness.

I talked to Betty-Ann about why she had trouble being assertive. She needed to learn to talk to her husband about his gambling with their money. If she didn't, her problems with her thyroid and breasts might get worse. Betty-Ann appreciated the input and told me that she would try to figure out a solution to her marital problems.

Two years passed and Betty-Ann called me for another medical intuitive reading. Since I don't remember names, I didn't recognize her name on the schedule. I did her reading like all the others, knowing only her name and age. My reading was essentially the same as the one I had done two years earlier. I saw a woman who was angry but numb because of a relationship in which she carried a huge financial burden. I also saw an increased risk of having hormonally sensitive lumpiness, which tends to calcify later in life, in her left breast.

At this time in the reading, Betty-Ann stopped me and said, "Okay, that's what you told me last time. I get it. . . . Now what do I do?"

Reminding me of my reading two years earlier, she told me she was still terrified about talking to her husband about her frustration with his financial losses. Over the last two years, she had just worked harder on her own business, where she seemed to have a measure of control. Recently, during a routine mammogram, a doctor had found a calcified lump that was biopsied and found to be cancerous. Betty-Ann wanted to know how to handle the paralyzing numbness she had felt for so long in her marriage and how to counter the chronic "emotional anesthesia." She also felt shame and blamed herself for having neglected her marital and financial problems for so long.

Betty-Ann's words, "Now what do I do?" echoed in my head for weeks. Betty-Ann had learned that her body was a source of intuition and was sending her the message that she shouldn't ignore her depression and anger at her husband. She didn't want a divorce, but she did not know how to create health in her life. Her emotional depression was also depressing her immune system, lowering the levels of natural killer cells, and increasing her risk for cancer. Her chronic frustration and anger influenced the estrogen and progesterone in her body to stimulate her breasts to become lumpy. To prevent her cancer from recurring, Betty-Ann *had* to address the emotional and relationship problems she was having. Now that she could hear the messages, she *had* to change her life.

Intuition Can Express Itself in Emotions

Most intuition comes to us through an emotion that really doesn't take a "psychic" to understand. But you do have to acknowledge the emotion you feel. Interestingly, the part of the brain that *generates* emotions such as fear, anger, sadness, love, and joy (the temporal lobe and limbic system) is also involved in *recognizing* intuitive input. This is the part of the brain that also registers clairvoyant or clairaudient experiences.

The temporal lobe is exquisitely sensitive to electromagnetic waves. Recently, medical treatments for mood disorders have included applying a magnet to an area in the head that overlies key mood areas in the brain. The magnet changes the electrical activity of the emotional circuits and improves mood. It seems amazing, but think how you can pick up on the magnetically charged quality of the air in a room in which an argument has transpired just before you entered. These waves can ultimately affect your own mood. Similarly, we often feel sad when we're around someone who is depressed or in pain.

This emotional sensitivity is intensified during the hormonal shifts of PMS, pregnancy, postpartum, perimenopause, and menopause. And emotional sensitivity can become chronic in individuals who were raised in a family environment that was chaotic and emotionally, physically, or sexually traumatizing. The emotional "gears" in their brain that control and stabilize their mood have gotten "stripped" by having to respond constantly to adults' ups and downs, and they can get stuck in anxiety or sadness. Rapid mood shifts from fear to anger to sadness to love to joy occur in children with a parent who is an alcoholic, a gambler, or a sexual philanderer. The child quickly learns to anticipate when something bad is going to happen—the next alcoholic binge, rage attack, or screaming scene. Unfortunately, many of those children feel that because they can sense that something painful is about to happen, it's also their responsibility to do something to prevent it. Trauma-associated emotional changes occur in their brains, and they develop the chronic mood problems, anxiety, and panic of posttraumatic stress disorder. Their emotional porousness can be both a curse and a gift. If untreated, they may have lifelong problems with mood, anxiety, attention, and memory, but they may also have an incredible capacity for intuition.

Cindy, forty-four years old, called me for a reading.

The reading: Although Cindy's voice on the phone sounded upbeat and pleasant, I intuitively saw a lot of tragedy in her life that she had worked very hard to overcome: an early childhood family environment that felt like a war zone, with people screaming at each other, kids cowering under beds, bottles flying through the air, and children trying to clean up the mess. Cindy seemed able to anticipate when these battles would occur. When she began feeling anxious or edgy, she would try to avert an impending attack by either separating the warring factions or creating a distraction. Cindy's emotional intuition helped her survive her chaotic, violent childhood, but it also seemed to increase her physical symptoms of illness when she was in an unsettled environment that scared her. Cindy's body seemed to have a hypervigilant, hyperactive immune system and several autoimmune problems. Her immune system would be triggered too easily by things that would not bother most people; for instance, when people at work or at home were not getting along, her body would make antibodies against her own tissues, especially her joints, thyroid, and reproductive system.

The facts: Cindy's mother was a heroin addict with a string of live-in boyfriends. Many nights, she had screaming fights and police officers had to break into the apartment to stop the violence. Cindy knew intuitively when her mother was getting "upset" and about to go on a binge; she would get an upset feeling in her stomach and feel jittery and panicky. Then she knew to look for the needles and try to hide them. She would also try to clean up the house to "make" her mother feel better in hopes that her mother wouldn't shoot up.

As an adult, Cindy became a divorce mediator and court-appointed advocate for children. She also developed psoriatic arthritis, an auto-immune illness that attacks the joints and skin. Cindy's joints and skin would "act up" when people around her were arguing. She was also diagnosed with posttraumatic stress disorder (PTSD), panic attacks, and depression.

Cindy had learned early on in her life that she couldn't be healthy and be around her mother. At a young age, she left home and had a series of surrogate mothers. From empathetic, supportive psychotherapists, she learned that she could always tell when she was in a bad relationship or un-healthy environment, because her body would intuitively signal her with fear. She would get anxious, arthritic, or psoriatic when a boyfriend was cheating or a client was lying. Eventually, Cindy learned how to stop her autoimmune illness from escalating into a full-blown attack by heeding the very earliest intuitive warning signs of worry, itchiness, or stiffness. She wasn't always successful, and during a painful divorce she had to go on high doses of steroids and antianxiety and antidepressant medicines, but she began to learn how to get the emotional, nurturing support she needed when she was entering a stressful time.

Cindy's emotional porousness and intuition were her genius, and they helped her help others in her work. Her intuition was expressed simulta-neously in her brain and body, and Cindy learned how to become con-scious of her emotional and physical wiring for intuition. Cindy developed a five-pronged approach to the successful treatment of her panic attacks, PTSD, depression, and psoriatic arthritis:

1. *Antianxiety and antidepressant medicines* during episodes of acute stress.
2. *Nutritional supplements and herbal combinations* to buffer her brain and body against developing excessive anxiety, depression, and immune system dysfunction.

3. *Cognitive and behavioral approaches* to help her maintain healthier emotional brain circuits for anxiety and mood, including exercise, yoga, and psychotherapy.
4. *Psychotherapy and other emotionally nurturing supportive relationships* that provide a corrective relationship with a surrogate mother.
5. *Keying into the intuition brain-body circuits.*

As Cindy was aware, applying only the first four approaches didn't help her brain-body disorder for very long. If she didn't address the precipitating event that ignited the first stages of anxiety, depression, and immune system dysfunction (intuitive or otherwise), the biochemistry in her brain and body would get progressively out of whack. Over time, medicines, vitamins, and herbs would have stopped working, even at higher and higher dosages, and the psychotherapy would have felt like a waste of time and money. Eventually anxiety and depression would have led to problems paying attention, learning, and remembering as the biochemical imbalances spread across her brain circuits. By using all five solutions, however, Cindy has been able to stay in a good mind-body balance.

Unexpressed Emotions Affect Many Areas in Your Brain and Body

Unresolved, unexpressed fear, anger, and sadness electrically and biochemically disrupt your brain circuits. This in turn hurts your capacity to pay attention, learn, or remember things. Your capacity to see or hear narrows and is distorted. You ruminate about other past upsetting events because your brain's attention and memory have been primed to focus on similarly upsetting situations. Let's explore further how this connection works so that you can identify if these patterns are affecting your health.

PROLONGED, UNRESOLVED ANGER INCREASES YOUR CHANCES OF DEVELOPING HEART DISEASE, STROKE, AND DEMENTIA

Like any emotion that's held too long, anger that is unresolved and unexpressed makes its way from the brain down into the body, increasing your chances of getting illnesses to which you are genetically predisposed. Neuronal pathways in the anger highway keep firing away, maintaining an elevation in heart rate, body temperature, and muscle tone in your blood vessels and heart, increasing your risk of atherosclerosis (hardening of the arteries), heart attack, or stroke. Anger (as well as sadness, fear, and other negative emotions) keeps the brain's sympathetic nervous system activated, which stimulates the body's adrenal glands to produce cortisol and epinephrine. Blood vessels all over the body constrict and elevated cholesterol levels set off a chain reaction of inflammation, a domino effect that increases your chances of getting coronary artery disease, a heart attack, or Alzheimer's disease. Chronically elevated cortisol levels increase your risk of developing cancer in a specific organ, which is in part determined by what upset you.

If you are unaware you are angry or unable to name what causes your frustration, the right brain's anger circuits stay activated. To stop the domino effect from working its way from the right brain to the body, you have to identify the external event, inner thought pattern, or intuitive event that precipitated the emotion in the first place. For example, anger is usually caused when:

a. you or someone you love feels a loss of power, status, respect
b. you feel insulted
c. things turn out in unexpected ways
d. you or someone you care about is physically or emotionally hurt
e. you do not get something you want

Alternatively, thought patterns or beliefs that reverberate in your head can also activate anger, including thinking that:

a. something is not fair, right, or just should be different than it is; or
b. your point of view in a conflict is the only correct one; others are not valid.

When you talk about a feeling, you're sending a right brain emotion across the "interbrain" highway, the corpus callosum, into the left brain. If you don't talk about it and release it, the emotion stays in the right brain and eventually "seeps" down into the body. Your body will experience it, express it, and act it out. So, when you're angry, you frown, yell, scream, clench your fists, tighten your neck or jaw muscles, or your blood pressure will go up. You'll eat, gain weight, and raise your cholesterol levels. In the end, you may not even remember what caused your anger, but you will notice its physical and health consequences. Whether it's fear, anger, or sadness, any negative emotion, if held long enough, will spread to the other negative emotional brain circuits, causing an "emotional goulash," in which you feel a lot of negative emotions simultaneously.

How People Describe Their Emotions When They Don't Know Exactly What They're Feeling or Why

Do you find yourself frequently saying the following phrases:

- I feel awful
- I'm overwhelmed
- I feel tired and exhausted
- I'm numb
- I'm in shock
- I'm dazed
- I feel out of control

If you find yourself walking around muttering these phrases, then you might be experiencing the aftereffects of having an unresolved feeling spread like wildfire to other brain circuits. They are, in essence, "gumming" up your brain, making it hard for you to think straight and feel healthier.

Turn the Beat Around: Find Out What You Are Really Feeling

If you feel a goulash of emotions, and can't think straight, how do you get a handle on what you are feeling so you don't get sick or so you can heal? You run your emotional right-brain/body pathways *in reverse*. Instead of following emotions as they travel from right brain to body, be a detective and trace back the evidence from your body to your brain. By identifying the symptoms in your body, looking at your face's expression, observing the position of your hands, spine, and limbs, becoming aware of the tone and volume of your voice and the content of your thoughts, you can identify the emotion and think back to the event that initiated it. Alternately, you can look at your body's health reactions, the speed of your heart rate, sense of either heat or cold in your body, and the behavior of other organs in your body. Your body's health reactions are a key part of your intuitive guidance system and point to an area in your life that is out of balance (see Emotional Feng Shui chart, fifth column, on the far night).

Because the brain circuits for emotions are closely intertwined, women are anatomically predisposed to emotional goulash, or amorphous combined emotional states. If something caused you to be angry, and you stayed that way for a sustained period of time, you may be more likely to spiral into other more confusing emotions, making it even harder to figure out what you're feeling. You may go from anger to sadness more quickly and cry and then feel shame for crying. Sustained, amorphous emotional confusion increases your chance of developing symptoms of pain and illness.

AMBIVALENT EMOTIONS: BEING STUCK IN GRAY

Opposite emotions can occur simultaneously in the feminine brain. Acceptance and disgust; joy and sadness; surprise and anticipation—each has a difference valence, that is, causes a different biological and behavioral response in your body. Anger makes you want to confront; fear makes you want to avoid. Usually any emotion leads to an action, but having opposite emotions in equal amounts is like putting the gas and brake on at the same time. They neutralize each other and lead to ambivalence—*ambi* (both) and *valence* (moving in the opposite direction) means you go *no*where and you are *stuck*. Nothing happens. Since women's brains are more interconnected, more than one emotional pathway is likely to fire at a time. And if the emotions are neutralizing, you are less likely to be able to know what's wrong and respond appropriately.

Censoring Intuition

Dora, age thirty-eight, had always known she wanted to be different from her alcoholic mother, who had been negative, angry, pessimistic, and demanding. So Dora decided always to see the good in a situation, and never get "negative." This required a lot of skill because Dora had experienced several traumatic events in her life: Her mother died of breast cancer when Dora was fifteen years old; she had a series of miscarriages in her early thirties; her oldest child had become a drug addict; and her second child was autistic. Through it all, Dora maintained her upbeat, sunny disposition and stiff upper lip even though she was chronically exhausted, had irritable bowel syndrome, and began to get embarrassing panic attacks at work.

Dora began using Klonopin, an antianxiety medicine, got acupuncture and traditional Chinese herbal treatments, and enrolled in a cognitive behavioral therapy class for panic disorder. For a while, Dora's fatigue and panic attacks practically disappeared. Even her irritable bowl syndrome calmed down. However, when her son, Elliot, came out of rehab and home to live, Dora began to feel the familiar uneasiness again. One day, Dora found a lump in her breast which the doctor diagnosed as cancerous. At this news, Dora's panic attacks and digestive tract both got completely out of control.

Breast cancer and other forms of cancer can be precipitated by extreme grief and loss. Women with breast cancer are more likely to hide negative emotions behind a brave, stoic face. Dora decided to turn her life around and dissect the emotions that were fueling her emotional and physical health problems. The only new event in her life was that her son had returned home from drug rehab. At first, Dora had thought that she was thrilled to have Elliot home again, since he had worked very hard to turn around his own life, but now she had to admit that underneath, she felt anxious. When she suspected Elliot had fallen off the wagon, she resisted her automatic impulse to convince herself that he was fine, and looked for facts to support her emotional and physical intuitive hunch: Money had been missing from her wallet. Elliot had been sleeping later and later, his eyes were watery, and he had begun to act jittery. Elliot finally admitted he was using cocaine again, and returned to the drug rehab facility.

Dora decided to rehab her own emotional and physical health. She went into a codependence recovery program where she learned that she had been denying her own painful emotions for years. With the help of her cognitive behavioral therapist, she learned how her body expressed emotions in the form of digestive symptoms or fatigue. Finally, Dora learned that she had always been very porous and sensitive to others' feelings, and that anxiety, panic, fatigue, and irritable bowel disorder were signals from her intuition that someone near her was in distress. Armed with this information, Dora learned how to respond to her emotions and her intuition effectively. Over time, with medical management and increased consciousness of her emotions, Dora's panic attacks and breast cancer went into remission. Every once in a while, Dora will begin to feel an emotional or physical pang of anxiety, but she no longer censors it. Instead, she explores it fully until she sees its source and can address it.

FEELING TWO EMOTIONS SIMULTANEOUSLY CAN BE CONFUSING AND PARALYZING

Women are more likely than men to say, "You hurt me." Hurt is a combination of sadness and anger. If her partner forgets her birthday or anniversary, a woman is more likely to simmer and "act hurt." And when her partner says, "What's wrong?" she is more likely to say "nothing," or "You hurt my feelings." It's harder to identify what's bothering you if you are hurt than if you are angry or sad, but knowing that hurt simultaneously involves anger (things didn't happen the way you expected) and sadness (anticipating losing a good friend) can help you. Disappointment is another "combined" emotion that can get you stuck. Women are more likely to say they are disappointed. Like hurt, disappointment is also a combination of sadness and anger. Jealousy is another difficult emotional blend, a combination of anger, sadness, fear, and love. Sometimes you might not even know you have fallen in love with someone until he falls in love with someone else and you feel jealous.

THE FEMININE BRAIN MAY NEUTRALIZE NEGATIVE EMOTIONS AND CENSOR INTUITION TO KEEP THE PEACE

In women and some atypical men, the left brain may mask a right-brain feeling by expressing its opposite emotion. For instance, to maintain goals in careers, to preserve the integrity of relationships, social standing, and status, a woman may act happy when she is really disappointed at a boss, husband, or partner. Feigning happiness doesn't get rid of the real sadness inside. In a similar fashion, the left brain may confabulate or create a reason to mask right-brain emotional intuition. Hiding emotions and censoring intuition may keep the peace. But détente comes at a price. Since neither the sadness nor the intuition has been dealt with, the body is more likely to react in the form of symptoms of illness.

We all have times when we are unable to mask our emotions. Before the age of seven, when the brain's frontal lobe inhibitory circuits aren't fully grown, we really don't have a "social facade." As children, if we felt frustrated, sad, or afraid, we were pretty obvious about it. At a sporting event, if you were frustrated, you were more likely to "lose it." In school, if a teacher looked at you harshly, you were more likely to cry. And when you were with your girlfriends and felt excluded, you were more likely to create a scene. As we age, the frontal lobe circuits for "fitting into society" come on board to help us determine how to mask, intensify, deintensify, and express our feelings directly and skillfully.

I have an author friend named Loretta LaRoche who is very, very funny. She says what everyone is thinking but is afraid to say. The problem is that when you're around Loretta, you end up losing your facade, because Loretta does not follow the rules of social appropriateness. She will act out what she's thinking and feeling and it's contagious.

Some women have what I call "emotional incontinence," that is, problems containing their feelings, which can sabotage their career, relationships, and goals.

We will learn what to do to soothe the five basic emotions of fear, anger, sadness, joy, and love in the next four chapters. You will also learn how your intuition is wired into your emotions and moods. Women have adapted to releasing their emotions in a socially appropriate way by talking about them, which reduces the risk that emotions will be impulsively expressed through actions that can get us in trouble. Alternatively, talking and then *transforming* your emotions prevents them from being funneled into your body to increase your risk of illness.

A woman is less likely to express an emotion if she thinks that asserting herself will jeopardize a relationship or career. Over time, she may become less conscious that she was even angry or sad in the first place. The emotion and its associated intuition will go "underground," be transferred into depression, chronic anxiety, panic, or symptoms of illness. But the skillful expression of emotions and intuition will keep you emotionally and physically healthy.

Using Emotional Feng Shui to Balance Emotions

When you have a healthy, balanced emotional landscape (good emotional feng shui), you keep all your channels open to intuition. Good emotional feng shui requires being able to have (a) a balanced daily emotional diet of the five emotions; (b) a capacity to contain and delay talking about your feelings when necessary; (c) a capacity to experience an emotion fully, comprehend its message, and respond appropriately, and then move on; (d) a capacity to express your feeling at an appropriate volume and intensity depending on the social situation; and (e) a capacity to express your feelings to the right person, at the right time. Having difficulty with any of these five emotional feng shui elements leads to biochemical stagnation in the brain and ultimately increases your chances of developing problems with the Big Four: depression, anxiety, attention, and memory.

Traditionally, men's and women's brains are wired differently in the intensity in which they experience and express emotions. Women tend to obsess about emotional issues longer than men. Brain areas for emotion, language, and behavior may have more connections in a woman's brain than a man's. As a result, women traditionally think about and talk about their feelings more intensely than men. With less connection between the right brain emotional areas and the left brain language areas, a traditional male brain is set up to compartmentalize emotions and not talk about them. The male brain more typically acts out emotions unconsciously or expresses them in health problems. All emotions use the body as their theater.

And our emotions can get unbalanced through emotional incontinence and emotional perseveration. All of us know when we become "emotionally incontinent": we "boil over," "blow up," or just plain "lose it." At times in our lives, especially during the hormonal changes of PMS, pregnancy, and menopause, we may be primed for "emotional inconti-nence." During these times, no matter how you try to stop thinking about emotions and their intuitive messages and box them away, you can't.

Getting stuck on an emotion is just like getting stuck in a gear while driving a car. We are meant to move fairly regularly and moderately from one emotion to another. Being sad for too long makes us depressed. Being angry too long makes us bitter and resentful. Staying fearful for too long causes us to be anxious and nervous. Remaining happy for too long or es-caping into love has its downsides as well if not balanced with the capacity to appropriately respond to new experiences.

In addition, the intensity of emotions can be either too exaggerated or too muted. If you don't attend to the initial, subtler forms of anger—that is, irritability, annoyance, and dislike and their associated intuition—your brain will turn up the volume and intensity until you find yourself expe-riencing fury and outrage. This, too, can lead to serious health problems and damaging consequences in your relationships and your job.

Assertiveness: Saying the Right Thing to the Right Person at the Right Time with the Right Intensity

Negotiating relationships daily, whether with a colleague, employee, ac-countant, husband, or partner, requires saying how you feel with the ap-propriate amount of directness and intensity.

Emotions like fear, anger, and sadness need to be expressed to some de-gree in every relationship. However, if your emotions or requests aren't bri-dled, toned down, or turned up in volume to the absolutely socially appropriate level of intensity, then your relationships will flounder, and you won't be able to successfully fit into society.

Assertiveness and emotional intensity are gender issues. Women may be socialized to deintensify an emotion, to make it more palatable to others so that they won't lose love, support, and financial safety. Having traditionally less power and status in the world, women have developed morality and so-cial bonding brain areas that inhibit or mute the direct expression of anger toward loved ones. This doesn't mean that a woman can't feel anger in-side—she may find it difficult to ask directly for what she wants. When she doesn't ask, she doesn't get, which makes her angry and frustrated. She may decrease the intensity of her request, *hint* that she needs something. "If it's okay with you, could you please call me next time and let me know you are going to be late, but if it's too much of an imposition, forget about it because I can always handle it." A woman is more likely to be apologetic, use a lot of words in a convoluted style that over time makes the listener feel confused and guilty. A woman is also more likely to wait a longer time before asking as well. Feminine behavior is modeled to do whatever we can to preserve a relationship, but unfortunately, over time our anger and disappointment are less likely to be heard clearly with such convoluted requests . . . and our relationships may devolve into a lack of boundaries and imbalance of power, with a higher risk for emotional and physical abuse.

Ultimately, a woman's emotional nature becomes a major source of intuition, wisdom, and guidance.

Create Your Own Brain Résumé

Now please look at the Emotional Feng Shui diagram (p. 70) and chart (pp. 71–72). What does your emotional landscape look like? Which of the five basic emotional circuits do you think your body slips into most easily? The emotional circuit in which you spend the most time is probably the one through which your intuition comes to you. What are your body's typical ways of reacting? Which emotional circuit best matches your typical health reactions under stress? You can find out what thoughts and feelings are overdeveloped in your emotional landscape.

Please now look at the Feminine Personality Style (Figure 5). Where do you tend to focus your emotions? Into personal goals, society, or into personal relationships? Let's see if what you think of as your feminine emotional and personality landscape matches how you are in real life.

Questionnaire: Circle any and all that apply

I. You have entered a crowded department store. What usually happens?

1.	Within an hour or two, I head straight for the snack bar to get coffee, soda, or a carbohydrate snack.
2.	I can go for hours without needing to eat or drink.
3.	If it's crowded, I usually leave. Why not catalogue shop or buy on the Web?
4.	My adrenaline and "juices" start to flow as I fight for position around the sale racks.
5.	I tend to impulsively buy things I don't need, especially if they're located by the cash registers.
6.	I usually have a shopping list and I follow it.

7.	I often forget what I needed to buy.
8.	I have the capacity to keep a mental list in my head of what I need to buy.

II. In a restaurant:

1.	It's hard for me to eat out alone since this makes me feel empty and alone.
2.	Dessert isn't that important to me. When it comes to chocolate, I can take it or leave it.
3.	Buffets make me a little nervous. You never know who has touched the food.
4.	If I see someone getting up to go to the buffet, I will subtly try to race to the plates so I don't get stuck behind them.
5.	After the waiter recites the list of salad dressings, I can usually recall only one or two types without having them repeat the list.
6.	I can usually recite the salad dressing list after I've heard the waiter announce it for the first time.
7.	Even if I've eaten there before, I usually can't recall where the restroom is.
8.	Where I've eaten before, I can almost always remember the name of the waiter or waitress.

III. In an airport:

1.	I almost always get irritable, frustrated, and in a bad mood. I can't stand all the rules, and there's invariably one aggravation after another.
2.	Despite numerous delays and inconveniences, I usually can find a magazine or other diversion to stay calm, cool, and collected.
3.	I am usually a little queasy, on edge, or uncomfortable before takeoff.
4.	I love the sensation and thrill of a great takeoff.
5.	I have to keep looking at my boarding pass because it's hard for me to remember the number of my departing gate.
6.	Once I get the number of my departing gate, I usually am able to keep it in mind even if I am distracted by stopping for a snack and newspaper before boarding the plane.

| 7. | In the parking lot, I frequently forget where I parked my car. |
| 8. | Once I've been to an airport a couple of times, I have a general idea of the location of the coffee shops, restaurants, and bathrooms. |

IV. At work:

1.	If my boss or co-worker is in a bad mood, it's hard for me to keep my attention on my work and keep my own spirits up.
2.	Although I notice when a boss or co-worker is distressed, I am able to focus on my responsibilities and be maximally productive.
3.	It's hard for me to work in a closed-in cubicle. If I can, I try to avoid giving oral presentations.
4.	I don't mind being near other associates as long as I have my own territory. The contact with others gets my "juices" flowing and can make me more productive.
5.	It's difficult to find something on my desk since it's usually disorganized. I tend to easily misplace files and important papers.
6.	When I get papers, I file them. My motto is: "A place for every thing and everything in its place."
7.	I have trouble remembering the names of colleagues and tend to forget important appointment dates unless someone reminds me.
8.	I usually try to remember a colleague or co-worker's name and can readily keep track of important business appointments.

V. Concerning the phone or on the Web:

1.	My home and cell phone bills are inversely proportional to my mood. The lower my mood, the higher my bill, or the more often I use my phone.
2.	My happiness isn't directly related to constant contact with friends and family. I can be happy alone or with others' company.
3.	If I'm home alone, which is rare, since I hate to be alone, I am frequently on the phone, or sending emails or IMs.
4.	Some nights, I prefer my own company and decide to return phone calls and emails another day.

5.	If I don't know a phone number, I tend to call 411 information. If someone tells me a phone number, I must write it down right away or it immediately leaves my mind.
6.	If I don't know a phone number, I tend to use the phone book to look up the number if it's available.
7.	I am rather hesitant to get a new computer or cell phone. I'd rather not have to learn and remember how to use new technology if I can get away with using what I am familiar with.
8.	Staying up-to-date with computers and other technology makes me feel like I am keeping up with what other people are interested in.

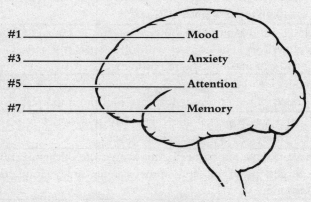

Figure 8. Questionnaire Key: Drawing of brain with #1, #3, #5, #7.

Now, please look at your answers to the questionnaire. If you repeatedly circled (1), then you have gifts of mood changes and challenges with moods. If you repeatedly circled (3), then you have gifts of anxiety and challenges with anxiety. If you consistently circled (5), you may have the gift of a fluid attention or problems paying attention. Finally, if you repeatedly circled (7), you may have problems with memory.

In the rest of this book, I will address the classic gifts and challenges of each of the Feminine Brain's classic emotional and thought styles. From problems with depression, anxiety, and anger, to concerns about eating, weight, and relationships, to problems with attention, learning, and memory, you will learn how to use the "head on your shoulders" and the intuitive wisdom in your brain and body to thrive in the face of common daily challenges.

FOUR

Blue Moon:
PMS, Depression, and Other Moods

When I first set foot on a psychiatric unit as a medical student, I noticed that most of the patients were depressed women. This made no sense to me, so I asked a psych nurse, "Where are all the men?" and he answered, "All the women are here; all the men are in jail. Women turn their anger inward and it becomes depression. Men turn their anger outward, into violence; they get in trouble with the law and end up in jail." Anger and sadness are related, which sets the scene for the New Feminine Brain's challenge with mood, depression, anger, and irritability.

Depression and moodiness are more common in women than men—depression occurs twice as often in women, most likely because of their unique dynamic hormonal makeup. If you get stuck in a negative frame of mind, either anger, sadness, or a combination of both, the depth of that bad mood and the length of time you are stuck in it have health implications. One in four women will have a major depression. That's right, 25 percent of all women will suffer at least one major episode of depression, compared with only 17 percent of the general population (all men and women) suffering from this disorder. By the age of thirty, over 15 percent of women will receive treatment for depression, and only 9 percent of men.

What Is a Mood, Anyway?

A mood is a pervasive, sustained emotion that colors your world and how you pay attention to what is around you. Moods can be sad, sullen, irritable, angry, euphoric . . . any prevailing emotional tone. A mood is a signal from your intuitive guidance system that something has changed, for good or for bad, in your life or in the life of someone you care about.

A "Normal Mood" Balances the Ups and Downs of Life

True emotional health—and brain health—involves moving regularly between the five basic emotions of fear, anger, sadness, joy, and love, and all the "mixed" mood states in between. What does it mean to have a "normal mood"? At any one time, you can be a little sad about having gained a pound in the last two weeks, a little angry that your favorite TV program was preempted for a ballgame, but also a little happy that you got a reasonably sized tax refund check in the mail, and finally, feel a little bit of love when that old college buddy called you on the phone.

Negative Emotions =		-1 sadness
	+	-1 anger
		-2 total
Positive Emotions =		+1 happy
	+	+1 love
		+2 total

Negative Emotions + Positive Emotions

$$-2 + 2 = 0 = \text{Normal Mixed Mood}$$

In a normal mood no one emotion is prominent—it's like a good sauce or soup, every herb or seasoning added in just the right blend so that it tastes just right. The regular experience of all five emotions is healthy for your brain and body, and keeps channels for intuition open.

The problem is that we have pathologized sadness and anger so much in our society that when we feel any of these emotions, we want to medicate them away, meditate them away, or dissociate them. When you don't allow yourself to feel negative emotions, you ultimately increase your chances of developing mood problems and mental and physical illness. You also deprive yourself of critical sources of intuition. If you are prone to bouts of depression, moodiness, and irritability, you need to learn to capture the intuitive information hidden in the mood.

Some Women Get Sad, Some Women Get Mad

Many life events that prompt sadness can also prompt anger. When we don't get what we want, some of us become depressed. Some people react to losing a relationship, getting betrayed, rejected, or abandoned with anger and outrage, while others become disappointed, dejected, and grief-stricken. Knowing your feelings is essential to healing the situation and moving forward.

Patsy Cline Seemed Sad, But She Was Really Mad

The woman in the song "Crazy," made famous by Patsy Cline, plaintively says that she thinks she's crazy for feeling lonely and blue. Obviously, she is sad because she has lost her guy, but she is also beating up on herself. She is disgusted or angry with herself for falling in love with him in the first place, and for still being "stuck" on him, unable to move into a new relationship. If this woman stayed stuck on that guy for several months, she might go to a psychotherapist or a psychiatrist, who might prescribe antidepressants. Her chronic self-deprecating thoughts and anger at herself would increase her chance of having hypertension and high cholesterol, disrupted hormonal metabolism, and menstrual and perimenopausal problems. Yet, if you asked her if she was angry, she'd say no, only sad, depressed, and low in self-esteem and confidence because she'd been left.

Janis Joplin Sounded Mad, But She Was Really Sad

When Janis Joplin instructs you take "another piece" of her heart, her singing sounds angry and bitter. She is also still in love with a guy who has left her, but the tone of the song is decidedly different. The tone of the music once again confuses the issue. Through the angry, dissonant-sounding rock and roll, and the furious, resentful, vengeful lyrics, we find the singer is crying all the time. This is a clue that beneath all the loud and bitter rage, she is very depressed. She gets so much of her anger out, it's no longer turned inward, but her depression still seems just as potent as her anger.

The New Feminine Brain's Mad-Sad Continuum

The reality is that a woman's anger circuit and her sad circuit are so enmeshed that when she experiences one of these emotions, the other is soon to follow. The anger and sadness brain circuits seem to have more anatomic similarities than differences.

Clearly, someone who is overtly sad usually acts different from someone who is obviously angry. Most often, depressed people have lower initiative and slowed movements; they walk slow, talk slow, think slow, and have problems with appropriate distance in relationships. They are either too distant ("Teflon") or lonely and craving too much contact ("Velcro"). In contrast, people who are irritated and angry move more quickly and intensely. They grit their teeth, bang things, get heated, slam doors, and talk in loud, sharp voices.

Both the sadness and anger circuits (1) activate an emotional and intuition area in the temporal lobes (called the insula) that has rich connections to the heart, blood vessels, lungs, and digestive tract; (2) activate the hormonal areas in the hypothalamus that control appetite, the menstrual cycle, pregnancy, and menopause; and (3) alter the activity of attention, learning, and memory areas in the brain.

The sadness and anger brain circuit connections to the body may illustrate why chronic anger and depression are associated with high blood pressure, high cholesterol levels, chest pain, menstrual irregularities, premenstrual dysphoric disorder, premenstrual syndrome, anorexia and bulimia, menopausal complaints, attention deficit disorder, and learning and memory disorders.

Your mood also affects what you remember and how you remember it. People with chronic depression complain of memory loss that appears to be similar to Alzheimer's disease. However, once the depression is successfully treated, their memory improves. The sadness circuit in the brain and body can actually disrupt the capacity to pay attention, learn, and remember. On the other hand, the joy circuit, with its release of neurotransmitter opiates, makes paying attention and learning rewarding and efficient. Excessive sadness and depression release norepinephrine and cortisol, which actually poison and block the hippocampal memory areas. In fact, long-term trauma and depression have been associated with measurable brain atrophy. The hippocampus shrinks in the setting of unrelenting, severe stress, chronic trauma, and depression—not as severely as it does in people with Alzheimer's disease, but still to a worrisome degree.

The Development of Mood in the Brain

Children and adolescents have particular difficulty differentiating between sadness and anger. In children, depression and chronic sadness don't usually have the same characteristics as in adults over the age of eighteen. Depressed adults display obvious behavior and body health changes; they think, talk, and move slowly; and have fatigue, lethargy, and problems with initiation and motivation. Not so with children and adolescents. Depression and sadness can sometimes present in children as irritable, brooding behavior that looks more like anger. In children's brains, the anger network isn't well differentiated from the sadness network, so sometimes when angry, hyperactive children are treated with antidepressants and other therapy for depression, they get better.

When little boys mature into men, these pathways traditionally differentiate, separate from one another. It becomes easier to see that when a man is mad, he's mad; when he's sad, he's sad. He may not talk about it, but his actions, thoughts, and body health reactions tend to stay in one emotional category or another (see Emotional Feng Shui in Chapter 3). When was the last time you saw a man cry when he was angry? Yet, many women cry when they are angry. No one knows if a woman's predisposition to cry when she is angry is biologically predetermined or due to social conditioning, or both, but women tend to hide their anger behind a sad face. A woman's brain may have evolved to mask anger with another facial expression that feigns sadness or fear. When our ancestors suffered a loss of power, status, or respect, failed to get what they wanted or had worked for, or felt emotional or physical pain, it may have been more socially adaptive for their brain to fire its sadness or fear circuits.

SURVIVAL OF THE SADDEST? SOCIAL STATUS AND EMOTIONAL EXPRESSION

Traditionally and still today, crying is more likely to get women a positive, caring response than anger, irritation, or annoyance. A woman who acts angry is more likely to suffer the social consequences of rejection, yet a man can more usually redirect his anger toward work and goals in the world, competing against other men on the battlefield, on the playing field, or in the boardroom. Today, women have other "frontal-lobe goals" available to them than the traditional homebound duties, and can pursue multiple vocations in business, medicine, scientific research, and competitive sports. There are also many more ways and situations in which women can potentially become irritated, annoyed, enraged, and outraged.

People who can express anger skillfully are usually considered healthy and assertive. People who have less status or power are more likely to show fear (or sadness) when they are angry. Women who show anger are considered more dominant. Yet a socially dominant woman doesn't always get what she wants. If she gets angry on a date, or with a group of people out socially, she may be considered whiny, high-maintenance, or bitchy. If she complains in an airport check-in line or in line while shopping, she is considered angry, demanding, or bitchy. If she is a CEO or supervisor and gets angry in a business situation, she's considered a "castrating bitch."

Ultimately, our culture doesn't condone a woman showing anger except in a therapist's office, where she learns words for feelings to help her get in touch with her anger so she can snap out of her depression. Women are taught to punch a pillow or write an angry note to the person they are upset with and then burn the note without mailing it. Sometimes women are taught how to express their disappointment skillfully to a loved one, but then they are often devastated if they receive a negative response.

If a woman gets angry at work, in today's competitive job market she is more likely to be replaced by another woman who's more of a "company team player" or a man who's "less emotional." A man in a high-level corporate position with anger is considered "Type A" or aggressive—a woman is considered "hormonal" or "irritable." Our society knows how to handle and accept direct, assertive comments from a man but not from a woman. When a traditional man loses power, status, or respect, or has some other reason to get angry, it may be easier for him to stay in the anger circuit, know he is angry, and communicate it in a straightforward way so everyone around him knows how he feels. Not so with a woman. Whether for sociological reasons or biological wiring, when a woman gets mad, she is more likely to experience and emote a mixture of anger and sadness. Her brain is not as compartmentalized as a man's and neither are her emotional networks. So traditionally, a woman's emotions are muddier; at first, it's harder for her to know how to respond—as a result, she is less likely to know what to do when she gets upset, when she loses power, respect, love, or when she experiences pain.

Women's anger is a biological and sociological problem. If women don't give voice to their anger and make the changes in their lives that the emotion demands, they risk getting ill. Anger is usually easier for you to express and resolve if you have confidence in your authority and status. Neither women nor society are comfortable with female power, and although anger and disappointment are part of any relationship or job, many old feminine brains genetically still react in a biologically murky way when they are disappointed and don't get what they want. One woman may cry when she's upset; another may brood and pace; another may complain, sulk, and withdraw; another, if she stays angry long enough, could gain weight, get attacks of angina, high cholesterol, hypertension, or other health problems. Since a woman may not know if she's angry, sad, or both, she will stay stuck in a negative murkiness that can create biochemical changes in her brain and body that are typical of the sadness and anger network.

In an extreme stuck case, the combined emotions become a mood disorder, an unmanageable constellation of feelings. Depending on the intensity of the depression, how often the mood goes up and down (called a cycle), and how long it lasts, as well as a lot of other associated symptoms, she may receive a diagnosis of either minor depression (dysthymia), major depression ("a nervous breakdown," a.k.a. a major depressive episode), bipolar I or II disorder-borderline personality disorder, PMS, or perimenopausal depression (see table). Each and every one of these mood disorders illustrates the many examples of the feminine brain's mad–sad continuum. Each presents unique situations in which a woman has to learn how to adapt her unique brain to an increasingly complex world.

Mood Disorder	Stable or Cycling	Usual Medical Treatment
PMS/PMMD	Irritability/depression during at most the last 2 weeks of menstrual cycle	SSRI, Bioidentical progesterone
Perimenopausal depression	Irritability/depression within 5–10 years of menopause	SSRI Estrogen Progesterone
Major depression	For at least 2 weeks a severely depressed mood with decreased pleasure and interest; change in weight and sleep; agitation; slowed thoughts, movement, fatigue; problems with concentration, memory; thoughts of death	SSRI and other antidepressants can have a significant effect
Minor depression (dysthymia)	Chronic "blah" depressed mood with disordered eating and sleeping, fatigue, apathy, low self-esteem, indecision, hopeless for at least 2 years	Medicine has only minimal effects
Bipolar I	Episodes of major depression interspersed with episodes of mania; abnormally elevated mood lasting for at least a week where one loses touch with reality; with decreased need for sleep, pressured speech, "speedy thoughts," lightning quick behavior, losing control of normal usual restraint in sex, spending, and behavior	Mood stabilizers have significant effect
Bipolar II	Episodes of irritability and impulsivity interspersed with depression and dysthymia	Medicine has some effect
Borderline personality disorder	Frequent rapid shifts in mood (within minutes to hours) that are environmentally precipitated. Unstable mood, unstable thoughts, unstable behavior, and unstable relationships. Erratic and dramatic behavior to avoid feelings of abandonment and emptiness. Intense anger with frequent displays of temper; frequent suicidal thoughts and behavior. Self-mutilation (cutting)	Medicine has only minimal effect

In traditional psychiatry, doctors tried to categorize women and men into the same aforementioned mood disorder categories, even though a woman's five emotional pathways are likely to be less well-defined than a man's, and it is harder to pinpoint the emotion and mood she is experiencing. Frequent mood shifts further complicate the issue, as do the constantly changing hormonal levels and concomitant changes in serotonin and other mood neurotransmitters that can change her diagnosis. Fitting a woman into traditional psychiatric categories of depression or mania just doesn't make sense, because the compartmentalization of distinct mood states fits a traditional man's brain more than a woman's.

Nonetheless, you need to pay attention to your moods.

You have to be able to:

1. Name the mood you have slipped into
2. Find out how it's expressed in both your brain and body
3. Figure out whether it's intuitively signaling a change in your life or a loved one's
4. Find out what event prompted the mood
5. Learn how to release the mood, and return to your "normal" state

Mood Disorders Lead to Physical Problems/Physical Problems Promote Mood Disorders

Long-term depression and mood disorders increase your chance of premature death. Depression increases your chances of having high blood pressure, high cholesterol, heart disease, and stroke. Long-term moodiness increases your chances of getting Alzheimer's disease and cancers of all kinds, including breast, lung, and colon cancer. Mood disorders are an independent risk factor for osteoporosis and severe debilitation from related fractures. Finally, long-term depression and other mood disorders increase your chance of having obesity, eating disorders, chronic pain from osteoarthritis, and other autoimmune disorders as well as increasing your chances of becoming addicted to alcohol, cigarettes, and prescription pain meds. Obesity and addiction to cigarettes and alcohol lead to diseases that are always the number one killers in the United States.

Clearly, if a woman doesn't attend to her biologically vulnerable mood circuitry, her physical health can be affected as well.

Many women who suffer from *chronic immune disorders,* such as lupus (systemic lupus erythematosis or SLE), scleroderma, sarcoidosis, rheumatoid arthritis, chronic fatigue/fibromyalgia, Lyme disease or other illnesses associated with an endemic pathogen (including Epstein–Barr virus [EBV], cytomegalovirus [CMV], and others), also suffer from mood disorders. Depression also plagues women who endure *chronic pain and inflammation* from osteoarthritis, headaches, migraines, temporomandibular joint (TMJ) disease, neck and lower back pain from disc disease, irritable bowel disease or ulcerative colitis, chronic pelvic pain from endometriosis or other uterine problems, vulvodynia, and other disorders. Over time, these chronic conditions wear down women and make them irritable, sad, and tense. Women with breast disease or hypertension or who have suffered a stroke (cerebrovascular disease) or heart disease are more likely to feel gloomy, grumpy, and depressed and have low frustration tolerance. Women who are obese or have eating disorders, addiction, or sleep disorders and insomnia also suffer from mood disorders and are more likely to be treated for depression.

All of these disorders ultimately will imbalance mood to one degree or another. It's not an issue of "Oh, it's hard to have this disease. I'm getting depressed being stuck with this problem." Depression or moodiness is not just about being sad or angry about being sick. Chronic health problems of any kind ultimately imbalance the five brain-body emotional networks, and lead to depression or mood disorder, which further imbalances the body's neurochemistry, ultimately making the chronic illness even worse. Ultimately, you should seek treatment for *both* your mood and your physical dysfunction. Interestingly, many of the medicines and supplements that effectively treat chronic immune disorders, inflammation, pain, sleep, and weight problems can also treat mood problems. We shall see why this might be so. Yet in spite of the range of severity of moodiness and mood disorders, modern psychiatry still attempts to fit the feminine brain's mood complaints into a few distinct disorders that fit the traditional masculine brain better than the New Feminine Brain.

PMS: The Canary in the Coal Mine of Mood Disorders

Alicia, age thirty-nine, called me for a reading.

The reading: I saw that Alicia was very bright and had a great capacity to see both sides of any conflict. She seemed to want to give birth to something personally in a relationship, and also professionally in a vocation, but her husband, with whom she wanted to have a child, did not have a strong sense of himself. He seemed to need Alicia to take care of him financially while he went from one educational program and job to another. Alicia could see what her husband needed, and had no problem providing it as long as he helped her have a child, but he seemed more focused on his own career development than on becoming a parent.

When I looked intuitively at Alicia's body, I saw cyclic problems with headache associated with severe carbohydrate craving, and melancholy and sadness associated with changing hormonal levels. I knew Alicia was concerned about her fertility.

The facts: Alicia was indeed concerned about depression and fertility. The first thing she said was, "My biological clock is ticking." Alicia was married to Ben, age forty-two, who also was very bright but had a "hard time finding out what he wanted to be when he grows up." He had completed two different master's degrees and was finally finishing a Ph.D. Alicia was looking forward to him finishing and finding gainful employment. Having supported him financially through his protracted education, she was also looking forward to him being the breadwinner for a while so she could have a child. But Ben was looking into a postdoctoral research position, which paid only a limited stipend, not the higher-paying industry job that Alicia had been planning for. Alicia had "dragged" her husband to a marriage therapist several times to clarify their long-range family plans, and they had spent many sessions discussing Ben's shame about his financial dependency on his wife. To Ben, it was only a matter of time before he was able to get the right amount of training and all the hard work paid off.

But Alicia didn't have all the time in the world. She was thirty-nine years old and was getting horrible migraine headaches that were worse in the two weeks before her period, along with terrible mood swings that caused her to crave sweets and gain weight. Alicia's periods had gotten irregular in the past few years, prompting her physician to put her on the Pill. Unfortunately, now her headaches and mood swings were worse than ever and she was fifteen pounds heavier.

Alicia suffered from a classic mood disorder called premenstrual syndrome, a cyclic disorder of mood instability. Beginning after ovulation, some susceptible women have changes in estrogen and progesterone levels that are associated with mixtures of sadness and anger. Most women get a milder moodiness that can range from fatigue and lethargy to irritability.

The temporal lobe areas for emotion and intuition and the frontal lobe areas that censor and contain anger and sadness have many receptors for both hormones (estrogen and progesterone) and mood-regulating neurotransmitters (serotonin, dopamine, and norepinephrine). Some women have an inborn weakness in their brain's circuitry for mood and impulse control, and when their hormone levels shift, so do their moods. During hormonally unstable periods such as pregnancy, the postpartum period, fertility treatments, and the perimenopausal/menopausal era, women with PMS/PMDD suffer from complex mixtures of nervousness, irritability, sadness, and anger.

What causes hormonal moodiness? Estrogen has an "antidepressant" effect on the brain, because, like Prozac and other antidepressants, it promotes serotonin activity. Progesterone stabilizes mood and prevents it from erratically shifting from sadness to irritability. Your mood and the frontal lobe that maintains its stability are dependent on predictable fluctuations of estrogen, progesterone, and serotonin. When estrogen and progesterone levels change abruptly, the frontal-lobe emotional censors become disengaged, and you are likely to become emotionally incontinent—irritable, sad, and angry. Without the maximal use of frontal lobe pathways to curtail or direct emotion, we feel unbridled, intense anger and sadness.

PMS: CYCLING HORMONES, CYCLING HEMISPHERES

For some women, like Alicia, feeling anger and sadness may be an intuitive signal that she needs to attend to a key area in her life: her marriage and her need to have a baby. PMS may exaggerate normal intuitive circuits of the New Feminine Brain that let women know something is out of balance in their lives.

Before ovulation, women are more likely to hear things through a positive mood filter. After ovulation, during the premenstrual time, a woman is more likely to hear negative emotions with her right brain/left ear. During these two weeks, the left-brain filter is disengaged and she can see and hear uncensored and undiluted intuitive information. Some women's changing estrogen and progesterone levels trigger them to express emotions inappropriately, but there are ways to find relief from this monthly pain by obtaining treatment with medicines, nutritional supplements, and cognitive behavioral therapy.

ALL EMOTIONS ARE NOT CREATED EQUAL

Although the right brain carries most of the responsibility for emotions, it takes both sides to give you a balanced emotional perspective. The right brain processes all five primary emotions (joy, love, sadness, fear, and anger), whereas the left brain processes social emotions, which are basically primary emotions that have had a kind of frontal-lobe judgmental "spin" placed upon them. For example: What would someone think of me if I got angry? If I acted scared, would people think I'm a wimp? When your left brain notices and identifies an emotion, you experience it consciously, in a way that you think is more acceptable to you and the people around you. So, the right-brain emotion of fear can become the left brain's shame, silliness, embarrassment, guilt, pride, or jealousy.

Both brains are ultimately involved in depression; a depressed individual can have left-brain and right-brain symptoms. Left-brain depression (social or "cognitive" depression) is characterized primarily by obsessive, ruminative thoughts of hopelessness, helplessness, guilt, self-blame, and worthlessness. Right-brain depression, called primary or endogenous depression, contributes somatic or body symptoms, since the right brain has more connections to the body. A right-brain so-called "vegetative depression" causes changes in sleep and weight and slowed thoughts, speech, and actions.

Eighty percent of women who experience PMS don't have any other psychiatric problem, but the symptoms of PMS do resemble a mild form of an episode of major depression (see chart, p. 103), but the symptoms occur only after ovulation and go away when menstruation begins. The moodiness, lethargy, fatigue, and slow thoughts, speech, and actions seem to be the product of an unbridled right brain that lacks the usual left-brain socializing, mood-elevating influence. Three to eight percent of women may experience these symptoms with such severity as to have it labeled a disorder.

PMS's raw, painful emotions are the downside of what may be an evolutionary advantage of the feminine brain—to have a monthly capacity to live in the right-brain dreams, and body wisdom. In our right brain, we enjoy and provide an exaggerated connection to intuition, learn things about our life that we're likely to want to censor at other times. PMS is a monthly email from a woman's intuitive guidance system letting her know that she must look at her life and make changes.

Scientists have not found abnormal levels of hormones in women with PMS, but their feminine brains are very sensitive to normal changes in their own hormonal cycles. Why then do hormonal changes affect these women's moods, personality, and behavior so dramatically? Frontal-lobe personality and behavior are uniquely sensitive to stress, especially if it lasts for a long time and is intense. Serotonin helps us respond flexibly and adaptively to jobs, relationships, and social-environmental stress. Long-term, inescapable stress (like Alicia's) "burns up serotonin," which promotes moodiness when estrogen and progesterone levels change.

For a very long time, Alicia had been angry at Ben for not getting a job, sticking with it, and helping her have a baby. She was terrified that she would soon be too old to have a child. Yet, she was still in love with Ben.

Love + fear + anger = ambivalence = stuck. In the first half of the month, Alicia could censor her right brain's negative emotions behind the dominating left-brain optimism; she would believe Ben when he said, "Things will be okay." But during the second half of the month, her right brain was dominant, and her intuition would scream at her through her low mood. The years of frustration of supporting Ben and stuffing her emotions about it were taking their toll. Stress-induced serotonin changes made her frontal lobe's censors more sensitive to hormones and less able to silence her fears and anger.

Alicia had other brain-body changes indicating that she had long-term serotonin dysfunction that the PMS had made obvious. In addition to her irritability, sadness, and emotional lability, Alicia suffered from an eating disorder in which she craved carbohydrates and gained weight, and she had painful monthly migraines.

If Alicia doesn't attend to her PMS—the monthly message from her right brain—her cyclic mood disorder could progress into a more severe, long-lasting one. The long-term stress of stuffing emotions and ignoring PMS warning signs and right-brain intuition has biological effects on her brain. Stress releases cortisol and epinephrine, and burns up serotonin, increasing the chances that her irritability and moodiness will get worse and more enduring.

CYCLIC TO STATIC: PMS CAN LEAD TO OTHER MOOD DISORDERS

PMS is the tip of the iceberg for other potential mood disorders in the New Feminine Brain. Its untreated mini-depressive episodes may upgrade the coach-class mood disorder (PMS) to a first-class, major depressive episode, dysthymia, or other mood disorder. PMS is really the canary in the coal mine: The exaggerated response some women have to the normal cycle of fluctuating hormones indicates something structurally unique about their brain, a biological vulnerability in their mood circuit. If they don't strengthen the circuit, their cyclic mood disorder can become sustained.

To shore up this circuit, you need to make changes in your thought patterns, emotions, behavior, and physical health. You can use antidepressant and mood stabilizer medicines and nutritional supplements for a time, but you must also attend to the other factors that can precipitate another depression. Your mood won't show any lasting improvement—and can worsen as you age—if you don't get in touch with the intuitive message your unstable emotions are sending.

Unstable Moods

Some feminine brains have a unique tendency for creating emotional drama. Because estrogen affects serotonin levels and serotonin levels affect mood, dramatic swings in estrogen with the menstrual cycle and other reproductive events can cause dramatic mood swings for some susceptible women. Emotional changes can be lifesaving when they draw attention to a crisis, but if a mood swing is not connected to a known precipitating event, it loses its functional advantage. This rubber-band flexibility in the brain's centers for personality and emotion can be an excellent quality for an actress, artist, or singer, but not as compatible with a nine-to-five job, or raising a family where children need a stable, safe, and secure emotional environment. A drama can be entertaining to watch but tough to live in, as Mary J. Blige says in her album title *No More Drama*.

Moodiness is a women's issue—almost every woman's concern. Many doctors today pathologize women's mood changes by labeling them bipolar II disorder. This is a major health problem for women today, similar to the health care crisis in the 1980s, when everyone seemed to be getting a diagnosis of ADD. In the 1990s, everyone seemed to have OCD (obsessive-compulsive disorder). In the twenty-first century, the "en vogue" diagnosis is bipolar II disorder. I can't tell you how many people call me to request a reading for a moody female relative who has received that label. More women than ever who have been given that diagnosis are also calling me for readings. I do *not* believe that all these women have bipolar disorder. Moodiness in response to life's problems, moodiness exacerbated by hormones, "doth not a bipolar make."

An emotion has a function: It tells you something about your life. It tells you something has changed and prompts you to respond. However, if your mood dramatically downshifts and you don't know why, you can feel as if you're a character in a poorly written soap opera. Chronically unstable moods do not have an adaptive advantage and are detrimental to your brain's and body's health.

In order to come to grips with your moods or moodiness, you need to know what phase of mood you tend to get stuck in.

THE BRAIN MOLDS TO THE MOOD

Being stuck in a single mood or having excessive shifts of moods affects your brain physically. Think of your brain as a muscle: If you overexercise one muscle group more than others, it gets hypertrophied and others become atrophied and fall into disuse. If you get stuck in one mood for too long, the parts of your brain that deal with that mood get larger, and the others that work with alternative moods shrink. Similarly, if your mood is constantly shifting from happy to sad to irritable and then back to happy again, the brain mechanism for stabilizing a mood shrinks. In some women, one mood or emotion may dominate another and part of that brain circuit will ultimately get larger anatomically.

When you're depressed and stay depressed, anatomic and physiological changes in the brain occur that make it easier for you to get depressed again. Similarly, if you swing in the opposite direction, euphoria or mania, and stay that way, your brain alters structurally, facilitating future episodes. Over time, it takes less and less environmental stress to cause your mood to shift. Like a spoon or piece of metal, the more you bend it, the easier it is to bend.

Even after the depressed or irritable mood resolves and you return to normal, or to a baseline mood, your brain can never really be the same. You have a type of "mood memory"—or kindling—in your brain's frontal-temporal emotional circuits. Even though the fire is out, the embers remain. You could have had the best round of antidepressant therapy, but the memory of the depression or mania remains in the brain, serving as kindling that can ignite and make it easier than before to slip into another depression or mania. If you don't stabilize the cycle, you start to cycle between sadness and happiness more and more easily. After a while, one mood is indistinguishable from another. You need less and less stress to shift between brain circuits, until one big, combined "bad" mood—a mixture of irritability, sadness, and edginess—results. Kindling causes plasticity—and not in a good way in this instance. The sprouting of nerve cells ultimately requires more oxygen and glucose, which helps that part of the brain grow and develop. In men with mania, for example, after repeated episodes, their left temporal lobe, important for positive mood states, becomes more active and gets bigger. The right temporal lobe, hypothesized to be critical for negative mood states, becomes less active and gets smaller. (The same study hasn't yet been done on women.)

HARDWIRED IN THE BRAIN: SELF-DEFEATING THOUGHTS CLOG EMOTIONAL AND INTUITIVE PATHWAYS

In a typical chronic depression, the initiation and motivation areas in the left brain go to sleep. This creates a real problem since your left brain lets you know if you are getting what you want in life. If your left brain interprets that you're not getting what you've been expecting, it lays down brain pathways that expect less and less. Hopefulness and other optimistic thought patterns of a normal brain are replaced by more depressive, pessimistic thoughts. It seems almost as if your brain is trying to protect you from disappointment. Optimistic brain synapses that scream, "I can do anything!" get erased slowly over time. Pessimistic pathways that whisper, "It's useless," "I can't change" get rewired in their place. When your brain holds an emotion long enough, be it sadness or happiness, depression or mania, your brain molds to it.

If this has occurred, you need to know how to alter your goals or get help to accomplish them, or helplessness and pessimism will set into the brain circuits. If you don't stop your brain from being infected and taken over by pessimistic thought "viruses," you are more likely to stay in a "bad" mood. No matter what dose of an antidepressant you are taking, no matter how often you go into therapy, you will find it harder and harder to "snap out of it" and return to a healthier frame of mind. And, when your emotional brain pathways are clogged by pessimism, you can't hear your intuition.

It may be easier for a woman than a man to rewire her brain pathways to create healthier moods. Because the classic feminine brain has more "connectivity," more white matter nerve cell connections, it also has greater plasticity and can adapt, learn, remember, and repair from injury. Although this can increase a woman's likelihood for kindling depression and moodiness, it also increases the likelihood of healing her mood—even in the face of today's nutritional, environmental, and societal challenges that can make it harder to manage mood.

MEDICINES AND SURGERY MAY AGGRAVATE MOODINESS

Oral contraceptive pills, hormone replacement, obesity, fertility treatments, and treatment for cancer can all change the brain.

The *oral contraceptive* pill contains synthetic, chemically modified estrogen and progesterone. If the Pill has too much estrogen and insufficient progesterone, you are more likely to suffer moodiness and irritability. Estrogen needs to be neither too high nor too low for appropriate mood. Even though it has antidepressant effects, more estrogen is not better in this case. In fact, in some women, too much estrogen, especially synthetic, chemically modified estrogen, causes depression: One of the major side effects of the Pill is depression.

Some women who have had their uteruses removed in a hysterectomy are given estrogen replacement but not progesterone, because many doctors erroneously believe that progesterone's only function is to prevent overgrowth of the uterine lining. These women may initially feel less depressed but, if they're susceptible to mood disorders, they're more likely to become moody or irritable because they don't have enough progesterone to stabilize mood.

If you are obese, you are more likely to have higher levels of estrogen stored in your fat in the form of "estrone," a condition called "estrogen dominance." Having inappropriately high levels of estrogen, like taking too much estrogen in the Pill or in hormonal replacement, raises your risk of depression.

Women who have fertility treatments are shot up with all kinds of medicines that stimulate the ovaries to produce eggs—and also cause hormone levels to fly all over the place. This can prime a woman biologically for depression, irritability, and moodiness, not just when she gets the hormonal fertility treatments, but also in the future. (The stress of infertility adds to a mood problem.) One well-known side effect of fertility treatments is depression.

An often-used treatment to prevent occurrence or recurrence of breast cancer—tamoxifen—lowers or blocks estrogen. Unfortunately, tamoxifen and other related medicines also have been associated with depression and some cognitive changes (see Chapter 10). Lowering estrogen in the brain lowers serotonin levels and increases the chance of developing depression and cancer. Depression weakens and imbalances the immune system by lowering NKs (natural killer cell activity) that help keep cancer cells at bay, and has been associated with impaired natural killer cell activity and increased risk of developing cancer.

Check Your Moodiness Quotient

Every woman must become aware of her New Feminine Brain's unique susceptibility to moodiness. To help you get a handle on your own moods, please look again at the questionnaire you filled out in Chapter 3. In scenarios I through V, did you frequently circle 1? If so, moodiness may be a concern and something you need to address to keep yourself healthy. For instance, do you head straight for the snack bar when you go shopping, foraging for carbohydrates and sweets? Do you always have chocolate chips stocked in your kitchen for that once-a-month craving? In a restaurant, do you read the menu backward, allocating what you are going to eat by first seeing what's on the dessert menu? You may use food, certain types of food, to medicate your mood.

Is your mood very porous? Will your mood easily plummet or escalate due to what's on the radio, or TV, or according to the weather? Does your mood seem to drop if someone in your life is suffering? Do you get a feeling of dread, a premonition, that something bad has happened to someone you love?

Can the smallest thing make you impatient and irritable, like someone taking too long in a bathroom stall or being too slow in traffic? Do environmental stimuli, noises, lights (especially fluorescent lights), or crowds in an airport make you irritable and edgy? Your feminine brain's circuitry may be vulnerable to mood problems.

Do you frequently use shopping, especially catalogue shopping, to improve your mood? If you don't exercise every day, do you get irritable and on edge? Do you feel empty if you're alone?

If other people in your family are predisposed to mood disorders, PMS, depression, or bipolar disorder, you may have genetic susceptibility to this temperament as well. If you have already had one run-in with a mood problem, by virtue of being a woman in today's society, you are more likely to have further, more severe events due to hormonal shifts and kindling. Your moods provide great opportunities to get messages from your intuition, but if you don't learn how to manage your moods and decipher their wisdom, they can turn against you and wreak havoc with your health.

This would be bad enough if the problem were contained in your brain, but it invariably moves into your body as well.

Can You Name That Mood?

Each mood tends to fire up a brain-body circuit that creates a series of *actions, thoughts,* and *body health reactions* (see Emotional Feng Shui chart in Chapter 3). Each mood phase has a profound effect on frontal lobe circuits for goals, what you go after in the world, including jobs and adventures. The specific mood also influences frontal lobe circuits for drives toward relationships and capacity to fit into the rules of society.

THE ANATOMY OF SADNESS

A feeling of sadness is precipitated when things turn out badly, when you lose love, acceptance, or an important relationship, or when you are in contact with someone who is sad. Sadness is transient, lasting minutes, days, up to a couple of months. You tend to act in slow motion; you walk slow, talk slow, think slow, and take a long time to make decisions. When your body feels tired, lethargic, and the chest feels hollow and empty, the sadness brain circuit may be firing. You are also more likely to experience chest pressure, shortness of breath, have a lump in your throat, feel grief and despair. If you have a source of inflammation in your body and your immune system is activated in the case of an allergy, infection, or autoimmune illness, the sadness brain circuit is more likely to be activated.

Normal Sadness and Bereavement: The Portuguese Funeral

I come from a Portuguese family, and a lot of my relatives are from "the old country." Many of their names are engraved on the wall at Ellis Island. I don't remember ever having a conversation with my grandparents, yet it never occurred to me that they didn't speak English. Our conversations were by eye contact, facial expression, and hand signals. Some of my aunts wore 1940s style clothing in the 1960s and '70s, including hairnets on their heads. Family social occasions were centered on baptisms, birthdays, weddings, wakes, and funerals and were always pretty emotional, especially the wake after the funeral of my Uncle Fernando.

Uncle Fernando died after a long struggle with prostate cancer, so my Tia Maria watched him waste away and dement when the cancer metastasized to his brain. She took care of him at home and continued to sleep in the same bed with him. Tia Maria never really looked particularly sad because taking care of my Uncle Fernando was a full-time job, and she didn't have time to "wallow." Eventually he died in his sleep and everyone in the Portuguese colonies in Rhode Island and neighboring Fall River and New Bedford attended the wake and funeral because that's what's done; first, second, and third cousins came from everywhere.

Immediately after Uncle Fernando's death, Tia Maria went into shock. His death was completely expected, but it didn't matter. Tia Maria sat at the kitchen table with a cup of tea and stared into space. People had to help her get dressed, and we cousins suspected she was heavily sedated. When she got up from her chair to go to the car to leave for the wake, she had to be assisted by two of her sons, one at each elbow, because she felt weak and faint. At the wake, when Tia Maria was sitting at the receiving line, she stared straight ahead with a numb look on her face until the nuns came to the line.

Our local Portuguese Catholic church somehow had not heard of Vatican II. Many of the services were still in Portuguese and people revered their priest, saying, "Father Correira, that man sits at the right hand of God." The nuns still wore habits with soaring headgear and huge starched yokes. They were very innocent and pious, and considered to be like angels, at least the two nuns were who approached my aunt at the funeral. One gently took Tia Maria's hand, and murmured, "You can be happy because your Fernando is with Jesus now." For some reason, that snapped Tia Maria out of her vacant, grief-stricken stare, and she looked right at her and screamed, "And you can go straight to Hell!"

We were stunned. We had never heard anyone swear at a nun before. People said it was the "medication" talking. Then the funeral began. Tia Maria started talking to the casket, and at the burial, when attendants began to lower it into the ground, she "came alive" again. Tia Maria broke free from both her tall, well-built sons and started running toward the grave. Just as she was about to fling herself on the partly interred casket, her sons were able to grab her from behind.

Tia Maria wasn't "quite right" for months after that. She wore all black and barely touched the food that people brought to her house. The doctor gave her sleeping pills, but she rarely slept. She lost weight and didn't want to leave the house. And then slowly she came back to herself. She started attending baptisms and birthdays after a couple of months, but she continued to wear black for two years (customary for the region of Portugal from which she had emigrated).

Was Tia Maria depressed? No. She had a culturally appropriate, normal level of sadness that was in line with a grief response to the loss of a loved one. Even though she had many of the symptoms of depression, including insomnia, poor appetite, and weight loss, her sadness was still normal. If Tia Maria had stayed stuck in grief for a very long time, however, it could have destabilized her brain's mood circuits and caused her to slip into a major depression. If her sadness had lasted longer than the two to six months considered normal for grieving, then we would have got her into some form of treatment. However, that didn't happen. Tia Maria slowly resumed her activities with the Portuguese church. She began to head bake sales and bazaars, and became a good friend to those nuns whom a year earlier she had told to go to hell.

Although Tia Maria had known for months that Fernando was dying, she was emotionally unprepared for the profound changes his death would precipitate. She had some idea that taking care of him up to the moment of his death would prevent a "total breakdown." She hated being dependent upon anyone and didn't anticipate how it would feel to be alone in her house, and single in a world, like Noah's ark, made for couples. Her grief wasn't just triggered by Fernando's death, but by the loss of familiar habits and emotions and of her place in a *social* network of people.

Interestingly, the emotion of sadness fires the same brain areas that are critical for intuition, areas key for mood, decision making, empathy, and the autonomic nervous system. Sadness changes the neurotransmitters that bathe the brain and the body. The levels of opiates, oxytocin, and prolactin are reduced. These are neuropeptides critical for feeling a sense of reward after successful activity, or feeling an emotional bond during childbirth, breast feeding, or social activity. Corticotropin releasing factor (CRF) is altered, something that also happens during immune system dysfunction and cancer. Transient changes in levels of norepinephrine and serotonin also occur, but these neurotransmitter levels change in many emotional states.

Depression Isn't Simply Excess Sadness

Depression is not a biochemical exaggeration of sadness. Sadness is a normal signal from your intuitive guidance system that things have not turned out the way you wanted. Depression has a similar intuitive message but with an added twist—that you've stayed "sad" for so long that that emotion is beginning to shut down other emotional channels in your brain. Depressive brain changes are the opposite of those seen in sadness. In sadness, the frontal lobe "lights up" on a functional MRI. In depression, those emotional pathways shut down and the frontal lobe "dims." This underactive frontal lobe is key to the severe apathy and profoundly retarded movement, thought, and speech of a major depression. It may also be key to the profound physical problems with sleep and appetite. When someone with severe depression is treated successfully, however, this area "lights up" again to normal levels.

Interestingly, when a sad person's transient mood corrects itself, the excessively lit up frontal lobe "dims back down" to normal levels again. It's as if it no longer has to work overtime to send out intuitive signals alerting you that a problem in your life needs attention. This frontal lobe area may get activated when you experience the initial sadness associated with a loss or a failed goal. However, if the "sadness" brain circuit fires away for too long, it's possible that the area "burns" itself out, and it becomes harder to make sense and respond skillfully to what your emotion and intuition are trying to tell you.

Whenever any area in the brain fires too much for too long, oxygen, energy, and glucose resources in that region are used up. The cells can't return to their normal resting state. For example, if the neural network for sadness stays "lit" up for a much longer time, as in depression, the brain can't keep up with the energy demand of the cells and a cascade of degenerative events occurs in the brain. Proteins in the cells get distorted, and free radicals, single oxygen molecules, are released. The lipids in the nerve cell membranes are oxidized, as are the proteins in the DNA in the interior of the nerve cell. The nerve cell ultimately dies an untimely death called apoptosis (see Chapter 10). Prolonged firing in a nerve network triggers an inflammation that also occurs in Alzheimer's disease and heart disease.

Body Depression: My Mood's Fine, But My Body's Not

Some women may not feel sad; they may only have the body symptoms typical of the sadness circuits in the brain. Dina, aged forty-two, had a long history of lupus (systemic lupus erythematosis). At age fifteen, she started to have bouts of fatigue and always felt like she was coming down with the flu. Her joints would ache, she would have problems focusing and paying attention, and she would have to push herself to go to school. Always very disciplined and a perfectionist, Dina got into a premed program at the state university. However, during the first semester final exam period, after a series of all-nighters, Dina ended up in Health Services. At first, she was thought to have a bad flu that wouldn't go away, then mononucleosis, but after a rash developed and a few joints swelled, Dina was diagnosed with lupus. Luckily, medicines and steroids put Dina into remission.

Despite the fact that her first bout of lupus put her behind in her premed studies, Dina pulled herself together, got back into her disciplined routine, and was able to graduate magna cum laude. She successfully completed medical school and residency. She adopted a strict whole foods diet, and exercised and meditated religiously. The few people who knew about Dina's health problem were in awe of her positive attitude and unflagging spirit. No matter what happened—some small irritation or a major disappointment—Dina's attitude was positive and unflaggingly optimistic. Dina credited her health and career success to her spiritual practice of meditation.

Then Dina hit a wall. The clinic where she worked was always out of control. No matter how disciplined she was, she always ran behind. The front desk was always fitting last-minute patients into a schedule already filled to capacity. Insurance companies and HMOs kept changing the rules, requiring her to spend more and more time doing paperwork. Although Dina stuck to her health regimen, she could feel herself getting more tired and run down. It was getting harder and harder to get up at 6:00 a.m. for her first appointment at 8:00 a.m., especially when she was working until 8:00 p.m. every night on paperwork. During her workouts, Dina tried to ignore the fact that she was getting out of breath and dizzy. She began to have problems with her jaw and neck, which her osteopath told her was TMJ (temporomandibular joint disease). Her optimism and enthusiasm slipped. The nonprofit hospital where she had worked for two years was bought out by a for-profit hospital system; more patients were jammed into the schedule, and she had more regulations to follow about how long to spend with a patient, what drugs to prescribe, and how often to refer a patient to a specialist for consultation.

It was getting harder and harder for Dina to "grin and bear it." Meditation and positive affirmations were doing little for the escalating fatigue and tension building up in her body. One Monday morning, Dina woke up so out of breath she called in sick and went to her doctor, who took one look at her and sent her to the emergency room. There she was found to be severely anemic with a raging kidney infection related to the lupus. In the hospital, she watched her body get more and more out of control. Her lungs filled up with fluid in reaction to the infection and her kidneys went into failure. After numerous antibiotic trials and steroids, Dina was back to baseline. She went back to the clinic more determined than ever not to let the job and the hospital system get the upper hand.

Over the next two years, each time the hospital administration made changes, which caused doctors like Dina to lose power and respect, Dina had a flare-up of lupus. Physician colleagues of Dina's began to leave the clinic, but Dina thought she needed to hang in there for the sake of the patients and for what she thought was her calling to provide health care for the disenfranchised. Dina persevered through her lupus, and refused to allow her mood to get "down," even though her career had turned into a disappointment and the new hospital administrators were taking away her authority to treat her patients in what she saw as an ethical manner. Through sheer force of will, Dina refused to feel angry, frustrated, sad, or disappointed. She kept her conscious thought patterns firmly in the pattern of the joy and love emotional brain networks.

Feeling optimism and enthusiasm is usually not associated with immune system dysfunction, fatigue, lethargy, and the tight muscles of TMJ. These body reactions are associated with sadness and anger. In fact, when we feel the positive emotions, opiates are released that improve immune system competency, decreasing our chances of getting infections. That wasn't happening with Dina, who could not circumvent her body's intuition that was telling her that her life was out of control by making her physically ill. Since Dina didn't allow herself to feel sad, angry, and disappointed about her work, and she tried to compartmentalize these emotions in order to continue functioning, her body would get her to feel these emotions instead, giving her an opportunity to change what wasn't working for her.

Like Dina, some women learn to compartmentalize their emotions so they can achieve career goals. This adaptation helps you fit into a man's world, but the structure of the feminine brain's emotional circuitry won't allow you to do this indefinitely. Ultimately, even if you try to convince yourself that you're fine, your body's health will let you know otherwise. You may never feel sad or angry, but you'll know that something is wrong through fatigue, lethargy, a hollow feeling in the chest, shortness of breath, dizziness, swallowing problems, a change in appetite or sleep habits—clues that your life is out of balance.

THE ANATOMY OF DEPRESSION

A full-blown episode of *major depression* (see table earlier in this chapter) may be preceded by weeks or months of simmering sadness, which then escalates to aberrant behavior, thoughts, emotions, and body symptoms, with incapacity at work and a deterioration of relationships and physical health. Appetite and sleep changes in major depression can include significant weight gain or loss of up to 5 percent of body weight in one month. People can die from major depression by starving or killing themselves. In most people with major depression, an untreated episode lasts four months or longer, but usually there is a complete resolution of symptoms and a return to a normal state. However, in 20 to 30 percent of people, a less profound depressed mood remains that can last for months or years, with some residual impairment in mood, thinking, and function in relationships and productivity.

Major Depression: Dragged Down by the Pressures of Life

Agnes was sixty-two years old when she called me for a reading.

The reading: I saw that Agnes loved a man who was in pain. He had always been driven, competitive, but something went wrong with his health that left him feeling angry, degraded, humiliated, and depressed. He was very hard to love right now because he was irritable and took out his frustrations on Agnes.

Agnes felt that she had always danced around her husband's moods, but she was getting tired of it. She could intuitively sense when her husband was about to be angry and she would get him what he needed to "calm down," but this was taking its toll on her body.

When I looked at her body, I felt a dizziness and a pressure in her head, either due to blood pressure problems or due to muscle tightness in her neck. The blood vessels in her body felt tight. I wondered if she had problems maintaining stable blood pressure. She seemed to have gained quite a bit of weight and to crave carbohydrates, especially at night. But more than anything, Agnes had tremendous fatigue; she felt like a pile of lead, but even though she was exhausted she had trouble falling asleep and staying asleep. This made it hard for her to be efficient at work, since she was always exhausted. There seemed to be a fog in her head, and she had problems with focused attention, sustained attention, and memory. Agnes felt depressed, but was stoic and didn't want to complain.

The facts: Agnes had been diagnosed with hypertension by the family doctor, who also noted that she had at least five of the symptoms of a major depressive episode. These include:

- A depressed mood
- Loss of interest
- Less pleasure in daily activities
- A change in body weight (up or down by 5 percent in one month)
- Change in sleeping; insomnia or hypersomnia
- Slowed or agitated movement
- Fatigue, loss of energy
- Self-deprecating thoughts
- Problems with concentration or making decisions
- Recurrent thoughts of death, or thoughts of killing oneself (suicidal thoughts)

Her husband, Rocky, had had several heart attacks and a series of incapacitating strokes. He had been a competitive lawyer, respected in his profession as a fearless, relentlessly driven litigator. Since his stroke, Rocky had few friends and few outlets to escape his daily frustrations, which were now considerable. He had been forced to take a medical leave from his law firm, which incensed him. More than usual, Rocky took out his anger on his wife and now needed her with him twenty-four hours a day to help him get in and out of bed, assist him in self-care, and keep him company.

Agnes felt trapped and miserable. On the one hand, she loved her husband and was sure she would never get over losing him. She knew he had a good heart under that tough, competitive exterior, but she was angry and frustrated that he couldn't see that his personality and lifestyle had driven him closer to the grave. She had pleaded with him for years to get help with his anger and depression, but he had brushed those pleas aside irritably. The sicker Rocky got, the more depressed and angry he became. And as Rocky's fury mounted, so did Agnes's blood pressure. After a while, the inescapably stressful situation wore out Agnes's nearly infinite capacity to adapt and her mind and body got worn down by this no-win situation. Agnes's brain and body hit the wall. She couldn't think clearly; she could only react. As days blended into the nights and Rocky got sicker, Agnes began to worry about her own health. Her severe depression made her slow, listless, and numb.

In major depression, the "slow motion" activity/sadness can progress to "no motion." Thinking and speaking can become so retarded that they become nearly "catatonic." Thoughts become fatalistic, catastrophic, and then entrenched and immovable. The occasional gray cloud in the sky of sadness slowly darkens and builds, finally progressing in the severest cases to a pitch-black darkness. Thoughts become devoid of optimism; there's no hope. Guilt and self-blame are unyielding; there is no escape. Thoughts then turn to suicide.

As in sadness, in major depression the body may feel tired, lethargic, but the fatigue and energy loss are deeper and more profound, making it nearly impossible to have goals, relationships, or any activity that gives pleasure. The physical sensations become more severe in major depression, which increases inflammation and immune system dysfunction so that the patient is more likely to develop angina, a heart attack, or other severe cardiovascular or cerebrovascular disease. The most enduring form of depression imbalances the immune system to such a degree that it can, over time, precipitate cancer or an autoimmune illness.

The So-Called "Minor Depression" (Dysthymia) Isn't So Minor

Some kinds of depression fall between a major depressive episode and the normal sadness we might experience here and there. These are considered minor depression or dysthymia, and are less intense than major depression but longer-lasting and stronger than the transient blues of sadness.

The reading: When Brenda called for a reading, I saw a past history of abuse and emotional rejection in adult relationships that mirrored the abuse and neglect of her early family life. She didn't remember many of the events that she experienced growing up, but her body sure did. To fit in so that "people would love her," even as an adult Brenda would avoid conflict at any cost, become submissive if there were a difference of opinion, and defer to others about money, child rearing, and day-to-day decisions.

Brenda hid her feelings of disappointment when she didn't agree with her husband. When Brenda was separated from a loved one, her physical and emotional health would destabilize; her body seemed physically to pine for contact with loved ones. Her need for "emotional connection" exhausted and drained her husband and everyone else. They had begun to avoid her, which made her feel rejected and abandoned.

When I looked intuitively at Brenda's body, I saw problems with attention and distractibility, melancholy and sadness that were made worse by changes in her hormonal levels. She seemed to have scarring in her pelvis and uterus and to crave pasta, rice, bread, or sweets, with occasional episodes of excessive eating. She also seemed to be fatigued and drowsy, with tenderness in the joints of her hands, wrists, shoulders, and upper back.

The facts: Brenda had suffered for years from depression, feeling gloomy and helpless for as long as she could remember. She had never clicked with her mother and always felt her mother got along better with her older sister because they were more alike. Since a very early age, Brenda had tried to earn her mother's love by being the perfect daughter, never disagreeing, always trying to do better to get noticed. But she was never able to do enough to make her feel as loved as her older sister.

Brenda married when she was nineteen. At first the marriage went well, but soon her husband, Steve, began to spend extra time at work. This terrified Brenda, who tried harder to please her husband. They began to fight about his need to withdraw emotionally; eventually, the fights got physical. Finally, Steve told her he was in love with another woman. Brenda wanted to work at the marriage in therapy, but Steve said he was tired of being "smothered."

Brenda and Steve got divorced, which reinforced her lifelong feeling of rejection. Her mind became more of a fog and her problems with attention, labeled attention deficit disorder, worsened even though she was taking the medicine Adderall. Her hormones started to get "all out of whack." Her doctor said that her thyroid was on the "low end of normal," but not enough to treat medically.

Brenda comforted herself with food: bagels with cream cheese, breakfast cereal and bars, especially at night when she was trying to get to sleep. Yet, despite an occasional "run-in" with a bag of peanut M&M's, she was pretty disciplined about her food intake. Nonetheless, she gained fifteen pounds in the two years since separating from Steve and was having a harder and harder time getting to sleep at night. Every day she was more and more exhausted, more achy.

From years of disappointment, hurt, and sorrow, Brenda had developed dysthymia, a depressed mood that persists for most of the day, almost every day, for longer than two years without periods of real, lasting relief. Women with dysthymia have a low opinion of themselves and a sense of futility and hopelessness. They may have trouble paying attention, remembering things, and ordering thoughts to make a decision. They may feel they have ADD or the beginning stages of senility, but their problems are due to the biochemical changes in their brain and body that are by-products of their mood disorder. Over time, these biochemical changes will make them feel exhausted; they may eat either too much or too little, have trouble getting to sleep and staying asleep, or, in some cases, sleeping too much. You can die from major depression either by starving yourself or killing yourself. In dysthymia, you're more likely to live in physical pain (see below) and emotional misery.

What Causes Depression?

Being born a woman is known to double your lifetime risk for depression. The increased risk starts at puberty and continues to menopause. Having a family history of depression, having a stressful life, lacking social support, or having physical illness predisposes you to depression. An addiction to alcohol or some other addictive substance increases your risk, as does a prior episode of depression or past suicide attempts. Depression's causes can be genetic, hormonal, environmental, or nutritional. Emotional stress and an accumulation of adverse life experiences and traumas can alter brain chemistry and anatomy to cause depression by disrupting the activity of serotonin, norepinephrine, and their building block, tryptophan. This may be true because antidepressant drugs like Prozac, Zoloft, and other selective serotonin reuptake inhibitors (SSRIs) can successfully treat 30 to 60 percent of people who develop major depression. But these particular medicines don't work as well for other types of depression, especially the kind that is even more common in women, the so-called *"atypical" depression,* which has symptoms of weight gain, hypersomnia (sleeping too much), and reactive mood (see below).

Neuroscientists claim that no single neurotransmitter is involved, since several very potent antidepressants (including tricyclic antidepressants [TCAs]) also affect the neurotransmitter acetylcholine, which plays a role in attention and memory. Many women, like Brenda, who suffer from depression also complain of attention and memory problems.

When you're stressed, your brain's fear and anxiety circuits begin to fire. If the stress becomes chronic, the fear areas in your brain become structurally altered, triggering the depression cascade of changing serotonin, norepinephrine, estrogen, and progesterone. Women's fear and depression circuits may be more closely linked than a masculinized brain's. Many women who have depression also have coexistent anxiety, which also has to be treated (see Chapters 6 and 7), or the anxiety will trigger a new round of depression and then the depression will trigger anxiety ... and around and around you will go.

Estrogen's antidepressant effect is directly related to serotonin function. Both serotonin and norepinephrine affect your hormone levels of estrogen and progesterone and probably testosterone. If you have a tendency toward depression, hormonal events like puberty, pregnancy, childbirth, postpartum, perimenopause, and menopause further amplify that tendency. Sparklers become fireworks.

So it is no wonder that women are more prone to depression and moodiness, since our emotional anatomy is more pliable. If your hormones normally go up and down regularly with your menstrual cycle, so do your neurotransmitters, and so will your moods.

All Stress Does Not Lead to Distress or Depression

Ultimately, if you find yourself blue and you don't know why, the sadness is a signal from your intuitive guidance system that you're not getting something you want or need in life. Or it may be a signal that someone you love is unhappy. The longer you let the signal persist without responding to it, the more likely your sadness will take the hormonal, neurotransmitter, and neuroanatomic nosedive into a minor or major depression.

Here are several kinds of stress that may be getting you down.

The "Black Flies" Type of Stress. In Maine, in the beginning of June, we have these Ambassadors of Evil called black flies. When I was younger (and probably more distractible), I used to hike on mountain trails all the time, crossing streams with a thirty-pound frame pack. The flies never bothered me and I rarely noticed them because I was always trying to focus on reading the map, staying on the trail, and not falling off a cliff. But now, my buffer for these tiny pests is nearly nonexistent. Even though one fly is harmless and annoying, the additive effect of being bitten over and over puts me over the edge. Depression is like that: Once you've had a run-in with a stress that puts you "over the edge," you're more likely to go off the deep end, but with fewer flies.

Even if stress from individual events seems to be mild, the unrelenting nature of them coming one after the other may overwhelm the buffer in your brain's mood circuits. Something "snaps" inside you. The neuro-chemical buffers in your brain, resources that keep you bouncing back, wear down. Transient sadness becomes fixed. Anger, hormones, your personality and temperament, past problems with depression, and mood problems all contribute to the strength or weakness of your mental buffer. The threshold sometimes lowers with age, but not always. Some people do become more resilient against the black flies of our lives.

Getting Sent Down to the Minor Leagues. Having a public failure or loss is very stressful and can precipitate depression. Declaring bankruptcy, being fired, divorced, or peripheralized from your social group reduces your status and can induce the biochemical change that leads to depression. If you become so defeated and dejected by the loss that you can't fight your way back up to the major leagues where you used to be, your risk of having severe depression, heart disease, and cancer climbs even higher. If your partner or a beloved family member has suffered this kind of loss, it is not uncommon for you to pick up on it intuitively and become depressed. This type of depression can be hard to treat, so you need to be particularly conscious of whether you are dependent upon another person and how.

Being Separated from the Mother Ship. Being prematurely separated from your mother affects your biological buffer for depression, moodiness, anxiety, and problems with controlling irritability, anger, and aggression. It can haunt you years later after suffering another separation. Get counseling; it can help.

The Catch-22 Environment. Not everyone develops depression from an environment of stress, pain, and chaos. The people who learn to escape the pain, whether through an inner mind-set, prayer, or meditation, are less likely to develop depression later in life. Perhaps they are spared by fate, some mystical "roll of the dice" of genetic selection, or perhaps they've inherited some soul quality of resistance. Some people, however, can't escape the pain, chaos, or trauma around them and their brain's circuits develop a pessimistic mind-set that learns to expect trauma. They feel that no matter what they do, they're going to suffer, so why bother trying? This is called "learned helplessness" and it's probably the leading cause of chronic depression. Women who suffer from physical, emotional, or sexual trauma and abuse are more likely to have their brains anatomically molded by "learned helplessness" into mood pathways that are vulnerable to chronic depression.

When I was a psych resident, I spent a lot of weekends on the psych unit on call. I would admit patients who came into the emergency room either suicidally depressed or mentally incapacitated in some way. I would also follow up on patients who were staying on the unit, or do consults on people in the hospital who had complex medical–psychiatric problems. The tricky thing about learning to be a psychiatrist was trying to absorb all the psychotherapy treatment theories of Freud, Jung, Klein, and others, learn all the neuroanatomy and neurochemistry of the brain that underpins both emotional problems and their medical treatment, and all the while balance these huge bodies of knowledge with some good old common sense.

One rainy Saturday, I hauled myself onto the unit. It was a cold, gloomy day, and I was physically and emotionally dragging anchor. As I worked on follow-up after follow-up, I noticed that many of the women were also at low ebb. Usually, patients brighten up from their depressions as they near discharge, but every one of these women was sleepy, snacking, or dragging herself around like a zombie. Hanging out in the psych ward made my mood sink even lower.

After my shift, I cheered myself up by going home, playing with my cats, and popping the comedy *Sister Act* into the VCR. Yet I found myself crying during the finale where Whoopi Goldberg and all these wonderful nuns are singing "I Will Follow Him" in front of the pope. I said out loud, "Mona Lisa, you're not right. You need to be evaluated."

The next day, I dragged my sorry behind out of bed to be in the psych ward on rounds, and again felt just as heavy as everyone else's mood, and as damp and lifeless as the weather. I said to one of the male nurses, "I can't wait for this weather to clear. It's a really dragging my mood down."

He looked at me and asked, "You're kidding, aren't you?"

I said, "No, why?"

Then he asked, "Are your moods really so keyed into the environment? Are you really that primitive?"

I was taken aback. He wasn't being nasty or snide; he was really a nice guy. I had a bachelor's degree, an M.D., and a Ph.D. in behavioral neuroscience and neuroanatomy. I was capable of abstract thought, walked on two legs, and read poetry occasionally. How could I be primitive? But twenty-nine years of formal education haven't changed the fact that I am a woman and, according to psychiatry and neuroanatomy, my moods and brain are "atypical," that is, they don't match the traditional compartmentalized male model. My moods, like everyone else's who has a hyperconnected feminine brain, are porous and react to what is going on inside of me as well as what's going on in my environment including the people around me. In a way, we women and some atypical men will always be more in touch, more responsive. Men and traditional psychiatry might label this "primitive," but we women know that we are simply more "reactive," more in tune with others and the world around us.

Even with this tendency, you *can* become conscious of when your mood is being dragged down and learn to keep it on an even keel. When your mood is starting to go off the deep end in reaction to something in your environment, there are a number of ways to shore up your emotional reserves so it doesn't make you suffer or get sick (see Chapter 5, "New Moon").

The feminine brain is more susceptible to seasonal affective disorder (SAD), another form of "reactive" depression that is frequently seen in the northern latitudes of the United States. This disorder is four times more common in women than men, and its symptoms include a depressed mood, increased appetite, weight gain, and hypersomnia, all of which are keyed into the weather and the length of the day. Symptoms usually begin in the fall, worsen in the winter, and dissipate as summer approaches. Women and men with this disorder are also prone to having other forms of "nonseasonal depression."

Being reactive may be both an advantage and disadvantage to a woman, especially as she gains more socioeconomic power and status. The downside is that being reactive to the feelings and criticisms of others can make you emotionally vulnerable, but being "keyed in" to the thoughts, feelings, and reactions of others can protect you if you skillfully respond to your perceptions. This is the challenge to women today. If you can capitalize on your hyperconnected brain's intuitions, you can thrive in any vocational environment or relationship.

The Chemistry of Joy/Love

We like the thrill of victory, but we hate the agony of defeat. And our actions reveal when we are happy even if we are unconscious of it or can't feel it inside.

The brain circuits for happiness, love, bonding, eating, and sex are structurally intertwined. Scientists have noted some difference between the sexes in certain regions of the joy/love brain networks. The changing amounts of estradiol, testosterone, and other steroids may shape these networks. Ultimately, how we act, think, and feel and how our health reacts to being happy and in love is determined by our genes, hormonal makeup, and past experience (traumatic, pleasurable, or otherwise).

When your love and happiness brain circuits fire, you may turn red, blush, your heart rate may go up, and your body temperature may rise as well. Some people *act* excited, energetic, and talkative when they are happy and in love, whereas other people get relaxed and calm. Some people smile and keep looking at what makes them feel happy and in love, whereas others look away. When you are happy and loving someone (or something), you tend to think about what you adore and what brings you joy. You feel safe, secure, lovable, accepted and have a sense that "this is where you belong." You focus on what you are good at; you feel powerful and strong.

If your brain's circuits for love and joy are firing, your immune system is more likely to be balanced. If your immune system is constantly on alert, as in chronic fatigue, or it's deficient, as after cancer treatment, you will have more trouble feeling happy and loving. An imbalanced immune system is likely to depress you because it releases neuropeptides and other chemical mediators (see below) that disrupt neurotransmitters (the inner opiates) that are key to feeling love and joy.

Other physical states can also turn on and off the brain's areas for love and happiness. Your happiness circuits light up when you achieve a goal, become successful at something, or get what you want, which ultimately raises your self-esteem. Whenever you even think about past successes, your brain releases happiness chemicals. Relationships, especially nurturing ones, can create the same mind-body elation. Neurotransmitters of love and happiness release when someone treats you well; abusive relationships deprive you of an uplifting neurochemical diet, erode your sense of self, and set the body-mind stage for depression. The same neurotransmitters for love and happiness can also relieve pain.

Oxytocin, another neuropeptide, is elevated during the initial stages of infatuation and love, and is key to the bond we feel during childbirth, sex, and breast feeding. Testosterone is also critical for joy, love, and relationships. When some women are unhappy or have lost a key relationship in their life, they may compulsively eat or have a pain disorder, a lowered threshold for feeling pain either from a previous injury or from a new one. These women may also obsessively ruminate about acquiring a new relationship as they try to reactivate the release of opiates. Postpartum women for a while have a lowered sex drive: In addition to just plain being exhausted from being pregnant, and from labor and delivery, a woman's bonding circuitry may be so taken up with falling in love with her newborn that all of her circuits are busy.

I'M OK IF YOU'RE OK: THE ANATOMY OF CODEPENDENCE, HAPPINESS
THAT IS DEPENDENT ON THE HAPPINESS OF OTHERS

Pregnancy, labor, delivery, and child rearing can make a woman hyper-connected and porous to the feelings of others. As some women say, "When you're happy, I'm happy." But if you are dependent on others' happiness, you've got a very big problem. Ultimately, you are going to strip the gears in your mood-balancing system from constant downshifting and up-shifting. Your loved ones may end up dependent upon you for happiness, and you all become unhealthily *codependent*. By compulsively trying to save people around you from their problems, you may accumulate more and more dependent people around you. You may get a high initially when you save someone who is unhappy, because opiates are released in your brain areas for mood, empathy, and bonding. But the chemicals you release when you compulsively "save" people are very similar to those involved in cocaine, amphetamine, alcohol, and other addictive substances. Your brain may become physiologically dependent on the neurotransmitters that are released during "search and rescue." This will become physically and emotionally unhealthy for you and them.

THE BIPOLAR DILEMMA

Some women with *bipolar disorder* (see table earlier in this chapter) bounce between extreme episodes of depression and happiness. They become so euphoric or manic that their frontal lobe's inhibition and judgment become lost entirely and they lose touch with reality. Other women with less extreme "highs," called hypomania, and "lows" of their mood will be labeled by psychiatry as having *bipolar II*. Still others carry the label of *borderline personality disorder* and have rapid shifts of mood, highs and lows, in reaction to perceived or actual separation and abandonment in a relationship. It is obviously beyond the scope of this book to discuss the controversial and, I believe, often arbitrary differences between these diagnoses. Some texts have come up with at least six different types of "bipolar" disorder, with erratic mood shifts associated with attention deficit disorder, addiction, the use of antidepressants, as well as a variety of other situations. The diagnosis of any type of bipolar disorder today has become so overused that the term has lost much of its original meaning and usefulness. Moodiness is a quality that is common among all of us, and its variation is dependent upon sex, genetic predisposition, history of trauma, and hormonal states.

Body Reactions

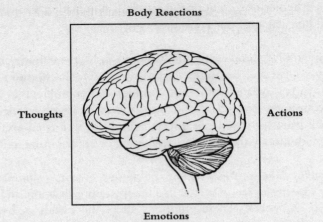

Thoughts

Actions

Emotions

Figure 9. Mood and Fear. Drawing of brain with body reactions, thoughts, actions, and emotions.

Learn Your Feminine Brain's Unique Language for Mood

I hope you are beginning to see in what side of the brain you tend to stay emotionally. Please try to determine if you tend to get stuck in one type of thought pattern. Examine your actions and behavior to find out what you are really feeling. Examine your body's health to see which emotional circuit in your brain it is reflecting. The following questions will help you. After you answer them, I'll take you through a story of one of my own clients to show you how she worked with her answers.

WHAT ARE MY MOODS TELLING ME ABOUT MY FEMININE BRAIN'S WIRING FOR EMOTION?

- ❏ *Do you tend to get stuck in one mood state?* If so, which one? Even getting stuck in the "normal mixed mood" may make you feel like your life is devoid of pizzazz, passion, and feeling, lacking the drama of the normal ups and downs of life.
- ❏ *Do your moods shift erratically?* If yes, do they shift in a cycle that is keyed into your menstrual cycle? Is your mood keyed to the seasons? Does your mood shift due to experiencing rejection? Is your mood overly porous to people's feelings in your environment?
- ❏ Maybe you feel your mood is okay, but you are still not happy and content with your life. To find out why you're still not happy, examining your thoughts, actions, and health may tell

you whether one emotional network is dominating your brain, and imbalancing your feminine brain.

Seven intuitive mood centers of the body can help you figure out what is causing you to feel sad, angry, happy, or irritable. Each emotional or mood center is associated with some common health problems in specific parts of your body. If you have one of the following health problems, say, lower back pain, see if you can discern a problem in a relationship or a problem with money that could be triggering or contributing to it.

- *The First Intuitive Mood Center: Safety and Security in the World:* The capacity to feel accepted in a family, an organization, and the world in general. These emotions affect the health of bones, joints, blood, and the immune system.
- *The Second Intuitive Mood Center: Relationships and Finances:* The capacity to feel good about yourself and confident in relationships and monetary matters. These emotions affect the health of the reproductive organs and lower back region.
- *The Third Intuitive Mood Center: Responsibility and Work:* The capacity to feel content about employment and commitment in your life. These feelings affect the digestive organs and weight.
- *The Fourth Intuitive Mood Center: Emotional Expression and Nurturance:* The capacity to have mutual partnerships and the emotions that go with them affect the health of the heart, breasts, and lungs.
- *The Fifth Intuitive Mood Center: Communication, Will, and Timing:* The capacity to communicate what you believe at the right time and with the right intensity affects the health of the mouth, neck, and thyroid region.
- *The Sixth Intuitive Mood Center: Perception, Thought, and Morality:* Feeling content that you and others have a variety of ways of seeing the world and a variety of opinions about them. Having a rigid outlook affects the health of the nervous system, eyes, and ears.
- *The Seventh Intuitive Mood Center: Life Purpose, Mortality, and the Spiritual World:* Feeling content about your life calling, accepting your mortality, and coming to terms with good, evil, and the spiritual world influences your ability to survive life-threatening illnesses.

What Do My Thoughts Tell Me About How My Feminine Brain is Wired for Mood?

Do you notice specific thoughts enter your consciousness more often than not? Unhealthy thoughts can distort your mood, and prevent you from hearing intuitive guidance and realizing your potential. These thoughts can also influence the physical regions associated with the mood center.

Sadness and Anger Thoughts

First Intuitive Mood Center (Bones, joints, blood, and immune system)
- ❑ I can easily feel rejected, abandoned, and betrayed in family and other relationships.
- ❑ I am misunderstood and underappreciated by a lot of people.
- ❑ I need people to help me since I feel weak and vulnerable.
- ❑ I feel empty and alone unless I am near someone strong.

Second Intuitive Mood Center (Reproductive organs and lower back region)
- ❑ People usually find me unattractive and unappealing. I am unlovable.
- ❑ Even when I fall in love with someone, it's hard for me not to focus on the negative aspects.
- ❑ Relationships usually end traumatically for me.

Third Intuitive Mood Center (Digestive organs and weight)
- ❑ I have trouble making decisions.
- ❑ I'm not smart enough. Mostly everyone is smarter than me, more attractive than me, more successful, loved, or appreciated.
- ❑ I blame myself for things that go wrong around me.
- ❑ I frequently look for faults in myself, criticizing myself all the time in school or work. I'll never be good enough.
- ❑ A lot of people have opportunities and gifts that I'll never get.
- ❑ Authority figures in my life have tended to be intrusive, demanding, controlling, and unfair. Being controlled and dominated by others is intolerable.

Fourth Intuitive Mood Center (Heart, breasts, and lungs)
- ❑ I am not valuable unless I am taking care of someone.
- ❑ I won't be loved and accepted if I get angry or sad.
- ❑ It's safer to take care of my own needs rather than accept help from others.

Fifth Intuitive Mood Center (Mouth, neck, and thyroid region)
- ❏ Even if I speak my mind, it never seems to change anything, so why bother.
- ❏ If only I could say it "the right way," maybe he'll change.

Sixth Intuitive Mood Center (Nervous system, eyes, and ears)
- ❏ I'm right and they're usually wrong.
- ❏ Things should be different in my life.

Seventh Intuitive Mood Center (Survival from life-threatening illnesses)
- ❏ I don't know what my true calling in life is.
- ❏ I'm not happy with what has happened so far in my life.
- ❏ I am afraid of death.

Ultimately, any of these thoughts can censor your intuition and distort your mood. You need to be conscious of them and do something about them, but you can't just cover them up with forced happy thoughts. Contrary to what you might think, if we think only positive "happy" thoughts, our mind and body will not be healthy. By not allowing ourselves to have a healthy, balanced diet of painful and pleasant feelings and thoughts, we deprive ourselves of intuition and inspiration that are key to surviving and thriving in the world.

Love/Joy Thoughts
- ❏ I feel successful about a lot of things in my life.
- ❏ I usually get what I want.
- ❏ I am usually accepted by others.
- ❏ I feel needed and appreciated.
- ❏ I feel physically attractive.

Mania/Overly Elevated Mood Style of Thinking
- ❏ Many people frequently find me sexually attractive; I have very frequent thoughts about sex.
- ❏ Everyone always moves too slowly for me; my thoughts race.
- ❏ I frequently think of funny situations and have trouble not talking humorously.
- ❏ People almost always like my ideas.
- ❏ I usually know best.
- ❏ I cannot lose no matter what.
- ❏ I am personally invincible; I live for today, for tomorrow *they* may not come.

WHAT DOES MY BEHAVIOR TELL ME ABOUT MY BRAIN'S WIRING FOR MOOD AND MOODINESS?

Do you or someone near you notice that you react in the following ways?

- ❏ I crave carbohydrates in the form of pasta, rice, bread, or sweets, or I maintain tight control over my carbohydrate intake.
- ❏ When I get upset, my computer crashes or I have trouble with electrical devices.
- ❏ I log in to the computer a lot to check my personal email.
- ❏ I constantly use my cell phone, and go into withdrawal if the battery runs out.
- ❏ I can't stand being put on hold.
- ❏ I hate automated phone answering services.
- ❏ I easily get impatient and irritated in traffic.
- ❏ I criticize other drivers' habits in traffic.
- ❏ I use certain music CDs to pick up my mood or calm me down.
- ❏ I am very sensitive to noise, papers rustling, babies crying.
- ❏ I am very sensitive to fluorescent lights or flashing lights.
- ❏ I get impatient and irritable, and have difficulty waiting in line for more than a few minutes.
- ❏ I shop or look through catalogues as a way to relax.
- ❏ I talk slowly, walk slowly, and my voice stays usually on one tone.
- ❏ I have slumped posture, with my neck jutted forward.
- ❏ I have droopy eyes.
- ❏ My posture is tight, tense.
- ❏ I frequently grit my teeth, or clench my jaw, fists, and hands.
- ❏ I slam things around.
- ❏ I have decreased eye control.

Love/Joy Behaviors
- ❏ Walking, moving, or talking with energy and excitement
- ❏ Straight posture with head up, shoulders erect
- ❏ Smiling, laughing
- ❏ Increased eye contact
- ❏ Looking relaxed and calm

Mania/Overly Elated Mood Behaviors
- ❏ Markedly decreased need for sleep
- ❏ Pressured, rapid-fire speech beyond normal regional dialect
- ❏ Increased participation in multiple goal-directed behaviors, occupations, political and religious activities

- ❏ Increased behavior that appears intrusive, domineering, or demanding
- ❏ Increased reckless behavior in spending, driving, or a sexual relationship that's not usual personal style

As you go through the above list of *feelings, thoughts,* and *actions* associated with the feminine brain's mood circuits, do you find yourself checking many of the items in certain mood categories? Are you spending too much time in one mood? That ultimately may impact your health and deprive you of optimal access to your intuition.

WHAT IS MY HEALTH TELLING ME ABOUT MY FEMININE BRAIN'S WIRING FOR MOOD AND MOODINESS?

Perhaps your health is giving you intuitive insight about the emotional mood circuits in your brain that are working overtime.

Health Patterns Associated with a Balanced Diet of All Five Basic Emotions
- ❏ I have healthy blood pressure and cardiovascular health.
- ❏ My immune system is generally healthy. I am less prone than most to coming down with the latest flu.
- ❏ I have not had cancer in the last five years.
- ❏ If I get injured, the acute pain of the injury soon goes away with minimal occupational therapy, physical therapy, or other treatment.
- ❏ I will fall asleep and stay asleep with ease.
- ❏ My weight pretty much stays within a normal range for my height, give or take ten pounds.
- ❏ I do not need sugar, chocolate, bread, or sweets to feel calm, happy, or contented.
- ❏ I don't have a first-degree relative with alcohol addiction or some other type of drug addiction, including prescription drugs like Valium, Ativan, Xanax, or Oxycodone.

HEALTH PROBLEMS THAT TEND TO PRECIPITATE MOOD PROBLEMS OR MOODINESS

Psychiatry calls these conditions *mood disorders secondary to general medical condition.* All of the feminine brain's emotional circuits for fear, anger, sadness, joy, and love have two-way connections through the brain stem to the body's organs (see Figure 7, "The Emotion-Disease Domino Effect").

Emotions can precipitate changes in the health of all the body's organs. Similarly, the health of your organs is transmitted back to the brain, and a change in your mood can be your intuition letting you know something's going on in your body.

- ❑ Cardiovascular and cerebrovascular problems: hypertension, angina, chest pain, palpitations
- ❑ Chronic immune system dysfunction: chronic autoimmune system disorders: rheumatoid arthritis, SLE (lupus), multiple sclerosis, Crohn's disease, ulcerative colitis, chronic infections or inflammation, chronic fatigue, fibromyalgia, Lyme disease, cancer of all kinds
- ❑ Chronic pain: lower back pain, neck pain, headache, and migraines
- ❑ Sleep disorders: insomnia or hypersomnia
- ❑ Eating disorders: bulimia, anorexia nervosa, obesity
- ❑ Addictions: alcohol, food, carbohydrates, prescription medications addiction

Your blood pressure obviously affects your mood: When it's high, you can be jittery or anxious; when it's low, your mood can be low. If you have chronic cardiovascular problems like hypertension, chest pain, angina, arrhythmias, palpitations, hot flashes, or even a heart attack, biochemical changes in the heart and blood vessels are communicated to emotional areas in your brain that ultimately may trigger sadness, melancholy, irritability, and anger. Immune disorders, and even colds and flus can make you blue. When your physical health changes, your mood is more likely to go up or down. Depending on your unique feminine brain wiring, certain aspects of your emotional brain–body circuits may be more "vocal" and others may be more silent.

Are You Sick, or Just Depressed?

Inflammation is created and cytokines are released when you are physically stressed by an illness in your body and when you are psychologically stressed by depression. So, it's pointless to ask someone who has chest pain, "Do you really have heart problems, or is it just in your head?" It would also be ridiculous to ask someone with chronic fatigue or fibromyalgia or a pain syndrome if she is *really* physically sick or just depressed. In fact, SSRIs (selective serotonin reuptake inhibitors) and antidepressants have been used successfully to treat chronic immune system syndromes like chronic fatigue/fibromyalgia, and pain syndromes. SSRIs inhibit the production of cytokines and other inflammatory mediators.

Nancy, age forty-nine, had a long history of depression and physical illness. Her mother was a therapist, her father a psychiatrist, and Nancy had always wanted to be a clinical psychologist. She worked hard in college to prepare for a prestigious Ph.D. clinical psychology program. To improve her chances of getting in, Nancy did extra research and a lot of networking, but she didn't do well on her GREs, and didn't get any interview requests. With unflagging optimism, she took classes to train herself to retake the exams, and improved her scores by 40 points, but still, on the next year's applications, she had no luck. Nancy married Bob, but didn't let their marriage distract her from her goal. She got a job as a research assistant in a psych lab at the local state university, worked hard, and focused on the professor's project with such determination that she earned the respect of everyone in the department. Nancy applied to the Ph.D. clinical psychology program at that university and was accepted.

Nancy was elated. Bob breathed a sigh of relief. At age twenty-eight, Nancy entered graduate school, but immediately began to have problems. At first, she thought that her academic difficulties were because she had been out of school for a while, so she got a tutor. But still, she almost always got the lowest grades in the class. She finished all of her basic courses with a C-plus to B-minus average. It took her two years to study for her qualifying exams, and to her dismay, she failed. The doctoral department committee voted to give her a "terminal master's degree," which meant that Nancy was out of the program.

Nancy was devastated and felt as if something inside her had died. At the age of thirty-two, she felt washed up. Her lifelong dream was dead in the water. She went to work at a local battered women's shelter, where she had worked earlier for a time, and the staff welcomed her with open arms. But it wasn't the same for Nancy. Without the dream of becoming a clinical psychologist on the horizon, she felt her life lacked focus. Her mood plummeted. She lost interest in her job and clients, and had to push herself through the day. Her life and mind slowed. She couldn't focus or pay attention. Her appetite diminished and she lost ten pounds in six weeks. She began to wake up at four in the morning, her mind racing, and she was exhausted.

Nancy was diagnosed with major depression, and after six weeks, improved on Zoloft. Even with supportive psychotherapy, however, Nancy was never the same. She gained sixty pounds. As she went to doctor after doctor to get something to help her sleep, her intense fatigue turned into an overall achiness in her body and a great dizziness and weakness. A sense of hopelessness set in. One therapist gave her a diagnosis of chronic fatigue/fibromyalgia. An internist found that her blood pressure was mildly elevated, as was her blood sugar. A neurologist evaluated her fatigue and dizziness by doing an MRI of her brain, which showed "mild ischemic changes" in the front. Nancy's doctors weren't concerned about the MRI, saying it was only "age-related changes," but they were concerned about her heart, now that she was mildly hypertensive, diabetic, and obese. She also had elevated homocysteine levels in the blood, which is associated with heart problems.

Nancy realized that she was dying of a broken heart. She had never really regained meaning in her life after she was kicked out of that Ph.D. program years earlier. The spark in her life was snuffed out that day. Even the word "terminal" in her master's degree felt like death. Although Nancy did not feel sad, her behavior reflected it: She walked slowly, talked slowly, her voice was low and scratchy, her posture slumped. Nancy's body was revealing very loudly that the anger and sadness brain/body circuits were firing away, and that she had to resolve the loss of her lifelong dream.

Loss triggers a chain reaction of physiological events in the body that, depending upon a person's genetic tendency, can result in immune system dysfunction and cancer, heart disease and stroke, pain syndromes, sleep disorders, and addictions. A *domino effect* was occurring between depression and disease in Nancy's body.

The Depression–Disease Domino Effect
1.   *Norepinephrine* is released from the brain stem.
2.   *Stress* causes too much cortisol to be secreted.
3.   The cortisol starts the *cytokine and inflammation* cascade.
4.   Inflammation initiates *chronic fatigue symptoms:*
         Fever-like feeling
         Weakness
         Depression
         Lethargy, slowed movements
5.   *Cytokine and inflammation* cascade literally "eats up" critical mood neurotransmitters *norepinephrine* and *serotonin*. Blood *homocysteine* levels rise, further lowering norepinephrine and serotonin and increasing inflammation. Disrupted norepinephrine and serotonin levels and higher levels of inflammation increase chances of having *pain* (headache, back pain, etc.), *sleep* problems (insomnia or hypersomnia), and ultimately *addiction*.

6. Person tries to self-medicate the loss of neurotransmitters by eating more carbohydrates, increasing her chance of having an *eating disorder.*

7. Person's *cholesterol levels* go up secondary to more dietary carbohydrates and increased stress levels (with increased LDL, decreased HDL).

8. Person develops *hyperinsulinism* and *hypertension* (called "Syndrome X").

9. *Inflammation accelerates,* cholesterol floating in blood gets oxidized, creates "free radicals."

10. *Blood vessels* and brain cell *cell membranes* constrict; omega-3 fatty acid levels go down.

In Nancy's case, her biological vulnerability was in the blood vessels of her brain. The domino effect of depression to disease increased her rate of developing inflammation, cytokine release, and elevated homocysteine levels that precipitated small vessel disease in her brain, which was readily seen by her doctors on her MRI. Interestingly, the abnormalities weren't everywhere in her brain randomly but were in areas related to the sadness network, the brain areas for assessing the success of goals and the areas for initiation and motivation.

In a classic chicken-or-egg debate, doctors question whether depression causes blood vessel disease in the brain, and white matter lesions on the MRI, or whether the cerebrovascular disease (blood vessel disease specific to the brain) causes the depression. When the blood vessels become diseased, they release cytokines that cause inflammation and depression. On the other hand, depression causes inflammation that precipitates the heart and blood vessel problems.

The brain has a mechanism to turn on inflammation and also turn off the disease-causing process: The neurotransmitter norepinephrine turns on the domino effect of depression to disease in the body, and acetylcholine turns off the inflammatory cascade. Many treatments that successfully beat depression, pain, heart disease, and autoimmune diseases turn on the body's innate inflammatory healing system.

If something turns out badly in your life or if you lose someone you love, your body's health may act out the emotions you feel through symptoms of illness. So what do you do then? You want to identify your *mood,* your *thoughts,* your *behavior,* and their associated *body health reactions*—all four sides of your emotional brain circuit. This is what Nancy began to do. First, she looked at how her brain and body had gotten out of control. She began to see that her body's health problems of weight gain, insomnia, intense fatigue, dizziness, weakness, chronic fatigue/fibromyalgia, elevated blood sugar, and blood vessel disease were all associated with mood problems. Nancy realized that the loss of her Ph.D. program gave her a problem in her *first intuitive mood center* (safety and security in the world [see above]) and her *seventh center* (life purpose). Nancy also realized that she had several thoughts that were associated with depression in these mood centers, including a feeling of rejection and betrayal by her Ph.D. committee (first mood center) and a feeling that she no longer knew what her new calling in life was (seventh mood center). Nancy also worked with a team of professionals to stop the depression–disease domino effect in her brain and body. She took medicines and supplements to correct her serotonin and epinephrine levels to improve her mood, sleep, and pain problems while taking other nutritional agents to stop the inflammation in her blood vessels and her brain. Finally, Nancy consulted with a therapist who knew cognitive behavior therapy to help her listen to the intuitive guidance underlying her depression and also correct the thought patterns that were preventing her from finding a fulfilling life purpose.

In the next chapter, you will learn how to tune up your feminine brain's mood area so that you can be more healthy and happy.

FIVE

New Moon:
Tune Up Your Mood Circuits

How would you know if your mood circuits and brain need a tune-up?

- Your mood tends toward being down in the dumps.
- Your mood shifts erratically from highs to lows.
- Your thoughts migrate toward things that are gloomy, irritating, annoying, or disappointing.
- You act impatient or on edge when you have to wait, or when in an environment where there is a moderate amount of people, noise, or bright light.
- Your health is very reactive to stress: You tend to have elevated cholesterol and high blood pressure. You easily gain weight, get migraine headaches, back pain, insomnia, or some characteristic problem for you.
- You are emotionally porous and intuitively key into other people's emotional and physical pain. You quite literally "feel for them." You get sick over their problems: you get an ulcer or you get physically tight watching your child compete in an athletic competition or seeing him struggle in school.

If you have any of these characteristics, this chapter can help you. You can address these problems biochemically, pharmacologically, and nutritionally. You can also learn to rewire your thought patterns *away* from being persistently pessimistic or self-depreciating and improve your mood by changing how you react to disappointing or painful situations. By treating physical health problems that are connected to the brain's circuits for sadness and anger, you can improve your mood. All of this becomes easier when you find the intuitive message behind the mood.

The Intuitive Message Behind the Mood

It's easy to understand how mood problems can increase your chances of getting sick, but it may be difficult to see how moodiness and depression can help you be intuitive. The following story might help you see how your intuition can come to you through a bad feeling.

April, age forty-eight, has suffered bouts of depression since adolescence, when she developed PMS and irritable bowel syndrome (IBS). April's mood problems began when she started to have arguments with her mother, who she felt was very judgmental and controlling. As soon as April turned eighteen, she left home and decided she would never be controlled again. During school vacations, April would try to have a peaceful visit with her parents, only to have to leave in despair with her stomach tied in knots. April learned to space her visits farther and farther apart until she was only going home once a year.

In college, she dated quite a bit, and eventually met Bob, who was so exciting to April that she felt weak-kneed. Rationally, April had sized up Bob as the "perfect catch": He was pre-law, didn't drink or smoke, and wasn't a womanizer—left-brain details that made him, to April, "Mr. Right." After their first "official date," however, April found herself in a very low mood and her stomach was "in agony." Even though April was excited about the potential of a long-term relationship with Bob, as the weeks passed, April's mood got worse and she had to see a doctor for her IBS. Several of her close friends didn't like Bob, and April passed it off as jealousy. But her right brain's mood and body language were drawing a very different picture from her left brain's. April's depression had gotten so bad that she had to resume taking Zoloft, which she had stopped after she left home to get away from all those arguments with her mother. Her digestive tract had gotten so bad, she couldn't tolerate many foods she had enjoyed for years.

Soon after Bob moved into her dorm room, April saw the similarities between her boyfriend and her mother. Bob began to insist on more and more of her attention. His demanding personality was identical to her mother's. He was judgmental, needed to have absolute control, and was never satisfied. Even though April's right brain had generated mood and health problems immediately during her first date with Bob to warn her of the lethal similarities between this potential boyfriend and her mother, it took six months for her left brain to add up all the warning signs logically to come to the same conclusion: Bob was bad news.

April ditched Bob and went into therapy to try to understand why she was attracted to a man so similar to her mother. She soon learned that her moodiness, depression, and irritable bowel syndrome could warn her when she was about to fall into this relationship trap. As April worked with a counselor, within a year she was able to stop taking the Zoloft and other medicines. Now, whenever her mood starts to dip, or her stomach starts to tighten, April checks in with her intuitive guidance system to find out who or what in her environment is silencing her voice or limiting her freedom.

How do you capture the intuitive genius behind your moods and at the same time minimize the emotional and physical pain that can result when they become unbalanced?

Brains Are Like Bras

There are as many ways to support your mood as there are types of bras. In a lingerie department, you can find all sizes, degrees of support, types of material, amounts of coverage. There are bras with single, double, or crossed straps, with or without underwire, and with "push-up" pads ("miracle" capability). The type of bra you need will vary depending on your age, size, or reproductive event, just as, during your monthly cycle, sometimes you'll need more support and other times less. During postpartum and perimenopausal times, your clothing needs change. At times of stress in your life you may put on or lose weight, and your emotional needs change. And, depending on whether you are on your feet in a stressful job, wearing evening wear, or relaxing, playing tennis, or jogging, the degree of support you need is different. You may need only mood support during critical hormonal events in your life, or a "mood splint" during times when life is bearing down on you—when you're in a bad marriage, a difficult job, taking care of someone who is sick or dying, or you yourself are physically ill.

The same holds for treating your moodiness. No two women have the same brain, and as a result, they need different kinds of support. The symptoms you get when you're depressed or moody will depend on how your brain assigns its duties between your left and right halves (see Chapter 1). As a result, the solutions that will help you manage your moods will be determined by whether your depression and irritability are expressed primarily as left-brain thoughts, right-brain feelings, body health reactions, or a combination of all three.

Factors That Determine If You Need Mood Treatments

> - Family history of mood problems
> - History of trauma: physical, sexual, emotional
> - Moods change depending on the season, length of daylight
> - Moods change with hormonal cycles
>   - Menstrual cycle
>   - Pregnancy/postpartum
>   - Perimenopause/menopause
> - Moods change with marriage, job, and financial stress
> - Moods change with a chronic illness, exacerbations/remissions
> - Moods that are intuitively keyed into mental/physical health of a loved one or some important person in your environment

The treatment you choose to support your feminine brain's mood circuits depends on other brain/body challenges. You need to take into consideration problems with attention, memory, sleep, fatigue, immune disorders, problems with pain, and digestive complaints. Many times, you can choose one supplement or medicine that treats all of your symptoms and has the welcome side effect of improving your other health problems.

Consider whether you have the following challenges:

- *Cognitive* problems such as attentional/memory problems
- Other *emotional* symptoms like fear, anxiety, and panic attacks (see also Chapters 6 and 7)
- Compensatory strategies you have adopted to cover up or "medicate" your moods including *eating disorders* like anorexia, bulimia, obesity, and *addictions* like alcohol, drugs, and gambling
- *Health reactions* that are keyed in to your mood problems
    Sleep problems: excessive sleepiness (hypersomnia) or trouble falling asleep (insomnia)
    Fatigue
    Restlessness
    Digestive concerns: constipation, diarrhea, nausea
    Sexual problems: low desire, impotence, anorgasmia
    Heart/blood vessel problems: arrhythmias, palpitations, high or low blood pressure
    Personal history/family history of cancer

Immune system challenges: HIV, hepatitis, chronic fa-
tigue/fibromyalgia, environmental illness/multiple chemical sensitivity, lupus, etc. Drug allergies or sensitivity to
stimulants

Dietary concerns/philosophies: macrobiotic, vegan, etc.

By now, from your work in Chapter 4, you know your own mood symptoms. You know when your thoughts, behavior, or health indicate that your brain's emotional circuits are firing overtime. You also know the triggers in your life and environment for mood problems. And, you have targeted other characteristics in your brain and body (see list above) that you need to take into consideration when supporting your mood.

Keep in mind that many medicines and herbal, nutritional, and hormonal supplements are only "mood splints." Many of these and other treatments (including light therapy, meditation, exercise, diet, or other similar modalities) can only hold your mood where it is or improve it for a short time—a year or two or even less. Ultimately, your brain will compensate, mold itself around the treatment you have chosen, and your moodiness, depression, and irritability will return—*unless* you balance all four sides of your feminine brain's mood circuit. You need to change your *thought* patterns, *actions and behavior,* and *health reactions* in addition to your *mood*—or your brain and body will fall back into their old painful pattern. If you don't attend to all four facets of your feminine brain, many treatments may not work at all. Whether you just "scotch tape your mood together" with medicine, herbs, or supplements, or "entrain" your neurochemistry into a healthier electromagnetic pattern with acupuncture, meditation, visualization, imagery, or exercise, you still need to figure out what your intuition is telling you is out of balance in your life. If you don't, no matter what treatment you pursue, your mood problems will persist, worsen over time, and recur.

Medicinal Mood Splints

Since 1987 (when I first entered medical school), 10 to 30 million people have been prescribed selective serotonin reuptake inhibitors (SSRIs). Some of us doctors wonder what these medicines are really treating, since they're used to treat so many different emotional and sometimes spiritual problems. By improving serotonin activity in the brain and body, medicines like Prozac (fluoxetine), Zoloft (sertraline), and Celexa (citalopram) are frequently used to improve *mood,* but they also affect *thought* patterns, *actions,* and *body health* reactions associated with depression and anger:

a. **Mood:** Depression, premenstrual syndrome, postpartum and perimenopausal depression, seasonal affective disorder, irritability, impatience

b. **Thought patterns:** Pessimism, lack of initiative, lack of motivation, problems with organization and planning, suicidal thoughts (although one side effect of SSRI that has been reported is suicidal behavior; see below)

c. **Actions:** Bulimia/compulsive eating, self-injurious behavior (cutting, self-mutilation), inactivity/hyperactivity, impulsivity, aggressive abusive behavior

d. **Body health reactions:** Obesity, carbohydrate craving, headache, insomnia, alcoholism, chronic pain, fibromyalgia/chronic fatigue, chronic immune system dysfunction

e. **Cognitive/learning problems:** Inattention/distractibility, ADHD/ADD

SSRIs like Prozac have been used to treat all types of depression, including major depression, dysthymia, and bipolar II. They also help mood problems associated with medical problems, including drug abuse (alcohol, sleeping pills, cocaine, and other stimulants), hormonal imbalances (thyroid disorders, PMS, postpartum depression, perimenopausal depression, and others), neurologic disorders (stroke, epilepsy, and dementias), and chronic viral syndrome (chronic fatigue/fibromyalgia, mononucleosis, and others). Prozac and other SSRIs also treat a variety of obsessional or anxiety disorders (see Chapter 7), including obsessive-compulsive disorder (OCD), panic disorder, posttraumatic stress disorder (PTSD), and social phobia. Finally, SSRIs have been used to treat impulsive and compulsive behaviors, including bulimia and anorexia nervosa, with mixed results.

PROZAC, THE PSYCHIATRIC PANACEA

When I was a medical intern, the following scenario occurred frequently. A sweet old lady, let's call her Mrs. Smith, would be brought to the hospital ER from her apartment or a nursing home. She had been found by a neighbor or health care assistant, either mildly confused or weak. In the ER, all tests were normal—vital signs, physical examination, the chest X-ray, and EKG.

No one could figure out why Mrs. Smith was weak, but she wasn't well enough to send home or sick enough to get a diagnosis. Frequently, we would reexamine the chest X-ray and discern some "vague shadow," which *could* be pneumonia . . . maybe. So Mrs. Smith would become a "twenty-four-hour admit," be sent to the medical floor, and given what was at that time the cure-all, the intravenous antibiotic Zinacef, affectionately called "Vitamin Z." In the morning, Mrs. Smith would seem much brighter and the order would be written to discharge her.

No one really knows what's wrong with patients like Mrs. Smith. There was no true shadow on the X-ray, no positive culture indicative of pneumonia, and no fever or elevated white blood cell count, typical signs of infection. It might have been better medicine just to admit the patient and passively observe her to see if she got better on her own, but if Mrs. Smith wasn't "actively treated" the hospital wouldn't be reimbursed and would have to eat the bill. At that time, Zinacef was used to treat a lot of people like Mrs. Smith who were weak or "not right." It would somehow "work," and make her stronger, but no one knew why.

Today, Prozac, Celexa, and other SSRIs have become similar panaceas in psychiatry. These drugs were originally thought to take several weeks to create a "therapeutic benefit," but people who are sad, melancholy, tired, irritable, impulsive, compulsive, or in pain often see some improvement in their symptoms within days, at least temporarily.

As you can see in the Antidepressant Primer for SSRIs (below), there are five basic medications: Prozac, Zoloft, Paxil, Celexa, and Luvox. Their immediate effect is to prevent serotonin from being "chewed up" (metabolized) in the brain and body, so this neurotransmitter is able to hang around longer and positively affect mood, depression, and other emotional and mental disorders (see "Uses" in the table).

Over time (four to six weeks), SSRIs true effects kick in. The receptors on the brain and body cells adapt to the extra amount of serotonin and somehow realign to produce a more elevated mood. The importation of serotonin into your brain releases an "internal brake" that keeps mood down in the dumps. Once your brain's mood brake is disengaged, your own brain cells can release more serotonin, thus elevating your mood.

Even though Prozac and its SSRI cousins hit all kinds of serotonin receptors in the brain and brain stem, these medicines aren't specific for just mood. As you can see in Figure 10 ("Serotonin Is Not Just for Mood,") they affect serotonin all over the body. In fact, 98 percent of the serotonin you have actually travels in the body; only 1 or 2 percent is in the brain. So when you take an SSRI (or an herbal nutritional supplement that affects serotonin receptors), it's not going just to your brain, it's also going to affect many organ systems in the body for better or worse, with side effects (see table).

Antidepressant Primer I: SSRIs

Medication	Generic Name	Uses	Advantage (neurotransmitter affected)	Side Effects	Dose Range (per day)
Prozac	Fluoxetine	• Major depression • Atypical depression (rejection sensitivity, excessive daytime sleepiness, fatigue, carbohydrate craving) • Bulimia • Obsessive-compulsive disorder	• Sometimes stimulating weight loss (serotonin)	• Nausea • Agitation, restlessness • Insomnia • Daytime sedation • Sexual dysfunction • Can precipitate mania • Increased amount of side effects of other meds • Suicidal behavior	20–80 mg
Zoloft	Sertraline	• Major depression • Atypical depression • Dysthymia • Panic disorder • Obsessive-compulsive disorder	• Less stimulating • Less drug-drug interaction (serotonin)	• More GI side effects than other SSRIs (nausea, diarrhea, esophageal reflux) • Agitation • Sexual dysfunction • Can precipitate mania • Decreased side effects with other meds • More constipating than other SSRIs	50–200 mg
Paxil	Paroxetine	• (Similar to Prozac) • Major depression • Atypical depression • Bulimia • Obsessive-compulsive disorder • Panic disorder • Social anxiety disorder	• Somewhat more sedating (serotonin)	• Insomnia • Sleepiness • Nausea • Fatigue • Tremors • Sexual dysfunction • Secreted in milk	10–30 mg
Celexa	Citalopram	• Major depression • Dysthymia • Obsessive-compulsive disorder • Panic disorder	• Less drug-drug interaction (serotonin)	• Similar side-effects profile as other SSRIs (above) • Fewer med-drug interactions	20–60 mg
Luvox	Fluvoxamine	• Major depression • Obsessive-compulsive disorder	• Decreases ruminating obsessive thoughts (serotonin)	• More nausea, vomiting than other SSRIs • Headache • Insomnia • Sedation • Sexual dysfunction (Antianxiety meds can cause further side effects if taken with Luvox.)	50–250 mg

The list of side effects of these drugs can make you dizzy and feel sick from just reading them. How do you and your doctor or other practitioner decide what antidepressant is good for you and will work best for your body?

Look at the body areas in the diagram: If you have problems with your immune system, heart, digestive tract, reproductive system/libido, or neurological system (i.e., pain), SSRIs can make those problem worse.

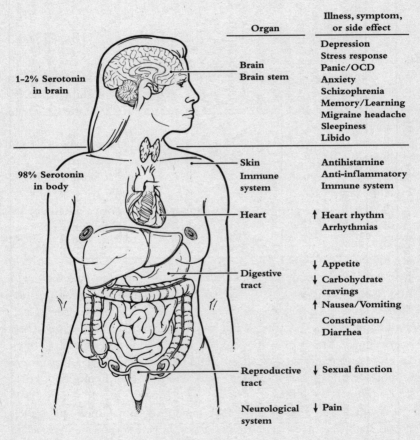

Figure 10. Serotonin is not just for mood. Many body areas are influenced by SSRIs and other serotonin compounds.

SSRIs Hit the GI Tract

Nearly every SSRI has an effect on your gastrointestinal tract, increasing your chances of having decreased appetite and nausea, and changing your bowel function. Your entire digestive tract, from esophagus to rectum, has serotonin receptors in it. So, if you also have an eating disorder or are over-weight, an SSRI may decrease your appetite and at least temporarily lower your weight. But if you have some digestive problems, including nausea, abdominal bloating, distension, gastroesophageal reflux disease (GERD), ir-ritable bowel syndrome, inflammatory bowel syndrome, or low appetite, SSRIs in general may be not good for you. The side effects may outweigh the benefits.

What's the Difference Between Prozac, Zoloft, and Other SSRIs?

For decades, neuroscientists have debated whether Prozac, Zoloft, Paxil, and Celexa are nearly the same drug made by different companies, or are really slightly different adaptations of a general, prototypical medicine. Es-sentially, SSRIs are like colas. Some people swear they can taste the differ-ence between Coke and Pepsi; others really can't tell.

To me, colas are the same. I can't taste the difference. My brain and body receptors for cola are broad and nonspecific, nondiscerning. Other people are more sensitive to the difference. Some say that Pepsi is more car-bonated, more gassy than Coke.

The same applies to SSRIs. Many people can't sense a difference be-tween these medicines, while others can pick up subtle features from one SSRI to another. Some are more activated, more stimulating, while others are more sedating (see "Advantage" column in chart I, p. 149). This can help you. If you are depressed, with fatigue and excessive daytime sleepi-ness, Prozac may be preferable for you, since it's activating and stimulating. Paxil is more sedating and could lessen your energy. On the other hand, if your depression is aggravated by irritability, nervousness, and a type of pan-icky edginess, Prozac may put you over the edge, and Zoloft or Paxil might be more calming. If your depression and nervousness are accompanied by an obsessionality, a compulsivity (gerbil wheel in your brain), then Luvox or Zoloft may be better.

If you are on a lot of medicines, including cardiac meds, painkillers, mood stabilizer meds, certain antibiotics, hormone replacement, or ta-moxifen, an SSRI can counteract these drugs' effects, making their levels dangerously higher or lower. You always have to take this into considera-tion. The SSRI Celexa has the benefit of having fewer interactions with other drugs.

But these generalizations aren't always true. Some women's brains are unusual and have an "idiosyncratic" or opposite-than-expected reaction.

Just as the stimulant Ritalin calms down people who have hyperactivity and ADHD, some people who take activity-enhancing Prozac have an unexpected side effect of sleepiness.

Gender may affect whether or not an antidepressant works or creates excessive side effects, in part due to hormonal differences. Zoloft seems to be overall more favorable for alleviating women's depression, including PMS and perimenopause-related depression. In contrast, the older, less selective antidepressant imipramine seems to have a more favorable effect in men.

Menopause may have something to do with antidepressants' effectiveness. Some SSRIs may be more appropriate than others, depending upon the woman's irritability or other mental state. This area of psychiatry is very controversial.

DANCING THE SSRI SHUFFLE: ONE DRUG STOPS WORKING, SO YOU SWITCH TO ANOTHER

One thing I noticed as a psych resident was that frequently people would be started on Prozac, Zoloft, or some other SSRI and it wouldn't work. Sure, 50 percent of the people who took it got better, but 50 percent wouldn't respond. And even if patients got better, the effect wouldn't last. About one or two years later, they would slowly slip back to where they were before, down in the dumps, with disordered eating and sleeping, not wanting to spend time with friends, unable to work. Even today, it really doesn't matter what type of antidepressant is used: Studies show that approximately 30 percent of patients will fully recover with an adequate dose of any antidepressant if it's used for at least six weeks. Ten to 15 percent will show no improvement, while the remaining 35 to 40 percent show partial improvement. Neuroscientists argue over why these meds stop working. Studies suggest that between 20 and 75 percent of the initial positive response may not be due to the rebalancing of serotonin levels in the brain's mood circuits. Scientists now believe that as much as 75 percent of the initial drug response is due to the placebo effect; that is, you could give the patient a "sugar pill" and get nearly the same result. Yet placebo effect isn't an imaginary improvement. When a patient develops a supportive relationship with a doctor or practitioner, the bond and expectation of a positive outcome releases opiates in the brain that can alter mood circuits, relieving depression (see "Different Strokes for Different Folks," page 181).

After two years of faithfully taking a drug, however, more often than not, the patient's depression begins to return and she is switched to another SSRI—very likely one that is brand new and has been brought to the hospital by a drug rep.

I can tell you I have no real faith in any of these pills for long-term treatment. If someone is mildly or moderately depressed, they work temporarily to splint the patient's mood, move the brain circuits into position, and give the patient energy, focus, and the capacity to tolerate being in a room with a psychotherapist—to change what's wrong with their life—which seems to have a more enduring effect than any SSRI. If a patient chooses not to engage in therapy, and doesn't change what is aggravating her mood, no SSRI will prevent the depression's return. SSRIs can't scotch-tape a woman's mood together for long if she is in an abusive relationship and doesn't do a "relationship-ectomy" or if she's spending forty hours a week in an irritating job that doesn't use her talents and skills.

Nonetheless, over the course of a decade or so, women may go through four or five medicines, called "dancing the SSRI shuffle." Sometimes when one SSRI stops working, another medicine is added on top of it—not substituted for it. After a short while, the patient feels better, but without other lifestyle changes, in a year or two, the depression returns yet again to be followed by other med additions. The med list can get longer and longer until it is very difficult to figure out which medicine is working and which is not.

Doctors, patients, nurses, psychologists, and psychotherapists—everyone does try to help women "fix" their depression and mood disorders. Unfortunately, few can honestly say that SSRIs are truly a permanent panacea for many people. A lucky few can stay on one of these medicines for more than a decade with continued successful mood support. Most women, however, will need to pursue other options sooner or later.

Newer, More Expensive Drugs or Older Cheaper Antidepressants?

Other atypical antidepressants are available when standard SSRIs don't work. (See Antidepressant Primer: Atypical Antidepressants below.) Atypical Antidepressants have a different structure from SSRIs and may function by hitting more neurotransmitters than just serotonin. Effexor (venlafaxine) may be more stimulating since it affects norepinephrine levels as well as serotonin, so it may also help women with attention deficit disorder and depression (see Chapter 9). However, in women with agitated or irritable depression, Effexor may be too stimulating.

Antidepressant Primer II: Atypical Antidepressants

Medication	Generic Name	Uses	Advantage (neurotransmitter affected)	Side Effects	Dose Range (per day)
Wellbutrin	Bupropion Zyban	• Depression • Dysthymia • Atypical depression (potentially useful) • Bipolar depression • ADHD • Can treat sexual dysfunction caused by SSRIs • May enhance libido • Rapidly cycling bipolar II • Smoking cessation	• Stimulating • Safest with heart disease • Fewer sexual side effects • Lacks significant drug interaction • Lower risk of precipitating mania than other meds • Appetite suppressant (norepinephrine and dopamine)	• Agitation • Restlessness • Insomnia • Seizures in some patients • Not appropriate in anorexia nervosa or bulimia • Headache • Constipation • Nausea • Dry mouth	100–300 mg
Effexor	Venlafaxine	• Depression • Dysthymia • Generalized anxiety disorder • ADHD • Chronic pain	• Useful with depression and ADHD • Useful in chronic pain (serotonin and norepinephrine)	• Anxiety or nervousness • Side effects similar to other SSRIs • Sedation • Dizziness • Constipation • Sweating • Increased blood pressure • Nausea • Fatigue • Loss of appetite	75–375 mg
Trazodone	Desyrel	• Insomnia • In dementia: decreases anxiety, agitation, aggression • Chronic pain	• Good for SSRI-induced insomnia (serotonin)	• Sedation • Low blood pressure • Weight gain • Dry mouth • Avoid in history of heart attack	50–600 mg

Older but very potent antidepressants called *tricyclic antidepressants* (see Antidepressant Primer III) can be effective in treating depression, but have a lot of side effects. Imipramine, desipramine, amitriptyline, and nortriptyline, all "tricyclics," can be sedating, constipating, and affect heart rhythm and blood pressure. As a result of their frequently dangerous side effects (especially at high dosage and overdoses), they aren't used as commonly today. But tricyclics can be very helpful with chronic pain syndromes including migraine headaches and lower back pain.

Nardil (phenelzine) and Parnate (tranylcypromine), called *MAO inhibitors,* may be an excellent, underutilized medicine for women with atypical depression, excessive daytime sleepiness, and obsessive eating. However, they require a very special, restrictive diet that makes many doctors shy away from prescribing them. For some women, an MAO inhibitor may be the only drug that makes a dent in their very hard to treat type of depression.

Antidepressant Add-ons

The other two antidepressants aren't new, but they're more controversial. Trazodone (Desyrel) can be added to another SSRI (like Prozac) as a type of sleeping pill, if these medicines help your depression but are so activating they make it hard for you to fall asleep at night. Wellbutrin (a.k.a. bupropion, Zyban) is now undergoing a revival in use for depression, but there is doubt whether this drug is truly a potent antidepressant when used alone, so it is frequently an "add-on" to Prozac, Zoloft, or another SSRI, since it has a somewhat weaker antidepressant effect and because some believe it counteracts sexual side effects of impotence and anorgasmia. When I was in medical school, psychiatrists often called Wellbutrin a drug "looking for a use." When it was used alone, we usually saw no effect, and for a while it fell out of favor. Maybe the drug company increased their marketing budget, because in the late 1990s, all of a sudden Wellbutrin was marketed under a new name (Zyban) and used to help people stop smoking. It is now used to treat simple depression.

Other Ways to Supplement Brain and Body Neurotransmitters

By discussing your daily medicine and nutritional supplement intake with your doctor, you can decide what is best for you. Every year, people get sick and in rare instances die of complications from the most common over-the-counter medicines, such as aspirin or Tylenol, or from prescribed

Antidepressant Primer III: Older But Very Potent Antidepressants

Medication	Generic Name	Uses	Advantage (neurotransmitter affected)	Side Effects	Dose Range (per day)
Tofranil	Imipramine	• Depression and insomnia • Chronic pain: headache, backache, etc. • Dysthymia • Anxiety disorders	• Lower cost • Better studied of all antidepressants • Also helpful for panic disorder (Tricyclic: serotonin, norepinephrine, dopamine)	• Moderately sedating • High tendency for lowered blood pressure • Moderate incidence of anticholinergic side effects: dry mouth, blurred vision, constipation, urinary retention, heat intolerance, increased heart rate, aggravate glaucoma	150–300 mg
Norpramin	Desipramine	• Depression • Chronic pain (as above) • Dysthymia • Anxiety disorders	• Less sedating • Less constipating (Tricyclic: serotonin, norepinephrine, dopamine)	• Lower incidence of sedation • High tendency to lower blood pressure • Lower incidence of anticholinergic side effects: dry mouth, blurred vision, constipation, urinary retention, heat intolerance, increased heart rate, aggravate glaucoma	150–300 mg
Elavil	Amitriptyline	• Depression and insomnia • Chronic pain (as above) • Dysthymia • Anxiety disorders	• Used in very low dosages for pain syndromes, esp. migraine headaches (Tricyclic: serotonin, norepinephrine, dopamine)	• Highly sedating • High tendency to lower blood pressure • High anticholinergic side effects: dry mouth, blurred vision, constipation, urinary retention, heat intolerance, increased heart rate, aggravate glaucoma	150–300 mg
Pamelor	Nortriptyline	• Depression • Chronic pain (as above) • Dysthymia • Anxiety disorders	• Less sedating • Less constipating • Fewer side effects than other tricyclic antidepressants • Good for older people (Tricyclic: serotonin, norepinephrine, dopamine)	• Lower incidence of sedation • Lowest tendency to decrease blood pressure • Low incidence of anticholinergic side effects: dry mouth, blurred vision, constipation, urinary retention, heat intolerance, increased heart rate, aggravate glaucoma	75–150 mg

Sinequan	Doxepin	• Depression and insomnia • Chronic pain (as above) • Dysthymia • Anxiety disorders	• Very sedating as treatment for insomnia • Anti-itch, for rashes, skin syndromes (Tricyclic: serotonin, norepinephrine, dopamine)	• Highly sedating • Moderate tendency to lower blood pressure • High incidence of anticholinergic side effects: dry mouth, blurred vision, constipation, urinary retention, heat intolerance, increased heart rate, aggravate glaucoma	150–300 mg
Nardil	Phenelzine	• Depression (when other drugs fail) • Panic disorder • Atypical depression • Anxiety disorders • OCD (obsessive-compulsive disorder)	• Very useful when other antidepressants fail • Atypical depression	• Dietary restrictions due to hypertensive crisis: avoid certain meats, pickled fish, vegetables, overripe fruits, wines, beers, chocolate, coffee, stimulants, allergy meds • Weight gain	15–60 mg
Parnate	Tranyl-cypromine	• Depression (when other drugs fail) • Panic disorder • Atypical depression • Anxiety disorders • OCD (obsessive-compulsive disorder)		• Drowsiness • Dry mouth • Sexual side effects • Insomnia	10–60 mg

antibiotics. In 1997, there were 8,986 reported adverse side effects from herbal preparations in Europe, but there were 2 million adverse side effects from prescription medicines that same year. You always have to balance the risks and benefits of everything you put in your mouth. Constant paranoia isn't good for your mood or the rest of your health, but neither is flying-by-the-seat-of-your-pants, uneducated, uninformed consumption of either medicines or nutritional supplements.

St. John's Wort

A relatively new treatment for depression in the United States, St. John's wort (0.3% standardized content hypericum perforatum) (300–600 mg 3x/day) has been used popularly in Europe for decades. In fact, more than 20 million people in Germany use St. John's wort regularly for mild to moderate depression (see table). St. John's wort works by many of the same mechanisms that make Prozac, Zoloft, and other SSRIs effective against mood disorders—it changes the serotonin receptors in the brain, making the brain more sensitive to the serotonin that's present. Higher doses of St. John's wort make the serotonin and other neurotransmitters that you do have hang out longer and not get metabolized. Sometimes, at higher dose levels, St. John's wort can be as effective as the tricyclic antidepressant imipramine.

St. John's Wort *(Hypericum perforatum)*

Uses	Side Effects	Drug Interactions and Drawbacks
Depression	Insomnia	Beware taking St. John's wort with gingko biloba
Dysthymia	Jitteriness	or other "blood thinners"
Anxiety	Digestive upset	Discontinue St. John's wort before surgery: may
Obsessive/compulsive	Sexual	increase bleeding
disorder	dysfunction	May be toxic with MAO antidepressants when
Menopausal mood	Dizziness	combined with stimulants
disorder	Mania in	Possible toxicity with other SSRI antidepressants
Pain disorders:	bipolar disorder	Increases photosensitivity effect of other drugs:
Migraine headaches		tetracycline, sulfa, or thiazides
Neuralgia		Lowers effectiveness of oral contraceptives; may
Sciatica		cause breakthrough bleeding
Muscle pain		Lowers effectiveness of HIV medicine Crixivan
		(indinavir)
		Lowers effectiveness of antibiotic cyclosporine
		Increases blood levels of Digoxin heart medicine,
		which may cause toxicity

Just because St. John's wort is an herbal supplement doesn't mean that it won't have side effects or interactions with other drugs such as pharmaceutically derived antidepressants. If you take St. John's wort with another SSRI like Prozac, you may experience a set of side effects called "serotonin syndrome," which include nausea, confusion, an elevated body temperature, unstable blood pressure and heart rate, tremor, stiff muscles, and in some extreme cases, seizures, coma, or death. Although this adverse effect has only been reported with Serzone, Paxil, and Zoloft, it theoretically can occur with all antidepressants that influence serotonin metabolism. Please consult with a psychiatrist before combining St. John's wort with other medications.

St. John's wort can alter the blood levels of other medicines you may be on, thus possibly making the other medical condition you have unstable. Specifically, St. John's wort or any other herb or drug can interfere with heart medicines, HIV drugs, antibiotics, and other medicines. Do not take St. John's wort with "the Pill": Oral contraceptives may disrupt "hormonal metabolism" and cause breakthrough bleeding. Women using St. John's wort should use another form of contraception. Always take supplements and medicines under the guidance of a physician or other licensed practitioner who can look at all the nutritional supplements/medicines you take.

Tryptophan

Serotonin is synthesized from the amino acid tryptophan (see Figure 11). Blood plasma tryptophan levels are found to be significantly lower in people who are depressed; in countries where suicide rates are high, tryptophan intake is low. So it makes sense that either altering dietary tryptophan intake or taking tryptophan supplementation might treat depression. In fact, it's possible to influence brain serotonin mood circuit function by altering dietary tryptophan, although this process may not be the most efficient way (calorie for calorie) of building up brain serotonin. Good sources of tryptophan are milk, cottage cheese, turkey and chicken, eggs, red meat, soybeans, tofu, nuts, and almonds.

A high-carbohydrate diet contains higher levels of tryptophan but fewer of the other amino acids. As a result, when you carbo-load (pasta, bread, rice, or sweets), tryptophan moves into your brain faster and more serotonin can be produced, elevating your mood. Because you're eating more calories, however, as you get more serotonin into your brain, you're also more likely to get more fat on your hips.

Taking six grams of tryptophan alone, or in combination with other antidepressants, treats depression, seasonal affective disorder, and premenstrual syndrome/premenstrual dysphoric disorder. However, because a number of people who took L-tryptophan in the late 1980s developed muscle and joint pain, fever, and weakness, and were diagnosed as having Eosinophilia-myalgia syndrome, the FDA outlawed over-the-counter L-tryptophan. There were 1,500 cases and fifty deaths. Scientists later found out that it wasn't the L-tryptophan itself that was making people sick, but a contaminant in two batches made by one Japanese company. Improvements were made in the production of L-tryptophan, but it's still only available by prescription from a formulary pharmacy.

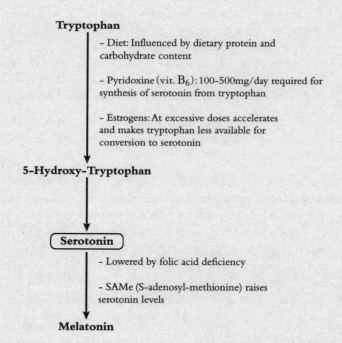

Tryptophan

- Diet: Influenced by dietary protein and carbohydrate content

- Pyridoxine (vit. B_6): 100–500mg/day required for synthesis of serotonin from tryptophan

- Estrogens: At excessive doses accelerates and makes tryptophan less available for conversion to serotonin

5-Hydroxy-Tryptophan

Serotonin

- Lowered by folic acid deficiency

- SAMe (S-adenosyl-methionine) raises serotonin levels

Melatonin

Figure 11. Diet-Serotonin Link: Tryptophan from a variety of sources influences mood by increasing the production of serotonin.

5-HTP

Tryptophan is converted to serotonin via an intermediary molecule called 5-HTP. Some sources say that in comparison to tryptophan, 5-HTP may be more readily taken into the brain to make serotonin, because it's more fat soluble. 5-HTP also raises levels of other neurotransmitters critical for mood function, including dopamine and norepinephrine. 5-HTP is rapidly taken up by serotonin-producing cells in the brain.

5-HTP at dosages of 50–100 milligrams, three times a day, has been shown to help patients with major depression and patients in the depressed phase of bipolar disorder. Few, if any, side effects were reported. Many patients improved within five to fourteen days, which means that 5-HTP can work faster than other types of antidepressants. 5-HTP worked as well as tricyclic antidepressants but caused fewer side effects; some people only experienced a little nausea. 5-HTP has helped some depressed patients for whom no other therapy or medicine had worked, including electroconvulsive therapy. 5-HTP is also effective in treating obesity, because it decreases appetite, and bulimia, because it reduces carbohydrate cravings. 5-HTP has also been helpful combined with other therapies for insomnia, headaches, fibromyalgia, and PMS, and may help depressed people who also have ADD or anxiety.

As with all herbs and supplements, consult a doctor before taking 5-HTP with other serotonin antidepressant medicines (including SSRIs), or with other drugs, because drug interactions may occur.

Gingko Biloba

Gingko biloba (240 mg/day) is an herbal supplement that increases serotonin levels in frontal lobe areas and hippocampal brain areas that are central to mood, depression, and memory. More commonly used for attention and memory, it may also interrupt the domino effect that depression has on the brain and the body by blocking the elevation of cortisol, a key component of this inflammation cascade.

Gingko biloba may help with depression that can occur with anxiety and attention deficit disorder. It may also help with the sexual side effects from other antidepressants. Gingko biloba has a similar mechanism to Viagra—it relaxes arteries in sex organs. In fact, gingko biloba may be more helpful for sex disorders in general, especially for women. Women who took this supplement noticed improvement in all four phases of the sex cycle—improving sexual desire, excitement, orgasm, and resolution—by increasing blood flow to the vagina and clitoris. Gingko biloba has been used for decades to treat Alzheimer's disease and cerebrovascular disease, for which depressed people have an increased risk.

Side effects include nausea, headaches, and occasional skin rashes. Because gingko biloba prevents blood platelets from clumping, it may promote bleeding and should not be taken with other blood thinners such as St. John's wort, heparin, Coumadin, and aspirin. You have to be especially careful about taking combinations of blood thinner medicines and herbal nutritional supplements before surgery. Studies suggest that all blood thinners should be stopped two to three weeks before any scheduled surgery to prevent excessive bleeding and complications with anesthesia.

Blood Thinners (anticoagulants and antiplatelet substances) —not a complete list—		
American ginseng	Garlic	Papain
Aspirin	Ginger	St. John's wort
Bromolin	Gingko biloba	Siberian ginseng
Danshen	Goldenseal	Stinging nettle
Dong quai	Guar gum	Vitamin C
European mistletoe	Heparin	Vitamin E
Fenugreek	Horse chestnut seed	Vitamin K
Feverfew	Omega-3 fatty acids/fish oil	Warfarin
Gammalinolenic acid	Panax ginseng	

Source: Therapeutic Research Facility (2000). *Natural Medicines Comprehensive Database.* Stockton, CA: Therapeutic Research Facility, p. 1427.

SIBERIAN GINSENG

Siberian ginseng (625 mg 2x/day) may have antidepressant activities, since it changes the metabolism of neurotransmitters that are important for initiation, motivation, and mood, notably dopamine, norepinephrine, and serotonin. This type of ginseng may make the brain more resilient to stress-induced, environmentally reactive depression and moodiness by buffering the brain against drops in serotonin. Siberian ginseng can also lower your risk for illnesses related to the brain's sadness and anger circuits. It normalizes high and low blood pressure, lowers cholesterol, improves atherosclerosis, chronic fatigue syndrome, fibromyalgia, and other chronic immune system disorders. Siberian ginseng stimulates the immune system, increases natural killer cell activity (an important defense against cancer), and makes other white cells act more effectively to neutralize bacteria and viruses.

Like gingko biloba, Siberian ginseng increases nitric oxide synthesis, which relaxes arteries, so it may also improve sexual dysfunction in depression or counteract the sexual side effects of taking other antidepressants. Ginseng also inhibits stress-induced elevation of cortisol, which may in part help block the adverse domino effect that stress-induced depression has on the brain and the body.

Often used to support learning and memory and help depressed people who have difficulty paying attention and remembering what they have learned (see Chapter 10), Siberian ginseng can help improve your mood with little risk of side effects. Since it has mild stimulating qualities, it can cause insomnia, a change in heart rhythm, and a rise in blood pressure in some susceptible individuals, but in others it causes the opposite side effects—sleepiness, melancholy, and anxiety. If you are taking other sedative or stimulant medicines or supplements, ginseng may augment the stimulating effect, so if you choose to try Siberian ginseng, start at one quarter of the usual dose (see above) and do so in close consultation with a physician.

Siberian ginseng may also "thin" the blood by preventing platelets from aggregating to form a clot, so you should avoid taking it with other blood thinners.

SAMe

SAMe (S-adenosyl-methionine; 800–1600 mg/day) improves brain levels of neurotransmitters that are critical for maintaining a healthy mood. It has been used by millions in Europe for depression and arthritis. Seventy-five clinical trials involving over 23,000 people have shown its usefulness. A critical enzyme that naturally occurs in your body, SAMe helps make neurotransmitters serotonin, dopamine, and norepinephrine, which are targeted by SSRIs such as Prozac and Zoloft, atypical antidepressants like Effexor, or more traditional antidepressants. SAMe also assists the nerve cell uptake of fats (called phospholipids), thus improving nerve transmission. Lower than normal levels of SAMe have been seen in the fluid surrounding the brains of patients with depression as well as Alzheimer's disease.

SAMe has been shown to decrease homocysteine levels, which are elevated in patients with depression and heart disease. It helps treat the pain and disability of fibromyalgia and chronic fatigue, and the emotional symptoms of sadness, despair, frustration, and grumpiness of major depression, dysthymia, and postpartum and menopausal depression. SAMe improves the associated behavioral symptoms of low initiation, motivation, lethargic movement, social withdrawal, and brooding. At appropriate dosages, it also treats many of the physical health problems associated with depression, including heart disease, Alzheimer's disease and other memory disorders, osteoarthritis, chronic fatigue, fibromyalgia, and other immune system disorders involving excessive inflammation. Because SAMe improves levels of serotonin, norepinephrine, and dopamine, which are important for attention and memory, it helps people with attention deficit disorder and learning and memory problems. So, like gingko biloba, if you have depression with inattentiveness and memory problems, SAMe may help you.

High doses of SAMe (800–1600 mg per day) are as effective as SSRIs like Prozac or tricyclic antidepressants like imipramine. The benefits of SAMe are that there are fewer side effects, especially no weight gain or sexual side effects that are common to other antidepressants. SAMe also works in half the time of most other antidepressants. The downside is that it is very expensive, and since it's an over-the-counter supplement, insurance companies will not pay for it, even though most prescription medicines cost more than SAMe.

When I've asked people about taking SAMe for their mood problems, they often tell me they tried it and it didn't do anything for them. When I ask what dose they took, they usually tell me it was only 50 to 200 milligrams a day, when they should have taken up to eight 200 milligram tablets a day (about $200 per month). Back in the 1980s and 1990s, in order to make the price more palatable to customers, manufacturers packaged SAMe in 50 milligram tablets, encouraging consumers to take three a day, even though that dosage did not match the published scientific studies suggesting that dosages of 400 up to 1600 milligrams a day were needed to treat depression successfully. Put this cost in perspective, though: When you consider the long-term costs of depression to work, productivity, and health (with the eventual risk of osteoarthritis, heart disease, dementia, and other disorders), it may be worth it to figure out how to manage the price in your budget, either through buying it online, on the Web, or through discount stores.

Generally speaking, you start by taking a very low dose of SAMe (200 mg/day) for a week. The next week, you add a pill (400 mg/day), and so on, until you start to feel a little jittery (or until you reach a dosage of 1600 mg/day). You keep the dose *below* where you feel jittery. SAMe may be inactivated if taken with food or on a full stomach and you must take it at least thirty minutes prior to a meal.

People who are ill, older, or have problems with anxiety may need to take lower dosages. Side effects of SAMe are few, but include mild transient jitteriness, loose bowels, and headache. People with bipolar/manic depressive illness may get manic on SAMe as they might on any antidepressant.

Why You May Need Supplements

I was not a vitamin taker until recently, even though when I was a kid, a close relative claimed to have cured her back problem (scoliosis) with vitamin C and chiropractor visits twice a week for years. She insisted she would be in a wheelchair if it weren't for the vitamin C, and tried to push it on me. At that time, in the 1960s, health food stores and the people who frequented them were an odd, peculiar lot, to be avoided if one aspired to be a "normal" doctor and scientist.

Then, as fate would have it, at age twelve I developed scoliosis (a very severe 120 degree curve in my spine) that required surgery, a fusion, and a rod. Twenty years later, because my back had begun deteriorating at an alarming rate, it had to be broken and re-fused, with the addition of ten rods, four-inch nails, and metal baskets. As my spine was curving into a pretzel, my brain was doing the same, developing a narcolepsy-like seizure disorder that caused me to fall asleep in the middle of walking, running, and every imaginable activity. At age twenty-two, I was asleep seventeen hours a day. Eventually, doctors found a medicine that worked, woke me up, and helped me graduate from college. To my horror, however, the medicine did not agree with my body, and after medical school I developed a very rare side effect in which the medicine started to wipe out my bone marrow.

No other medicine could prevent these sleep attacks, so I had to resort to a variety of healing methods to get my health back on track. I got acupuncture and traditional Chinese herbs. A friend was studying for the Oregon State Board of Acupuncture licensing exam, so I reviewed and drilled her on the entire four-year curriculum. I learned a lot, and the multiple medical and psychiatric application of this form of medicine impressed me. I also worked with the emotional and thought patterns that aggravated my brain and spinal problems with a medical intuitive and psychotherapist.

In the 1990s, Dr. Christiane Northrup introduced me to vitamins, although I resisted them then as much as I had in the 1960s. She put me on vitamin C, calcium, and magnesium to help both my spine and my brain. For the first few days, I spent most of my time in the bathroom with diarrhea, so I stopped taking them. Chris then gave me intravenous pharmaceutical-grade vitamins and the results were amazing, but after a while, I got sick of having a needle put in my vein and decided to investigate alternate ways of getting vitamins into my system. I went to that dreaded health food store, where the dizzying "alphabet soup" on the vitamin bottle labels gave me vertigo.

After much research, I learned that the only vitamins I could tolerate were those with pharmaceutical-grade ingredients—the same grade that a pharmacist puts in an IV vitamin prep. I now take a little baggie of vitamins, Chinese herbs, and nutritional supplements daily, at breakfast, lunch, and dinner. If I leave the house without the baggie, I go back home and get it. I could never get from my diet what I have in that baggie: I'd have to eat enormous quantities of high-quality whole foods, and spend most of my day looking for that food. I'd feel like a locust or a caterpillar, and would probably be one hundred pounds heavier.

Are they expensive, all these vitamins, Chinese herbs, and nutritional supplements? Absolutely. However, falling asleep in heavy traffic or having a spinal injury is also expensive in more ways than I care to enumerate. If all these supplements didn't work, I wouldn't take them.

If you want to make the biggest, most cost-effective difference in your health, take a good multiple vitamin, with mineral supplementation. Call the manufacturer and ask if the raw ingredients come from pharmaceutical-grade vitamins and minerals. If they don't know what you're talking about, you probably need another brand.

D-PHENYLALANINE AND PHENYLETHYLAMINE (CHOCOLATE)

D-phenylalanine and phenylethylamine (100–400 mg/day) (PEA) are chemically related to mood neurotransmitters norepinephrine and dopamine. Chocolate contains high levels of PEA. Both neurotransmitters pump up the frontal and temporal lobe mood circuits for initiation, motivation, relationships, bonding, and empathy, as well as soothe sadness and anger areas. There is evidence that medicines and supplements like phenylalanine and PEA that affect dopamine activity are effective antidepressants. PEA and phenylalanine may also help some of the chronic health conditions that people with mood disorders develop. PEA and phenylalanine may enhance the pain-relieving effects of acupuncture on chronic lower back pain and other pain disorders.

It's a brave soul who stands between a woman and her chocolate. I have a gumball machine in my kitchen that dispenses peanut M&M's as my portion-control device for PEA-laden chocolate. I could graph how many pennies I put in the machine, and the line would go up the week before my period and down during the days after my period. Quite literally, I am medicating my premenstrual moodiness, irritability, and fatigue with the high levels of stimulant-like, pseudo-amphetamine properties of PEA in the peanut M&M's.

You can get the same or similar effect (without the calories or carbo-hydrate grams) by taking D-phenylalanine (100–400 mg/day) with vita-min B_6 (100 mg 2x/day), which the body converts to the mood neurotransmitters dopamine and norepinephrine. Phenylethylamine or D-phenylalanine and vitamin B_6 can have side effects, though, including transient mild headaches and nausea, constipation, insomnia, anxiety, ele-vated blood pressure, and in some unfortunate individuals, irritability and aggressiveness. For some, chocolate use can become excessive and lead to binges.

MULTIPLE VITAMINS AND MINERALS

B Vitamins		
	Vitamin B_1 (thiamine)	27 mg
	Vitamin B_2 (riboflavin)	27 mg
	Vitamin B_3 (niacin)	40 mg
	Vitamin B_6 (pyridoxine)	27–40 mg
	Vitamin B_{12}	60 mg
	Biotin	300 mg
	Pantothenic acid	90 mg
	Folic acid	1000 mg

To maintain stable levels of serotonin, you need adequate levels of the B vi-tamins listed here. Folic acid and vitamin B_{12} help convert 5HTP (above) to serotonin. Frequently, vitamins B_2, B_6, and B_{12} are low in depressed people.

Excessive estrogen levels (found in obesity and with taking oral con-traceptive pills) may promote depression by blocking vitamin B_6's role in serotonin synthesis. Women on "the Pill" have an increased risk of devel-oping not just depression, but also lowered libido, and vitamin B_6 relieves these symptoms. Low folic acid levels have also been associated with a poorer response to antidepressant treatment, including treatment with Prozac, Zoloft, or nortriptyline.

MINERALS

Low and high blood levels of calcium and magnesium are associated with depression (see p. 179). So taking a regular supplement of calcium citrate and magnesium is a good idea.

Mood Stabilizers and Anti-Kindling Agents

Most antidepressants elevate your mood, but don't prevent you from shifting from one mood to another, erratically "stripping the gears" in your brain's mood circuitry. Mood stabilizers help put out the long slow burn that depression causes to brain cells. These neuroprotective agents prevent the repetitive cycling of brain cells firing in and out of depression and so interrupt the inflammation domino effect that depression causes in the brain and the body.

MEDICATIONS

Medicines like lithium, Tegretol, and valproic acid all put out these brain-cell "brush fires." Specifically, lithium and valproic acid increase proteins that protect brain cells. Lithium can actually reverse brain shrinkage (or atrophy) in people with bipolar disorder. In addition, both antidepressants and mood stabilizers enhance brain cell *growth,* as may newer medicines like Neurontin, Lamictal, Topamax, and others. However, as you can see in the table Mood Stabilizer Primer, these medicines are "big guns." They have significant, possibly dangerous, side effects on many organ systems. If you can't figure out how to stabilize your mood by a number of other available routes, they can be used safely under very close regular supervision by a trained psychiatrist, who may have to monitor the drug's effects by regular blood tests. Depending on the medicine, you'll have to get your liver, thyroid, kidney, or heart examined at regular intervals to make sure you are not having serious side effects.

Many of these medicines also have multiple drug interactions. They can change hormonal levels if you take oral contraceptive pills, tamoxifen, or hormone replacement therapy. They interfere with cardiac medicines. Many antibiotics, antidepressants, and other medicines too numerous to list here are affected by mood stabilizers. However, these medicines can be emotional or physical lifesavers if your mood problem gets out of control.

DHA

In contrast to these medicines, DHA (a specific type of omega-3 fatty acid, a.k.a. docosahexaenoic acid) is a mood stabilizer, an antidepressant, and prevents inflammation in the body with few side effects. DHA increases brain dopamine, norepinephrine, and epinephrine levels like many of the

Mood Stabilizer Primer (anti-kindling agents)

Medication (Generic)	Brand Name	Uses	Advantage	Side Effects	Dose Range
Lithium	Eskalith Lithonate	• Mania • Bipolar I + II • Augment antidepressant therapy in depression • Cyclothymia/rapid cycling mood disorders • Borderline personality disorder	• Buffers explosive angry behavior in some patients with depression and bipolar disorder	• Digestive complaints • Nausea/vomiting • Tremor • "Fuzzy thinking" • Frequently drinking with frequent urination • Low thyroid function • Heart rhythm problems • Change in kidney function • Drug-drug interactions	300–1200 mg/day depending on blood tests
Carba-mazepine Oxy-carba-mazepine	Tegretol Carbatrol Trileptal	• Mania • Bipolar I + II • Augment antidepressant therapy in depression • Rapid cycling mood disorders/ cyclothymia • Borderline personality disorder • Epilepsy	• Most effect in rapid cycling mood disorders	• Drug-drug interactions • Digestive complaints • Nausea/vomiting • Diarrhea/constipation • Sleepiness • Dizziness • Rare cases—life-threatening loss of white blood cells and platelets • Change in liver function • Heart rhythm problems • Rash: can be severe	200–1200 mg/day depending on blood tests
Valproic acid Divalproex	Depakene Depakote Depakote ER	• Bipolar I + II • Treats depressed phase in bipolar I + II • Augment antidepressant therapy in depression • Cyclothymia/rapid cycling mood disorders • Epilepsy • Borderline personality disorder	• Most effective in rapid cycling mood disorders • Very effective in "mixed mood states" • Buffers explosive angry behavior in depression/bipolar disorder	• Sleepiness • Dizziness • Nausea/ vomiting • Rare liver and pancreas problems • Low platelets • Tremor • Drug-drug interactions • Hair loss • Weight gain	500–2500 mg/day depending on blood tests
Gabapentin	Neurontin	• Bipolar I + II • Rapid cycling mood disorder • Treatment-resistant depression • Epilepsy • Anxiety disorders • Panic/social phobias • Pain disorders including migraine headache	• Fewer side effects • Fewer drug interactions • Don't need blood level monitoring	• Sleepiness • Nausea/vomiting • High blood pressure • Change in appetite and weight	300–1800 mg/day

Medication (Generic)	Brand Name	Uses	Advantage	Side Effects	Dose Range
Lamotrigine	Lamictal	• Bipolar I + II • Rapid cycling mood disorders after failing other treatments • Treatment-resistant depression • Pain disorders • Epilepsy		• Rash: can be severe • Drug-drug interactions • Dizziness • Sleepiness • Headache • Weight gain • Nausea/vomiting	100–400 mg/day
Newer Drugs:					
Topiramate	Topamax	• Treatment-resistant mood disorders • Seizures	• Weight reduction	• Sleepiness • Dizziness • Weight loss • Change in speech and language • High number of side effects • Anxiety/mood changes	25–400 mg/day
Tiagabine	Gabitril	• Bipolar I + II	• No known drug interactions	• Weakness • Dizziness • Sleepiness • Tremor • Change in concentration • Depression	
Vigabutrin	Sabrol	• Mood disorders with adduction	• Treat? addiction to cocaine and nicotine	• Weight gain • Sleepiness • Depression	

Sources: Data from E Perucca (1996). The new generation of antiepileptic drugs. *Brit J Clin Pharm,* 42:531–543; N Sussman (1998). Background and rational use of anticonvulsants in psychiatry. *Cleveland Clinic J Med,* 65:Sup1–7; JR Calabrese et al (1999). A double-blind, placebo-controlled study of lamotrigene monotherapy in outpatients with bipolar I depression. *J Clin Psychiatry,* 60:79–88.

antidepressants discussed earlier. It has an effect on attention and attention deficit disorder, memory problems, dementia, and Alzheimer's disease, but studies suggest that people who have problems with anger, aggression, and depression have lower omega-3 fatty acids levels.

Omega-3 fatty acids and DHA may inhibit excessive nerve cell firing the way lithium and valproic acid do but without the higher risk that these medicines pose to the liver, kidney, thyroid, and bone marrow. They also provide mood stabilization in bipolar disorder and rapid cycling mood disorders.

DHA inhibits inflammation in the brain and body, and suppresses cancer cell formation, stabilizes mood, and increases bone density. Remember, depression is an independent risk factor for both coronary heart disease and osteoporosis, so taking DHA can treat both simultaneously.

Supplementing with DHA (omega-3 fatty acids, 100–3400 mg/day) may help lower depression, improve moodiness, irritability, and hostility, especially when associated with PMS and perimenopause. DHA (up to 3 grams) a day improves joint function in rheumatoid arthritis, an autoimmune disease. A similar dose was shown to improve colon function, and reduced relapse rates in Crohn's disease and ulcerative colitis, both autoimmune illnesses. Other studies report improvement in patients with psoriasis. Studies report few side effects to DHA/omega-3 fatty acids, except for mild "digestive side effects."

You have to be careful of taking DHA with aspirin, other NSAIDs, garlic, or gingko, because it can increase bleeding. Some people, including me, burp up a fish taste when they take DHA derived from fish oil, so if you are "fish sensitive," you can take DHA derived from soy (Neuromins— see under Omega-3 Fatty Acids/DHA in Resource Guide).

A note about flaxseed: Flaxseed contains high levels of *alpha-linolenic acid (ALA),* which can be converted by most people's bodies to omega-3 fatty acids and DHA. However, if you are under a lot of stress (as people with mood disorders frequently are), the enzyme (called delta-6-desaturase) that is involved in this conversion doesn't work so well.

How do you increase DHA in your brain and body? Three ounces of salmon contains 2000 milligrams of DHA, so my friend Chris Northrup eats "free range" (wild) salmon once a day. I don't think I can do this without growing gills and having the urge to swim upstream once a year. The other available options are tuna (3 ounces contains 1000 mg DHA), egg yolk, and organ meat.

Omega-6 fatty acids may have the opposite effect in the brain and the body. Omega-6 fatty acids are prevalent in the American diet (and in borage and evening primrose oils). Omega-6 fatty acids increase inflammation if not balanced by appropriate levels of omega-3 fatty acids/DHA and actually may increase the brain cells' capacity to fire. So, trying to get your omega-6 fatty acids from evening primrose or borage oil without taking equivalent amounts of DHA/omega-3 fatty acids may not help your mood disorder, and in fact may aggravate it over time.

Since a higher ratio of omega-6 fatty acids is associated with depression, and you get plenty of omega-6's in your diet, you may want to consider staying away from evening primrose and borage oils if you have a mood problem.

LECITHIN

Many patients who respond to lecithin did not respond well to any other antidepressants. There is some evidence that a component of lecithin, "phosphatidyl-choline," which is sometimes recommended for PMS, may control mania or rapid mood shifts. In combination with lithium, it was shown to treat rapid cycling bipolar disorder in patients who weren't helped with other medicines.

Like DHA, lecithin (15–30 g/day) provides oils that become incorporated into cell membranes all over the body, including brain nerve cell membranes. This may strengthen the membrane and possibly mood stability as well. Lecithin may also be helpful for treating memory problems and Alzheimer's disease. It is important to take this supplement under the care of a physician or other medical professional, since lecithin can worsen mood problems in some people.

INOSITOL

Taking between 12 and 20 grams a day of inositol may also improve mood disorders since, like DHA, lithium, and other mood stabilizers, it affects the nerve cell's internal signaling machinery. Inositol has successfully treated depression with minimal side effects and can help people with anxiety, panic disorder, agoraphobia, obsessive-compulsive disorder, and insomnia. It may also improve cognitive disorders, attention deficit disorder, and Alzheimer's disease.

BIOIDENTICAL ESTROGEN AND PROGESTERONE HORMONES

Having a healthy mood depends in part on the antidepressant effects of estrogen and mood-stabilizing effects of progesterone. Too little or too much progesterone increases the chance of depression. Most doctors do agree that PMS, postpartum, or perimenopausal depression are not a simple deficiency of any hormone, either estradiol, testosterone, or DHEA.

Bioidentical estrogen (Estraderm patch 100 mcg/24 hours) (beta-estradiol) increases brain cell firing (called excitability) and causes cells in specific brain emotional and memory areas to sprout. For women whose estrogen drops suddenly and precipitously (after a hysterectomy and oophorectomy, or postpartum), supplementation with bioidentical estrogen (which matches the receptors in your brain) may prevent depression. However, they must also take progesterone to prevent moodiness and anxiety.

Some women with PMS in perimenopause have excessive estrogen levels but an inappropriately low progesterone buffer, which sets the scene for irritability, anger, and moodiness. For women who are perimenopausal with irregular periods and low thyroid function, some doctors prescribe a 17 beta-estradiol 100 mcg patch/24 hours transdermally for dysthymia and major depression.

Bioidentical progesterone (either progesterone solution transdermal, or oral progesterone, in the form of Prometrium) may help treat irritability, moodiness, and anxiety in PMS and perimenopause. Interestingly, progesterone may also treat pain disorders that have increased chance of becoming a problem with the lowered serotonin levels of depression. Progesterone may play a role in repairing and replacing the protective myelin covering of peripheral nerves that may be damaged in people with spinal and other chronic orthopedic problems.

What's Wrong with Synthetic, Non-Bioidentical Hormones?

Taking synthetic estrogen and synthetic progesterone (Provera) is not as good for women's mood or memory as bioidentical hormones. *Synthetic conjugated estrogens* or *synthetic progesterone* do not match the brain cell receptors and over time may aggravate mood problems. Synthetic progesterone (Provera) may cause a number of side effects in women, including major depression, obsession, compulsions, irritability, and anxiety disorders.

Do Tamoxifen and Other Drugs That Lower Estrogen Affect Mood?

Tamoxifen and other SERMs (selective estrogen receptor modulators) have been reported to produce depressive symptoms. It may be that any drug that alters hormonal levels causes mood problems in women who are predisposed to them during their menstrual cycle, postpartum, or menopause. If you have had serious irritability and depression during these hormonal events, and absolutely have to take tamoxifen or raloxifene, then you need to shore up your brain's mood circuits and improve your mood with some of the medicines or nutritional supplements in this section.

Are Estrogen and Progesterone Hormone Replacement Safe?

The short answer is that no one really knows. In 2002, the Women's Health Initiative stopped synthetic estrogen and progestin treatment ("artificial" estrogen and progesterone, including non-bioidentical Provera) for participants in its study because they found a "significant increased risk in breast cancer, stroke, and cardiac events." Some argue that the increase in death in some of the women was because they were in their late sixties and hormone replacement was started too late in life. Scientists hypothesized that their bodies' blood vessels were already diseased, and, since estrogen encourages blood clot growth and development, clots and strokes might have been inevitable. However, the doctors believe that if the women had been much younger (say, late forties, early fifties) with less atherosclerosis in their blood vessels, estrogen would have caused fewer strokes and cardiovascular complications.

The Women's Health Initiative study tells us nothing about the potential safety or danger of bioidentical 17-beta-estradiol or bioidentical progesterone, because it didn't test either hormone.

As a result of the Women's Health Initiative study, women and their doctors or other health practitioners have to look at the risks and benefits of taking hormones for mood or memory problems. Do you or a first-degree relative have a history of breast cancer or other hormonally responsive cancer? Do you have a history of stroke? If so, you may want to avoid bioidentical and synthetic hormone supplementation and try the numerous other nonhormonal methods for dealing with your mood problems.

OTHER HORMONAL REPLACEMENT: DHEA, TESTOSTERONE, AND THYROID HORMONE

DHEA levels decrease with age and drop even more precipitously in women than men. Menopausal women who have had their ovaries removed also are especially prone to lower DHEA, as are older women who are debilitated or have severe chronic physical illness. Some studies suggest that the precipitous drop of DHEA in middle-aged women may have a role in the onset of depression. DHEA has successfully treated depression and midlife dysthymia. Many patients who responded favorably had depression that was somewhat resistant to other forms of treatment. DHEA's positive effect on mood may be via its capacity to be converted into estrogen and testosterone. After DHEA treatment, some women have increased energy and motivation, and less sadness and anxiety.

Some studies suggest DHEA slows the aging process and prevents, improves, or reverses cancer, heart disease, obesity, and osteoporosis. If your depression occurs with anxiety, edginess, and irritability, however, DHEA may be too activating for you. DHEA can be so stimulating that some people become addicted. In addition, DHEA can be converted in your body to excessive estrogen levels, or of testosterone, which can cause "masculinizing" side effects like hair growth, so if your medical history makes you want to avoid estrogen, you want to avoid DHEA as well.

Depending upon your unique genetic makeup, weight, body fat content, and level of stress in your body, hormonal supplementation of DHEA and progesterone can have different effects. For some, DHEA and progesterone supplementation may calm and stabilize mood, acting as an antianxiety hormone. However, for others, the progesterone or DHEA will have an energizing, antidepressant effect. This variation in female response to hormones may explain the great diversity of opinions about whether hormones should be used to treat mood disorders in women.

Testosterone

Although no one has studied extensively how testosterone affects women's mood, there have been extensive studies on men, and we do know that women must have testosterone for libido, strength, energy, and well-being. A woman's ovaries and adrenal glands produce testosterone throughout her life, but some produce it in insufficient amounts. Women who have had chemotherapy, radiation, or surgery may have lower than normal testosterone levels, and ultimately feel their mood and energy dip. In one study, more than half of menopausal women with low testosterone levels who received supplementation had improved libido and a sense of well-being. According to Dr. Christiane Northrup, however, testosterone supplements won't help a woman's sex life if her relationship isn't healthy. If the relationship has problems that are being "swept under the rug," this hormonal supplementation probably will do little to override a "situationally appropriate" loss of interest in sex.

You can find out if your testosterone levels are low by getting your doctor to check your unbound (free) testosterone (and/or DHEA) levels.

If they are low, you may want to try a prescription of natural testosterone either in a capsule or cream. Doses begin at 1–2 milligrams every other day.

Some women who take a lot of progesterone or DHEA supplementation may see their testosterone levels and estrogen levels improve along with their mood and libido. After high levels of DHEA (1600 mg/day), a woman begins to develop high blood levels of testosterone.

Thyroid Hormones T_4 and T_3

When a woman gains weight, sleeps a lot, and has low energy and a depressed mood, the first thing she usually wants to know is whether she has a thyroid problem. The fact is, many symptoms of hypothyroidism (low thyroid function) overlap with the symptoms of depression, but thyroid function involves more than mood.

Symptoms of Hypothyroidism	
Mild: Increased TSH only	More Severe: Increased TSH, Decreased T_4 and/or T_3
• Moodiness • Depressed, anxious, panicky • Poor sleep • Fatigue • Exhausted • Lowered enthusiasm • Feeling hot or cold • Bothered by mild changes in skin or hair • Inexplicable change in weight	• Depression • Psychosis • Lethargy • Stupor • Mental slowing • Motor slowing • Cold intolerance • Dry skin • Loss of eyebrow hair • Brittle hair • Edema • Swollen tongue • Anorexia • Weight gain • Constipation • Menorrhagia • Enlarged heart

A high percentage of women in perimenopause and menopause have thyroid problems. While severe hypothyroidism affects about 2 percent of the population, milder forms, including subclinical hypothyroidism, are much more common, affecting nearly 26 percent. Since hypothyroidism and depression share so many symptoms, it is important to figure out if a component of your mood problem is due to a change in thyroid function.

For centuries, doctors and scientists have seen the link between low thyroid function and depression. Hypothyroidism is classically defined as low T_4 and T_3 hormones, and *elevated* TSH, the neuropeptide produced by the pituitary gland. In subclinical hypothyroidism, levels of thyroid T_4, T_3 hormone are normal (thus the term "subclinical"), but TSH, the brain's hormone that signals the thyroid gland to pump out more of its own hormones, is elevated. Studies don't agree about whether or not subclinical hypothyroidism is associated with depression, but it is associated with problems with attention, memory, and moodiness.

Even if thyroid hormone is supplemented to treat the garden-variety hypothyroidism or the subclinical type, depression doesn't always immediately improve. Frequently, antidepressant therapy is also required. If you are depressed and suspect hypothyroidism, have your doctor or other practitioner test your blood for pituitary TSH and thyroid hormones T_4 and T_3. If you or your doctor think you have *some* form of hypothyroidism, you might want to try thyroid replacement to see if it can improve your mood. Combinations of T_4 (Synthroid) and T_3 (Cytomel) seem to be more effective in treating hypothyroidism than T_4 alone, and yield greater improvements in mood, attention, and memory.

The depression associated with "subclinical hypothyroidism" (normal T_4 and T_3, with only an elevated TSH level) is much less likely to respond to conventional antidepressants than the garden-variety hypothyroidism. Even if a woman's blood test indicates completely normal thyroid function, adding small amounts of thyroid hormone to her antidepressant medication may greatly improve her mood. T_3, 25–75 milligrams a day, can "augment" tricyclic antidepressant therapy. Interestingly, adding thyroid hormone to antidepressant therapy works better in women than in men, and seems to make the antidepressant take effect in a shorter period of time. Neuroscientists believe that adding thyroid hormone T_3 may treat some subtle thyroid deficiency.

Excessive estrogen replacement may repress thyroid function, promoting hypothyroidism. So, if you take estrogen replacement, you should get your blood estrogen and thyroid hormones tested to make sure that both are at normal levels for your age. You don't want to replace one hormone only to repress another.

Herbal Mood Stabilizers

Women use a variety of herbal nutritional supplements for the depression, moodiness, and irritability associated with PMS, perimenopause, and menopause. Many women use these herbals because they feel uncomfortable taking estrogen replacement or other bioidentical hormones.

Chasteberry (Vitex agnus castus) *as Directed on Preparation*

Chasteberry (or Vitex) alleviates PMS and menopausal irritability, moodiness, and depression. Vitex reduces excess estrogen, elevates progesterone, and ultimately eases hormonal moodiness, breast tenderness, fluid retention, constipation, headache, and fatigue. Vitex also improves depression by influencing the mood neurotransmitter dopamine. Side effects can include headaches, diarrhea, abdominal cramps, increased menstrual flow, and rash.

Vitex is frequently used in combination with *black cohosh, licorice, dong quai,* and other herbs (see below).

Black Cohosh (Cimicifuga racemosa)

Black cohosh (60–120 mg 2x/day) has been used in Europe for more than sixty years to treat hot flashes and other menopausal symptoms. It has a mild estrogenic effect on the brain and the body, binding weakly to estrogen receptors. Its antidepressant effects have been shown in a variety of studies for PMS and menopause. It can also lower blood pressure. Black cohosh has few side effects, but it can cause excessively low blood pressure in women who take antihypertensive medicines. Remifemin is a standardized preparation of black cohosh and has been extensively studied.

Licorice Root (Glycyrrhiza glabra)

Licorice is one of the most extensively studied herbs. It has both antiestrogen and estrogen effects, and contains phytoestrogens and isoflavones (see "Soy," below) which ultimately balance the estrogen levels in your body and brain. If estrogen levels are high, licorice (1–4 g powdered root/day) blocks their action. If estrogen levels are low, licorice potentiates their activity. In addition to acting as an antidepressant, licorice may also stabilize mood by increasing progesterone. It may also inhibit the breakdown of norepinephrine, a key mood neurotransmitter, and it blocks inflammation that depression promotes.

Licorice is benign, although in high dosages it can cause high blood pressure, headache, and sodium and water retention. It can lower testosterone levels and at very high dosages cause a loss of libido. Licorice is a "blood thinner" and may promote bleeding if combined with other herbs and medicines, so keep to the suggested dose. Pregnant women should not take licorice.

Dong Quai (Angelica sinensis)

This herbal supplement has anti-inflammatory, analgesic, and antihypertensive effects, and has successfully treated menopausal symptoms. Dong quai (4.5 g/day) has some "estrogen-like" activity and may also have anti-inflammatory effects that can help prevent diseases linked with depression, notably heart disease and stroke. However, like many other herbs, dong quai is a blood thinner and should be avoided with other antiplatelet medicines or herbs.

Red Clover (Trifolium pratense)

Rich in phytoestrogens, red clover (40–80 mg/day, or as directed by your practitioner) somehow affects the estrogen receptors in the brain and body to give a mild antidepressant effect. It also improves osteoporosis, and red clover may block the proliferation of estrogen-stimulated cancer cell growth (i.e., breast cancer).

Red clover may cause rash in some women. It may cause bleeding when combined with other "blood thinner herbs" (see gingko biloba section). Since it can enhance *or* block estrogen, red clover, like other phytoestrogens, may interfere with hormone replacement therapy or other phytoestrogen herbal supplements.

Soy

Soy (40–60 g/day) has "isoflavones" that act as phytoestrogens. Though not a "bioidentical estrogen compound," soy binds to and stimulates some estrogen receptors and may block others, ultimately preventing breast cancer and hot flashes in some women as well as peri- and postmenopausal heart disease, hypertension, high cholesterol, constipation, osteoporosis, and dementia. Eating whole soy does give some women constipation, bloating, nausea, or a rash.

Even though some Western practitioners are concerned about the safety of prolonged use of soy because of its estrogen receptor activity, this whole food has been a staple in the Asian diet for centuries, and fewer than 20 percent of Japanese women have hot flashes. Many companies have tried to take the active ingredient out of whole soy to make it a more potent menopausal nutritional supplement, but this isolated isoflavone, genistein, does not have the same activity as whole soy and may compromise soy's safety. Whole soy contains genistein at much lower concentrations, balanced biochemically with many other compounds.

MOOD-STABILIZING MINERALS: MAGNESIUM AND CALCIUM

Magnesium supplementation stabilizes mood in some individuals, although at low or high levels it can predispose you to depression. Low levels are seen in women who complain of PMS, and oral magnesium supplementation can successfully relieve their irritability and moodiness. Magnesium may be a mood stabilizer because it is important for the electrical stability of cell membranes, including nerve cells. Magnesium citrate (900–2500 mg/day) and calcium work together in the body: Magnesium is relaxing and soothes nerve conduction, calcium stimulates it. Magnesium blocks nerve cell irritability without side effects.

Low magnesium levels are not uncommon in our culture, caused by diabetes, excessive alcohol intake, thyroid disorders, "malabsorption syndromes" (i.e., diarrhea), and drug side effects. You get magnesium by eating a lot of dark leafy vegetables, but you may want to consider taking a magnesium supplement, too. Calcium/magnesium supplements are especially effective for treating osteoporosis, hypertension, diabetes, and asthma. Magnesium deficiency may in fact increase the incidence of all these illnesses.

Calcium supplements may stabilize mood in some women, especially those with PMS, but excessive levels *or* low levels of calcium can lead to depression. Low calcium levels, which are also common in our culture, cause social withdrawal and irritability, depression, fatigue, and obsessiveness. Some people who have sensitive digestive tracts have to "start low and go slow" with calcium and magnesium supplements, since they are more likely to develop diarrhea, abdominal bloating, and distension. Taking calcium buffered with citrate and carbonate (900–4100 mg/day) and magnesium buffered with citrate, amino acid, and oxide may help your bowel tolerate these supplements (see Resource Guide).

It is important to take magnesium in two different forms each day: Take a combination mineral pill containing calcium (3210 mg/day total) and magnesium (2100 mg total) *with food* since this supplement is important for bone health and mood. In addition, if you have problems with irritability and anxiety, take an additional supplement of magnesium without calcium (100–300 mg a day on an *empty* stomach for maximal absorption). Apart from bioidentical progesterone, magnesium is the most important supplement I take. I take 100 mg three times a day on an absolutely empty stomach. It has had a tremendous effect on my perimenopausal irritability and anxiety and all but eliminated my seizures. My brain feels like a peaceful kingdom . . . most of the time, which is a huge improvement.

Balancing the Feminine Brain: Inner and Outer Treatments
Traditional Chinese Medicine: Acupuncture and Herbal Nutritional Supplements

As part of a complete treatment plan, you can use Traditional Chinese Medicine to balance your moods. Acupuncture and Chinese herbs (see Traditional Chinese Herbs table, p. 182) are great for irritability and physical problems related to moods. Just as there are five different emotional circuits in the feminine emotional brain (joy, love, fear, anger, and sadness), there are five elements in Traditional Chinese Medicine (earth, wood, air, water, and fire). When a trained acupuncturist figures out which element/emotion is excess or deficient in you, he knows the acupuncture points to needle and the herbal blend to give you. It's an amazing, effective treatment and it really does not hurt.

Acupuncture Mood-Meridian Translations				
Mood	Emotion	Meridian	Element	Acupuncture Diagnosis
Depression	Sadness	Lung/large intestine	Air	
Irritability/Moodiness	Anger	Liver/gallbladder	Wood	Stuck liver Qi
Mania/depression	Joy	Heart/small intestine	Fire	Heart fire rising
	Love	Kidney/bladder	Water	Deficient kidney yang
Anxiety	Fear	Spleen/stomach	Earth	

Acupuncture has been proven scientifically in many studies to relieve pain disorders (headaches, back pain, etc.), problems with sleep, and addiction. Acupuncture and traditional Chinese herbal supplements can also improve hypercholesterolemia, hypertension, immune system dysfunction in arthritis, HIV/AIDS, and improve recovery from stroke, among other physical health problems.

Different Strokes for Different Folks

In a study comparing running (an "active outward" approach) and meditation (the calm inward form), both treatments improved mood. Even though one approach involved vigorous movement and the other stillness, both created identical changes in brain chemistry. Whatever exercise or practice you choose, make sure it is something that has meaning for you and you genuinely enjoy. Otherwise, your treatment approach will add more stress than relieve it.

Traditional Chinese Herbs

Mood	Health Problem(s)	Available Chinese Herbal Supplements
Menopausal irritability and depression	Palpitations Insomnia Hot flashes	Codonopsis Angelica Scleratium Polygalae Tenufulbine ZiZiph Spinosa Seutellariae Rehmanniae Discecoreae
Depression	+ Constipation	Sm. Biota
Depression	+ Skin problems	Cinnabar
Depression	+ Asthma	Lumbricus
Depression	+ Eye problems	Concha halitodis
Depression	+ Headache	Scolopendra feverfew
Depression	+ Hypertension	Scorpio
Depression	+ Tinnitus	Magnetitum
Depression	+ Insomnia	Os Draconis
Depression	+ Gastroesophageal reflux	Concha ostea

Sources: Data from MA Naeser (1990). *Outline Guide to Chinese Herbal Medicines in Pill Form with Sample Pictures of the Boxes,* Boston Chinese Medicine; E Ernst et al (1998). Complementary therapies for depression. *Arch Gen Psychiatry,* 55:1026–1032; G Liu et al (1992). Electroacupuncture treatment of presenile and senile depressive state. *J Tradit Chin Med,* 12:91–94; SE Polyakov (1988). Acupuncture in the treatment of endogenous depressions. *Zh Neuropat Psikhiatr Korsakova,* 21:327–329; X Yang (1994). Clinical observations on needling extra channel points in treating major depression. In: L Tank and S Tang, eds. *Neurochemistry in Clinical Application,* New York, Plenum Press, pp. 104–122; H Luo et al (1985). Electroacupuncture vs. amitriptyline in the treatment of depressive states. *J Tradit Chin Med,* 5:3–8; H Luo et al (1990). Electroacupuncture in the treatment of depressive psychosis. *Int J Clin Acupuncture,* 1:7-13.

MOVEMENT AND MIRTH

Women who are melancholic, sad, lethargic, sleepy, crave carbohydrates, and have problems with initiation and motivation may respond better to a more stimulating, active treatment.

Laughter and Humor

Everyone knows that seeing a funny movie or watching your favorite sitcom can lift your spirits and improve your mood. I was first introduced to the healing power of humor when I ran across Norman Cousins's book, *The Anatomy of an Illness.* Mr. Cousins had been hospitalized with a severe autoimmune illness. During his treatment, he watched funny movies and TV programs like

Candid Camera reruns and spent his day laughing. The more he laughed, the better he felt, and soon the symptoms of his illness waned. As a result of many scientific studies on the healing power of humor, hospitals all over the United States incorporated humor and laughter as part of their treatments to improve immune response during cancer treatment and relieve pain.

Laughter inhibits the depression-disease domino effect and keeps stress from turning into inflammation, immune system dysfunction, depression, and disease. Stress lowers immunoglobulin IgA, one of the first lines of defense in the immune system, but people who are rated high on a "humor scale" do not have a drop of IgA during stress. People who are able to laugh or keep a wry perspective during a stressful event are less likely to become depressed, angry, tired, or tense.

Humor alters the the brain's mood circuit and, even if you're sad, buffers pain and makes you more resilient. Humor has been used to help patients prepare for surgery and medical procedures: Patients who saw a funny film were less anxious and their spirits were in better shape to deal with medical care.

EXERCISE

Physical activity of all kinds rewires and biochemically balances all four parts of the Feminine Emotional Brain.

1. *Mood.* People who are inactive or sedentary are twice as likely to have symptoms of depression. Regular exercise, five days a week, has a true antidepressant effect, especially in mild or moderate depression. Movement therapy is also relatively inexpensive—in some cases, free—and lacks the side effects and stigma associated with taking medicine. Regular exercise that challenges you but doesn't exhaust you or bore you releases the same neurotransmitters—beta endorphin, serotonin, and norepinephrine—that Prozac, Zoloft, or St. John's wort affect. Aerobic exercise for at least twenty minutes also releases these neurotransmitters that decrease anger, elevate mood, create a feeling of euphoria, and relieve tension. Many women don't get a mental benefit from aerobic exercise like running and biking and find them boring and painful, but as long as you move and love what you're doing, you'll reap the physical and emotional benefits.

2. *Thought patterns.* Consistent exercise and physical activity have been shown to improve self-concept and self-esteem. Even if you exercise for twenty to thirty minutes a day, the physical activity distracts your thoughts from stressful things in your life. Regular, challenging exercise makes you feel more effective at handling difficult situations.

3. *Behavior.* Many people with depression suffer from fatigue, lethargy, and inactivity. Exercise and movement therapy "jump-start" the frontal lobe areas for initiation and motivation, and get the neurochemicals flowing through the emotional brain circuits. People with depression frequently tend to withdraw socially and remove themselves from friends and loved ones. Taking a daily walk or working out regularly with a friend is beneficial for at least two reasons. Your friend, in a way, donates the initiation brain circuitry that your depression has temporarily unplugged. Even if it's hard to get out of bed, the fact that someone is on your doorstep ringing your bell can be very motivating. In addition, social contact in itself releases beta-endorphin and oxytocin, neurotransmitters that elevate mood and improve a sense of personal reward.

4. *Body health.* Regular exercise improves many health conditions that increase your risk of becoming depressed and for which you are at risk if you are depressed, including cardiovascular disease and osteoporosis. Regular exercise also helps the immune system fight viruses (colds, flus, and cancers), although exercising to exhaustion can actually weaken your immune system. Start your exercise under the direction of a physician, physical therapist, or skilled trainer. Some women's exercise can get out of control, notably in anorexia, or other eating disorders, or during the manic phase of bipolar disorder.

Physical activity improves your physical response to stress: After twelve to sixteen weeks of aerobic exercise, your heart rate and blood pressure don't rise as much when you get irritated. It improves insomnia, which is both a symptom and a cause of depression. Exercise helps you get to sleep and helps you achieve a deeper, more restful sleep. Regular exercise, under the direction of a physical therapist, can improve lower back pain, osteoarthritis, and other pain disorders. Finally, physical exercise and activity help you live longer and healthier. Physical inactivity in older adults, is associated with poor health and earlier death.

I exercise seven days per week. When I started running at age eighteen, I felt a "clarity" in my brain. Aerobic exercise made me calmer, more alert, helped me get fewer colds, and made me feel better about myself. Unfortunately, my scoliosis and rod fusion probably weren't compatible with this form of exercise and after thirteen years and thousands of miles of pounded pavement, I had blown more than ten spinal discs, and had had four surgeries to insert ten metal rods and nails. I could no longer get my serotonin, norepinephrine, and beta-endorphin high through running, and I went into withdrawal. I had to find another way to get exercise. Tai chi makes me fall asleep and yoga isn't possible with all the surgical hardware, but God knows I tried. (In one class, the teacher said, "Hey, Mona Lisa, try to relax. You look like you have a rod up your _____.") So, every morning I exercise on an elliptical trainer for twenty to thirty minutes. Every afternoon, I walk for forty-five minutes outside or on a treadmill if it's raining or snowing. Both create the same feeling in my head that running did, without my back falling apart. I also do ballet stretches and pushups, and I pull rubber bands to improve my joints and general spinal health. Every day, after exercising, I feel alert, awake, in a good mood, and am more or less pain-free.

Inward Treatments: Massage, Meditation, and Mindfulness

If your depression causes you to seclude yourself, isolate yourself away from loved ones, friends, and family, you may be drawn to meditation and mindfulness, but they could actually *exacerbate* your depression, irritability, and moodiness. You most likely need to combine calm inward treatment approaches with active ones. Women who are agitated, irritable, insomniac, and anxious may respond to the structured, stimulus-minimizing features of massage, meditation, and mindfulness treatments.

Massage has been shown in more than sixty-three studies to improve depression, PMS, and a variety of pain disorders, addiction, asthma, diabetes, fibromyalgia/chronic fatigue, lower back pain, headaches, and other immune problems including cancer. Massage relieves depression directly by increasing serotonin levels and indirectly by stimulating the immune system, and relieves pain by releasing endorphins.

A note of caution: For someone with a history of physical, sexual, or emotional abuse, massage may not be the best therapy in the initial stages of treatment for depression and posttraumatic stress disorder. Even if done skillfully by a practitioner who has a depth of experience with trauma patients, the physical touch may evoke flashbacks and reenact trauma. It's best to consult your therapist, psychiatrist, or physician about whether to get massage and other somatic touch therapies.

Meditation and prayer and other intentional practices improve mood disorders and physical disorders for which depression increases the risk, including hypertension, psoriasis, chronic pain, angina, and insomnia. It does this by interfering with the biochemical cascade in the depression-disease domino effect. Meditation may also stimulate the immune system.

Prayer may have just as positive an effect on mood in the feminine brain as it has on the blood cells and the immune system, because blood cells have many of the same neurotransmitter receptors as the brain. Many studies show that engaging in prayer, meditation, and imagery can help the health of others, and has helped to bolster red blood cells, protect people in a coronary care unit from infection and minimize their need for antibiotics, and in fact seems to prevent death (fewer people who were prayed for died during the study). Prayer is recognized as a complementary therapy by the NIH, and funded studies are currently underway.

Yoga has successfully treated mild depression, dysthymia, PMS, menopausal dysfunction, severe depressions, and bipolar disorder. It can also improve low initiative, motivation and libido when practiced regularly. However, in severe depression, it may be very hard to have enough motivation to begin such a program in the first place, so you probably need a combination of other therapies, too.

TREATING DARK MOODS WITH LIGHT THERAPY

Daily bright light exposure alone or in combination with antidepressant medical therapy is effective in treating seasonal depression, major depression, PMS, as well as depression during and after pregnancy. You can get light from going outside or indoors from a "full-spectrum" light source (see Resource Guide). In some people with bipolar disorder, light therapy can precipitate mania. Winter seasonal depression has been effectively treated with an ultraviolet-screened diffuse white fluorescent light source (see Resource Guide). You sit at a distance of 33 centimeters, with the light tilted downward toward the head, and use the light for sixty minutes daily within ten minutes of awakening in the morning.

Light therapy can help treat cyclic hormonally sensitive mood disorders if you want to avoid estrogen hormonal replacement. Light will not stimulate estrogen-responsive breast, ovary, and uterine tissue as hormonal replacement therapy will. Light therapy advances your circadian rhythm, and has an antidepressant effect on hormones and the immune system.

By this time, you have learned all the biochemical and environmental routes to improve your mood. In Chapter 8, "I've Got a Feeling," you will learn to rewire your thoughts that increase your chance of being depressed and you'll also learn how to get in touch with the intuitive genius behind your moods.

SIX

I'm All Shook Up:
Fears and Phobias, Anxiety and Obsessions

I have worked in the field of medical intuition for almost two decades and the number one question that people ask me is, "How can you tell the difference between anxiety and intuition?" If you feel uncomfortable or troubled, or you sense that someone important to you is in trouble, how do you know if you're just being neurotic or you've had an intuition? When are you intuitive and when are you just being a worrywart?

Anxiety, intuition, and the feminine brain go hand in hand. An anxiety disorder of some kind or another affects over 30 percent of women, and anxiety can be as paralyzing as depression. Yet only 19 percent of men have it. How can this be?

The hormonally altered New Feminine Brain puts us at greater risk for anxiety. This risk is compounded by oral contraceptives, fertility drugs, tamoxifen, other antiestrogen drugs, and synthetic high-dose hormone replacement at perimenopause and menopause.

Although modern medicine has made great strides in treating depression, it hasn't yet come up with truly effective, nonaddictive medicines for anxiety. We women who suffer from nervousness, chronic worry, and panic have tended to suffer in silence. Social pressures forced us to hide our anxiety for fear we would be labeled wimpy or weak. Anxiety is an insidious problem for women. If you have a problem with anxiety, you tend to avoid what makes you nervous. Left untreated, anxiety tends to grow and intensify. Like a weed in the garden, one seeds and leads to many; one thing that makes you nervous turns into two things, and so on. Over time, you tend to avoid more and more situations and your life becomes more and more restricted. Some women try to self-medicate their anxiety with food, alcohol, cigarettes, and other addictions and compulsions that themselves can negatively affect their physical health.

However, the *emotional pain* of anxiety isn't its most debilitating feature. The more paralyzing symptom of anxiety is *avoidance*. To avoid panic, women often try to control their environment so tightly that they restrict their lives severely. Ann-Marie's story below demonstrates how anxiety can rob a woman of her freedom, intellectual potential, and self-esteem, and at times cause her to stay in a loveless, sometimes abusive relationship.

Anxiety, Perfectionism, Control, and Avoiding Risk

Ann-Marie was a perfectionist. Her father was a Nobel laureate physicist and her mother had always encouraged her to do her best. The classic overachiever, Ann-Marie pushed herself to excel in every class. After graduating from Vassar with a major in English, Ann-Marie married her high school sweetheart, Bruce, because it seemed like the "logical thing" to do. Ann-Marie and Bruce had two kids, ages twenty-three and sixteen, both of whom Ann-Marie homeschooled.

Although Ann-Marie had always known she was a little anxious, she had been able to hide it through conscientiousness, and being what others called a little bit of a "control freak," as she tried to impose order on the outside world. Other neighborhood homemakers admired her impeccable order in housekeeping and yard work. Her marriage was "functional," but Ann-Marie turned her passion into organizing her children's education and social lives. She had a Daytimer organizer that she carried like a bible. She kept meticulous files on each of her kids and got a great sense of security being a soccer mom in the suburbs.

Ann-Marie's life started to unravel at midlife at age forty-five. Her stomach had always been "easily upset," but now she suffered from severe attacks of nausea and stomach distress, especially in the morning. She was getting "hot flashes," pressure in her chest, and heart palpitations. An EKG was performed, which showed an occasional PVD "pre-ventricular contraction." The cardiologist wasn't particularly concerned, but he gave Ann-Marie a beta-blocker, which made her dizzy and weak. Ann-Marie went to her gynecologist and asked for treatment for "perimenopausal symptoms," but the low-dose estrogen patch she was prescribed made her feel irritable, and bioidentical progesterone nauseated her. Finally, her gynecologist offered her Xanax for what she thought might be panic attacks and anxiety.

Ann-Marie's lifelong tendency toward anxiety was now becoming unleashed at midlife. For years she had "medicated" her worrying and nervousness through perfectionism and control. Having a low tolerance for risk or being alone, she married her first and only boyfriend to create a safe haven. Bruce gave her a home, a steady relationship, and a financially secure future. Her identity as a soccer mom helped her create a suburban utopia—she could control every aspect of her family's life. However, she was about to lose this control. Both kids would soon graduate college and it would be just Ann-Marie and Bruce, which terrified her. The idea of getting a job or going back to school also terrified her. Even though she had an IQ of 148 and a multitude of talents, Ann-Marie's anxiety and fear of failure had emotionally and physically paralyzed her. For years, she had also avoided the problems in her marriage. She now realized she couldn't imagine living forever with Bruce, but she couldn't figure out how she could live on her own without him. Ann-Marie had created a stress-free, anxiety-free, controlled life that avoided everything that made her panic, but that life was changing, and she felt out of control emotionally and physically. Ann-Marie knew her body's anxiety and physical symptoms were telling her she was stuck and needed to change her life, or get sicker, but she couldn't quite tell if her fear of getting sicker was really intuition or just her anxiety causing her to worry.

Ann-Marie was living proof of the connection between anxiety and intuition. She was sick with worry, and needed to work to clarify the intuitive message in her anxiety.

What Are Fear and Anxiety?

When you feel *fear,* you are responding to an actual threat that you directly perceive with your five senses. In contrast, when you feel *anxious,* no real threat is present, but you are anticipating one in the future. With more brain-body connections, and an exaggerated tendency toward putting words to emotional experience, the traditional feminine brain may also be more biologically primed to giving voice to fear, anxiety, and intuition.

Women tend to prefer shared experiences. Many women see the world through their own eyes but at the same time watch others' emotional reactions. Going to a movie, the supermarket, class, or work, they are constantly intuitively plugged into the emotional experiences and reactions of others around them. A woman's brain is so well-adapted for empathy that it functions almost like an environmental emotional barometer, constantly assessing and registering the stress and distress in others. For some women, the most obvious signs that their brain's fear circuits are active are changes in right-brain unconscious behavior or health problems, *not* a change in emotions, moods, or thoughts (see Emotional Feng Shui chart, pp. 71–72). For example, fear can generate anxious behavior like nervous-sounding speech, a shaky voice, crying, running, hiding, or avoidance. Some get cold chills or hot flashes. Others will sweat, get jittery or shaky, have heart palpitations, shortness of breath, or muscle tension. Still others may develop allergies, colds, asthma, a lump in the throat, thyroid dysfunction, abdominal pain, nausea, diarrhea, constipation, or skin problems. In women who exhibit anxious behavior, fear gets "stuck" in the right brain, unable to gain access to left-brain language to be spoken and released.

The Brain-to-Body Emergency Broadcast System

When your brain's amygdala—the watchdog organ in your brain—determines that something is threatening you, it initiates an emergency or stress reaction. It sends a signal to the hypothalamus-pituitary-adrenal system. This signal goes through an important area in the hypothalamus called the *bed nucleus stria terminalis,* which is the I-95 of the brain, the stress superhighway. In men's brains, the amygdala and the bed nucleus are twice as big as in women's brains, although we don't know why that is significant. With brains, bigger isn't better and smaller isn't worse—it's just different. But the amygdala and the bed nucleus do have estrogen and testosterone receptors, so hormone fluctuations may affect how women respond to fear-provoking situations. A woman's hormonally goosed-up anxiety circuits may make her more susceptible to anxiety and related specific medical problems. The feminine brain's unique wiring for fear and anxiety may also be the highway for what our society calls "women's intuition"—the instinctive ability to know things about others, especially loved ones.

After traveling through the bed nucleus, right-brain fear and anxiety set off other alarms in the body: The heart rate speeds up, blood pressure rises, and the digestive system gets in an uproar. Changes in estrogen and progesterone may turn up the volume of anxiety symptoms, which may help explain why physical symptoms (panic attack, heart palpitations, elevated blood pressure, nausea, and digestive upset) are more common in women than men.

The Female Health Emergency Broadcast System may be more developed than men's due to her enhanced brain connectivity and hormonal cycles. For example, when men have a heart attack, the first symptoms are usually "para-sternal" crushing chest pain and jaw pain radiating to the left arm. In contrast, some of the first signs of a woman's heart attack are emotional, such as feelings of anxiety, uneasiness, and apprehension—signs of the brain's fear circuits firing away. (As a result, for many years women's heart attacks were missed, because doctors just thought that the women were nervous.) Other physical illnesses also send you a sense of tension, nervousness, or edginess, but if you aren't aware that the emotion is caused by a change within your body's biochemistry, your brain may interpret the fear as caused by your external environment. You will then interpret the uneasiness and foreboding as a portent that something bad is going to happen, that you are losing control of your life, or that someone or something is threatening you.

THE FEMININE ANATOMY FOR COURAGE, FEAR, ANXIETY, VIGILANCE, AND INTUITION

Input from your five senses, your "gut," and heart sense converge in the brain stem. There the emotional motor system broadcasts the information to brain areas, that, like a panel of judges, determine whether there is a real emergency. They compare the present perceptions and situation to past experiences that were painful or harmful. In a way, the brain areas vote whether you sense danger or something else to get worked up about, or something harmless and to be ignored.

AC or DC: Cycling Hormones, Cycling Hemispheres

The rise and fall of estrogen and progesterone in PMS, pregnancy, postpartum, and perimenopause may predispose some women to anxiety disorders in those phases of their lives. Some women who have excessive estrogen levels with inappropriately low progesterone levels have an enhanced capacity to be receptive to others' feelings and an increased risk of anxiety and nervousness. Progesterone is an "antianxiety," mood-stabilizing hormone. If you are deficient in progesterone, your chance of having an anxiety problem is increased. If the anxiety and intuition get too intense, the emotional excess can prevent you from achieving career goals, maintaining relationships, or fitting into society in general. You could get to the point where you're anxious even when things are okay or numb when things aren't. The anxiety warning can go off at the smallest provocation, like an overly sensitive smoke alarm in your kitchen that responds to heat instead of smoke. You can begin to feel that no one, not even your family, is safe. Ironically, if you have a history of abuse, your wires may get crossed and you may trust the wrong people and end up being traumatized repeatedly in relationships.

In the first part of a woman's monthly cycle, she is more likely to have greater left-brain processing of thoughts and emotions, more likely to feel on an even keel with positive emotions. But, during the second half of her cycle, after ovulation, she is more likely to experience the right-brain's "negative" emotions, including fear, anxiety, and panic. They may come from her hormonal intuition rather than from external danger, but they probably indicate that something in her life is off-kilter. For some women, this intuition runs in a *DC current,* that is, PMS with *D*epression *C*ycling in and out throughout the month. Others' intuition runs on an *AC current: A*nxiety *C*ycling in and out throughout their monthly menstrual cycle. In either case, if they don't address the stress and resolve it, the anxiety (or depression) episodes will become more frequent and severe. The physical illnesses associated with anxiety are also likely to occur and worsen.

Check Your Anxiety Quotient

Please look again at the questionnaire you filled out in Chapter 3 of this book. Now look closely at answer 3 in each scenario. If you frequently circled 3, you may have inappropriately high levels of fear in your life. Do you tend to leave public places like malls or stores if they're even a little bit crowded? (See Question I.) Do certain types of environments consistently make you nervous, edgy, jumpy, or panicky? Do you spend an inordinate amount of time avoiding these situations, elevators, bridges, crowds, or closed-in spaces even if it is a tremendous inconvenience?

If you are alone at home (Question V), are you more likely to import "virtual" companionship by being on the phone or on the Web? Do you have a lot of "performance" anxiety and get easily overwhelmed, tense, or worried if you have to prepare a meal for someone, give a public talk, or perform an individual athletic feat in front of several people, such as shoot a basketball, or putt in golf?

Do you have a lot of "food anxiety" (Question II)? Are you more tentative than most people you know about putting anything in your mouth? Do you avoid eating in public, in crowds, and in most restaurants? Are you able to eat at a buffet knowing that several other people, other than the chef, have been around the food?

Are you frequently edgy and nervous, or worrying about people in your family? Is it nearly impossible for you not to obsess about potential danger that can occur in the lives of the people you care about? Do you frequently get a "bad feeling" that something painful is going to happen to someone you love, only to find out later that your concerns were well-founded? If you frequently endorsed number 3 in the various scenarios in the questionnaire or you seem to experience intuitive anxiety about others' lives, then you may have an anxiety problem.

If, however, you more consistently answered number 4 in the questionnaire, in a variety of specific environmental circumstances you may have *inappropriately low levels of fear;* you may have a tendency to be "numb" to the inherent physical danger or social opinion of others in certain circumstances. You may also have trouble listening to intuition as it speaks to you through your brain-body fear circuits.

Are you drawn to competitive situations where there is limited space? That is, do your competitive juices start to flow in heavy traffic and do you begin to get caught up in vying for "lane" position (Question I)? Does a lot of environmental stimulus, such as noise and flashing lights that overwhelm other people, make you feel calm? Is it easy for you to make requests and demands from waiters? If you are drawn consistently to stimulating situations and noisy, busy areas and crave competition, you may have a tendency to an extreme fearlessness or "numbness" in the face of unsafe, potentially dangerous situations.

Some individuals are stimulus seeking and risk taking because the stimulus or thrill helps pump up their brains—specifically, their attentional circuits. People with ADHD may appear to have this brain style and tend not to pay attention to their fear or rational brain's warning in dangerous situations, increasing their chances of injury or accident.

People who have a risk-taking, stimulus-bound, driven, apparently fearless personality are labeled Type A in our culture. If you truly have this personality, it may be hard for you to be receptive to others' emotions in a relationship, let alone intuit them. People with this personality style are especially prone to heart attacks and stroke, and have a lot of relationship fallout.

Other individuals who are excessively drawn to stimulus and are inappropriately numb to danger or others' feelings often tend to break rules to accomplish their goals. These people may be *sociopaths* and, while their *antisocial behavior* makes the people around them suffer physically and emotionally, they tend not to get physically ill from their own harmful behavior.

A Round Peg in a Square Hole: Modern Psychiatry and Women's Anxiety Disorders

Just as it does with depressive illnesses, traditional psychiatry tries to categorize women's anxiety disorders in the same way men's are classified—even though women's brains are not like men's. Most women don't experience anxiety in a way that fits into distinct categories. Nor do they experience an emotion in separate modalities. For women, an emotion is not just an emotion. But doctors try to pinpoint anxiety as a *feeling state* (anxiety or fear), a *behavior* (a compulsion: a need to hand-wash, count, make lists, pace) or a *thought pattern* (obsession to think about failing, being rejected, criticized, or shamed), or a *body reaction* (panic attack, sweating, shaking, lump in the throat, heart palpitations, shortness of breath, digestive disturbances, hot flashes, cold chills, or other symptoms). Even if a woman's experience did fit neatly into one of the diagnostic categories (generalized anxiety disorder, obsessive-compulsive disorder, panic disorder, or a specific type of phobia), she can develop one or more additional types of anxiety over time. For instance, a woman who initially had an elevator phobia may find her anxiety spread into additional environmental conditions, including heights, closed-in spaces, airplanes, trains, and long car drives. Eventually, it can progress into full-blown panic attacks. It can also change at different times of life as constantly shifting hormone and neurotransmitter levels prime her brain to be anxious, edgy, or plain overwhelmed. Women's problems with anxiety just don't fit into the "neat" diagnostic labels that traditional psychiatry has devised.

The Anxiety-Depression Continuum

Many women who have anxiety ultimately develop problems with anger and depression. Similarly, many women with depression develop anxiety and panic. Because the five basic emotional brain circuits of the feminine brain are not as distinct as men's, women are more likely to experience blends of several emotional states. For instance, women more than men suffer from hard-to-treat combinations of anxiety *and* depression. In the 1950s, many depressed women were treated with Valium, then believed to be an antianxiety drug, and their depression improved. To make matters even more complicated, when women who had suffered from long depressions—and undergone multiple, unsuccessful trials of medicines and therapy—were treated for a "latent" or hidden anxiety disorder, their depression would remit.

If you get treatment for anxiety and panic without addressing imbalances in your other mood circuits—depression, anger, and irritability, or unbridled intuition—the treatment might not work. It could even increase your chance of developing health problems. To have true mental health, you need to balance all five emotions (see Emotional Feng Shui diagram on page 73), and become conscious of the language of your emotional intuition. If one emotion is imbalanced, other emotional and physical imbalances are soon to follow.

Camouflaged Anxiety

Many women suffer from anxiety that is camouflaged by other emotions. The following story illustrates this syndrome. In an airport check-in line, I noticed a couple in front of me. The man, I'll call him Ralph, was a sweet-looking, skinny guy, but his partner, Alice, was a large woman who seemed to be edgy and restless. She kept haranguing him, "I knew we should have allowed two hours to get here. Look at this crowd! Do you have all the bags? Did you lock the car?" The man kept saying, "Yes . . . yes . . . yes . . . everything will be fine." Alice, Ralph, and I headed to the same gate and waited for the our flight. During the forty-five-minute wait before boarding, Alice sat motionless in the chair, while Ralph tried to get her beverages, snacks, magazines. Finally, she snapped at him, "Do me a favor. Don't talk to me . . . leave me alone!" I looked around and saw others also eavesdropping on the "honeymooners," and everyone around had the same look on their faces as if to say, "What an angry bitch!"

Once on the plane, Alice, Ralph, and I were seated in nearby seats. As I settled down, I noticed that Alice and Ralph were already buckled in and were sitting silently, staring straight ahead. While the plane was taxiing down the runway, Alice leaned forward, hands clenched, and started to sweat. She started to fan herself with her hands as if to cool herself down. Right in front of me, in the bulkhead seating, Alice was having a full-blown panic attack. By 25,000 feet, her panic attack stopped. She opened up a box of cookies and started to talk to her husband. It wasn't until then that I realized that Alice was really very anxious, camouflaged by her anger.

Many women with anxiety also suffer from irritability and depression, a syndrome I call "the cows are restless." Before a huge storm, domestic animals do get restless and look very irritable. You can observe the same phenomenon in a veterinarian's waiting room. Some animals are irritable, and when the vet tries to take them out of their cages, they may even snap at the vet's hand.

Like Alice, many women who experience anxiety as irritability and anger may snap at those around them who are trying to help. They may not even know they are nervous until after the anxiety-provoking event has passed. Then, of course, they often are remorseful and depressed at how they acted. Like the animals in the vet's office, their anger is a defense, a wall of protection that covers up anxiety in an attempt to gain control over their environment. Alice may have carped at Ralph to stop talking because she needed silence to cope—to decrease the stimulus that was aggravating a growing inner panic. If a woman with anxiety feels as if she can control the anxiety or what's making her anxious, she will try to control her environment. Some women may start to clean, wash, dust and vacuum as a way to create a soothing sense of order. Others need to make lists. However, if their environment can't fit into their rigid control system—if someone talks to them, if a cat sheds fur on the rug, if someone messes up their desk or makes them late—they lose it. Just like Alice, they snap.

It's not surprising that Alice began to binge on a box of cookies after her panic attack. She was medicating her anxiety and irritability by overeating, which explained her appearance. Many women who suffer from anxiety (complicated by mood problems) tend to be obese.

Walking Around with a "Mad-On": The Anger-Anxiety Connection

Many people use a "prickly," irritable facade to keep others at bay because they are quite anxious inside. The first patient I saw in the ER as a psychiatry resident was in "quiet room one," the euphemism for the holding tank for patients who need a psych evaluation. I walked into the room with my hand outstretched and said politely, "My name is Dr. Schulz. How can I be of help?" A small woman, Bea, said, "Get the hell out of here!" I ran out of the room and got my attending, who told me that Bea had severe anxiety and posttraumatic stress disorder, and was hoping that her anger would repel me; it was her way of keeping people, even well-meaning professionals, at a distance, because she was terrified of everyone. I went back to "quiet room one," stood at the door, and said, "I understand you might be quite anxious to be in a hospital right now, but I'm not going to hurt you. I would like to know how I can help you." Bea's angry facade melted, she eased back in her chair, and began to tell me how a past boyfriend had committed suicide in front of her and how her current boyfriend was physically abusing her.

People who have had severe trauma, witnessed a murder or suicide, been attacked, or suffered some other catastrophe are left with a form of anxiety, PTSD (posttraumatic stress disorder), which causes their body to be hypervigilant, always aroused to keep away potential threats. In addition to other symptoms (see below), people with PTSD can appear irritable and angry. Others have been a source of trauma to them, so their wall of anger protects them by keeping people away. Women with PTSD may have had one relationship after another, until they start to say "never again." They walk around with a "mad-on"—a bitter facade. They gain weight. Their anger and weight serve as protective insulation that keeps away men or anyone who resembles someone who harmed them in the past. But they also keep out opportunities for healing, growth, and development.

Many women with hidden traumas have a lot of trouble losing weight with the normal methods. And the usual antidepressants don't help women with the irritable bad mood. Painful though it may be, these women need to realize that they have an *anxiety problem,* or they are likely to get angrier and heavier.

Trauma Rewires and Activates the Brain's Fear Circuits

Being in a threatening situation overwhelms your coping mechanisms and rewires how you experience fear emotionally, mentally, and physically. Traditionally, PTSD is a brain-body disorder that involves excess fear and anxiety after a traumatic event. The traumatic experience is wired into the brain's and body's memory circuits and something that evokes a memory of the trauma triggers emotional and physical symptoms of anxiety.

Characteristics of PTSD

1. *Involuntary flashes of memory of the trauma.* Memories can occur in images (flashbacks) and thoughts about the trauma that replay over and over in their head like a CD with a skip.

2. *A compulsive need to avoid any memory or reminder of the trauma.* Individuals characteristically avoid talking about the stressful event or shy away from being in any situation reminiscent of the trauma. Over time, they have to avoid more and more situations to escape anxious memories. This leads to restricted career goals, relationships, and social activities in general.

3. *A constant feeling of anxiety and being keyed up leads to "burnout" and a numbing of emotions.* They may not *feel* nervous and they may not *think* that anything around them is anxiety provoking. To the casual observer, they don't *act* nervous, either. Trauma has altered their emotional memory circuits, diminishing their capacity to talk through and release anxiety. Instead, anxiety is shunted from the right brain down into the body, and experienced primarily in physical symptoms of illness. Yet, still, with

only the slightest provocation, they may feel extreme panic, ruminate and worry for hours, and act terrified.

Studies show that children may not experience intense fear, anxiety, or numbness after a trauma. Instead, they may act out the trauma by behaving in a disorganized or agitated manner. In addition, instead of having involuntary memories or flashbacks, children may reenact the trauma while playing with toys or friends. Women, too, are less likely than men to have flashbacks and are more likely to reenact trauma in relationships and in a job setting. Who a woman is attracted to, who she is likely to have a relationship with, and who she is repelled by are in part determined by past traumas.

A Star Burning Out on Broadway

Cathy came to me after her third failed marriage. A dancer on Broadway, Cathy's passion and dramatic personality made her someone you "couldn't take your eyes off" on stage. But her life was spiraling out of control with panic attacks, asthma, reflux, and pain.

Cathy had had a traumatic childhood. Her mother was an actress who brought boyfriend after boyfriend into their home. At age fourteen, Cathy was molested by one of them, a situation that went on for two years until Cathy ran away. By age seventeen, Cathy was getting paid to dance, and by nineteen she was on Broadway. The awards accumulated, and Cathy enjoyed over a decade of stable work. Her relationships, however, weren't so successful. Her first husband turned out to be abusive and a drug addict, her second husband turned out to be gay, and her third husband was having an affair. Cathy's friends told her that she was a bum-magnet: If there was an abusive, addicted, philandering man within ten miles, Cathy would be dating him and living with him in less than a month.

All of Cathy's friends would panic when she began going out with another "bad news" guy, but Cathy was "numb" to their vocal, anxious warnings. She could always see the guy's "good heart," his potential, and she would turn a blind eye to his difficult side. Each time Cathy landed in one of these "dead end" relationships, she would start to get nervous and anxious the week before her period. Her asthma would get worse, causing her to have to use her inhaler more and more between acts when she was working on stage. Cathy would get a lump in her throat and become dizzy and nauseated. Soon after, her "reflux" would cause her to vomit, which made her exhausted and unable to perform. Cathy would also binge and purge after performances, and her panic and anxiety worsened as she watched herself put on the pounds.

Cathy had posttraumatic stress disorder. The sexual abuse that she suffered as a teenager had altered her feminine brain's anxiety circuits. The normal emergency warning system that signals fear when danger is imminent had disconnected. Although everyone around her worried when Cathy met someone whose personality resembled her abuser's, Cathy's own right-brain fear circuits could not send the warning of the danger to the left brain. Instead, the right brain's fear signals would travel down into her body, giving her shortness of breath, asthma, a lump in her throat, nausea, digestive distress, and exhaustion. To numb her physical distress, Cathy would binge on carbohydrates, which ultimately led her to purge and gain weight.

Thankfully, Cathy began to learn the intuitive language behind her body's symptoms, which were essentially panic attacks. She learned that her body could signal when she was making a poor choice in a man, even if her mind was blind to his problems. With nutritional and herbal supplements and medicine (see Chapter 7, "In the Still of the Night"), Cathy learned how to buffer her brain–body fear circuits and build a sense of inner calm and self-confidence.

POSTTRAUMATIC RELATIONSHIP DISORDER

For women, posttraumatic stress disorder (PTSD) is more likely to occur after painful personal relationships than after impersonal trauma like combat or natural disaster. So I generally call this condition posttraumatic relationship disorder (PTRD), since this term more accurately describes how a traumatic relationship has warped the woman's brain circuits for fear, mood, and future relationships.

Childhood sexual abuse, incest, or adolescent rape can rewire brain circuits for love, bonding, trust, and intimacy, so that women tend to love, bond to, trust, and be intimate with people they should in fact fear, people who resemble the perpetrator of their trauma. And they tend to *fear* those they could *love,* those with whom they could actually have a trusting, secure, healing relationship. In effect, with PTRD, the fear and love circuits get *crossed*.

The same can happen with monkeys that have had both amygdalas removed, a key temporal lobe area that is important for encoding and detecting fear, anxiety, and intuition. When monkeys have had a bilateral amygdalectomy, they lose the capacity to feel fear in frightening situations. The monkeys run and hug laboratory workers in white coats—people they should be frightened of. They also try to have sex with inappropriate partners. These monkeys, called Kluver-Bucy monkeys, are said to have psychic blindness, a numbness. Their fear and love emotional circuits have switched: They lose the capacity to make correct choices even though all the indicators are clearly in front of them, right before their very eyes.

Posttraumatic relationship disorder alters the amygdalas and other brain areas so that women tend to have "psychic blindness" to dangerous situations, especially relationships.

NOT ALL WOMEN WHO EXPERIENCE TRAUMA EXPERIENCE POSTTRAUMATIC STRESS DISORDER

Not all women suffer from PTSD or PTRD after a trauma. Women are less likely to experience a posttraumatic rewiring of their feminine brain's fear circuits if they:

1. Are raised in families with healthy patterns of trust, intimacy, and boundaries
2. Have a great capacity to tolerate fear and threat
3. Have demonstrated an ability to cope with emotional loss
4. Know how to recruit social support from friends and family during stressful times.

However, women are more likely to experience long-term emotional, mental, and physical effects of trauma if they were raised in a family that didn't deal well with stressful changes in the environment. Caregivers play a key role in appropriately responding to a child's fear. A responsive parent who soothes the child, letting her know she's safe and secure, will help entrain appropriate frontal-lobe skills to soothe fear and calm emotional and physical reactions to stress. However, if no one appropriately responds to the child's fear, her brain circuits become more and more sensitive to environmental stress, and appropriate, lifesaving emotional and physical fear reactions are replaced with the maladaptive symptoms of PTSD. In response to even the slightest changes in her environment, a woman with these rewired fear circuits has either overreactive or underreactive emotional, mental, behavioral, and physical reactions.

Prostitutes are more likely to have survived childhood sex abuse. Rape victims are more likely to be raped again. Women who have experienced physical abuse as a child are more likely to be in a physically abusive relationship as adults. Pain and stress are more likely to be recorded in body memory by the temporal lobe's amygdala, where it evokes physical health reactions, like digestive complaints and heart palpitations. The hippocampus, the memory system that puts fear into words and creates conscious thought, is less apt to lay down traumatic memories. When a woman has had a life-defining, emotionally traumatizing experience, the frontal lobe–hippocampal circuits are disconnected in a way so she is less likely to talk about it. She will, however, reenact the trauma—not in art or play therapy as a child would—on the biggest playing field: relationships.

Previous traumatic experience is very likely to shape your unconscious behavior, and your personal choices in mates, jobs, and social contacts. You are less likely to understand why you feel the attraction that you feel, because during traumatic stress, stress neuropeptides norepinephrine and cortisol disconnect the left-brain "talk" memory systems, but simultaneously turn up the volume on the right-brain "action" memory system. Your brain and body are primed emotionally to return to the relationship "scene of the crime," and react and reenact that past traumatic relationship over and over again.

Baby mice who are raised in a locked box where they are repeatedly shocked tend to return to that box when set free as adults. Despite the genetic differences between a woman and a mouse, unfortunately, we do tend to act similarly when it comes to trauma.

Previous traumatic experience preheats and warms up the brain pathways, increasing your chances of having the same type of relationship again and again. Even if you try to think it through, and say to yourself, "I am never going to fall into that trap again," you may be pulled back toward it like a moth to a flame. Your frontal-lobe reasoning circuits will murmur, "Think this through. You don't want to go through all that pain, do you?" But your temporal-lobe amygdala, body-memory circuits will scream louder. What would you be more likely to hear?

"He's so exciting."

"She really just understands me."

"Being in his arms feels like I've come home again."

"I feel like we've known each other for years and years, even though we just met."

The greater the trauma, the more inescapably stressful it seems, the longer it lasts, and the greater its intensity, the more likely the feminine brain-body circuits will be shaped into creating a chain of relationships that mimic the trauma. Unlike the male combat veteran who has flashbacks, visual memories of the trauma, a woman will replay the memory over and over again in the cinema verité of her life until she gets the proper help to stop the pattern. Alone, she can't prevent herself from being attracted to reenacting the trauma any more than an alcoholic can stop drinking by himself without proper treatment.

Each time she chooses the "loser," the "creep," that "bum," whatever "prototype" can play the part of the perpetrator, the deeper the pattern gets engraved in the memory networks of her brain and body.

In fact, the brain's visual and attentional pathways that could actually direct her to healthier mates fall into disuse. Abused women are attracted to the same people who mistreat them because their brains become molded in such a way that that's the only kind of person they tend to *notice*. The nicer, normal men and women don't seem ever to make it on the screen of their relationship radar.

The Anatomy of Numbness: Disconnected Emotional and Intuition Circuits

During the intense stress of a traumatic experience, the brain releases opiates and painkiller molecules. When a woman is physically, sexually, or emotionally abused, her brain has the capacity to release the equivalent of 8 milligrams of a natural opiate that is just like the morphine you get after a painful surgical procedure. The PSA morphine pump (patient self-administered pump) releases only 3 to 5 milligrams of morphine during the acute recovery period from a surgical procedure. So, during the intense stress of the trauma, or its reenactments, a woman can actually be unaware of any fear, since her emotional circuits have been numbed. Yet the fear circuits can still communicate quite loudly that there is danger through noticeable changes in her health.

Palpitations, shortness of breath, abdominal crampy pain, hormonal changes, hot flashes, cold chills, rashes, hives, and a variety of other symptoms may be the first and only signs for some women that something is threatening in a relationship. Their physical intuition is letting them know that they are in a familiar situation in which they or someone they love has been threatened or hurt in the past. In one woman I treated, her body's outbreaks of irritable bowl/ulcerative colitis were the first intuition that her husband was once again having an affair.

Have you ever been told you were "too sensitive"? Perhaps you're one of those women whose brain's fear circuits have become supersensitized to even the most minute environmental changes. Even the most bland, minimally stressful change in their environment makes their body scream with bladder, gut, and eating disorders. This exaggerated sensitivity can be quite disabling. Symptoms in your heart, lungs, GI tract, and immune system can actually, over time, metamorphose into illness that can be serious. Women with a history of abuse may suffer for years from these problems, unable to make the connection because their left brain's capacity to talk about it has been muted.

PTRD may also leave a woman unable to (1) articulate what she's feeling, (2) know when she is afraid, (3) know who she should be afraid of, and (4) know when she has an impending health problem. Yet, ironically, she may have an enhanced intuitive capacity to sense when someone she loves is in a dangerous situation or has failing health.

Every Woman Has a Blind Spot

Our "blind spot" is in love and relationships about which we don't have a good perspective. All women's brains, especially our amygdalas, are shaped to one degree or another by painful and stressful experiences, whether it's a conflicted relationship with a parent, brother, sister, or relative, or someone who challenged our capacity to cope. Some of us have a "mother complex," others have a "father complex," or problem with bosses or teachers, but we try to master this history over and over in our lives. We may not see how we are falling into the same problematic relationship pattern again, but often a close friend or relative can have painful but astute insights into this core problem.

Don't Put Me Through This Again: I've Suffered Enough!

On the 1970s *Mary Tyler Moore Show,* Mary's friend Rhoda's mother was always "kvetching" and worrying about something. As Mary and Rhoda experienced the normal problems faced by adult single women in a big city, Mrs. Morgenstern would say, "Don't put me through this, I've suffered enough!" Mrs. Morgenstern was "pre-worrying," picking up intuitively when something could or would go wrong and experiencing anxiety. As the classic "Jewish mother," Mrs. Morgenstern used guilt instead of Valium to get relief from anxiety, thinking that if she could influence Mary's and Rhoda's choices, she wouldn't get sick with worry. The cycle of maternal caring, mother's intuition, guilt, and control is not exclusive to a single religious tradition. In *Moonstruck,* Olympia Dukakis played an Italian mother who was skilled in using "Catholic guilt," and the mother in *My Big Fat Greek Wedding* worked in a restaurant, giving her children a "side dish" of guilt as well.

Like a Geiger counter, which can detect dangerous levels of radioactivity, the feminine brain can easily pick up "hot spots," the danger in the lives of her loved ones. Women for centuries have been intuitively plugged in to the growing pains of their children and have carried the suffering by getting sick with worry. Often, a daughter is "guilted" into curtailing the part of her life that's provoking her mother's anxiety. And if she *doesn't* curb her behavior, the daughter herself may intuitively pick up her mother's anxiety and become a nervous wreck.

Our feminine brain's enhanced connectivity makes it difficult to ignore or distract ourselves when an anxious intuition is screaming at us that someone we care about is making a dangerous mistake. By being an emotional environmental barometer that registers stress and distress in others, the feminine brain may anatomically have an evolutionary advantage of perceiving potential danger to others, but also may predispose women to excessive levels of anxiety and anxiety disorders. Normal cyclic changes in progesterone may enhance this protective ability. Lowered progesterone during the menstrual cycle may amplify our ability to intuitively feel fear and anxiety when there's danger. Elevated levels of progesterone may give us a break from being so plugged into the lives of loved ones.

Most women who experience anxiety have clusters of symptoms that may involve several traditional diagnoses, but the feminine brain doesn't usually fit the rigid classification seen in psychiatric diagnostic manuals. Essentially, every one of the classical anxiety disorders has excessive activity in one or more components of the fear circuit. In either panic disorders, phobias, obsessive-compulsive disorders, anxiety due to health problems or addictions, or generalized anxiety disorder, you have:

a. Excessive *feelings* of nervousness or fear
b. Excessive *thoughts* (obsessions), i.e., worrying
c. Excessive *actions,* behaviors associated with anxiety *(compulsions)*
d. Unpleasant *health reactions* that are biochemically associated with the brain's fear circuits

Panic disorder is mostly the product of hyperactive *health reactions* associated with the fear circuit. Like a seven-alarm fire, seven organs scream out warning signals even if you aren't aware there's anything to feel frightened about:

1. Your *heart* has palpitations, you feel chest pain.
2. Your *lungs* feel like someone is sitting on your chest. You feel shortness of breath. Your allergies and asthma act up.
3. Your *digestive tract* gets "upset," you feel nauseous, you may vomit or easily gag. You have a hard time swallowing pills. You

may get abdominal cramps, diarrhea, constipation, abdominal bloating, and distension.

4.   Your *temperature regulation* system goes on the fritz. You develop hot flashes, cold chills, and sweating.

5.   Your *muscles* tend to tremble and shake. You feel keyed up and jittery *or* weak and exhausted.

6.   Your *brain and nerves* become hypersensitive to small sounds, sights, and sensations; "little" things like lint, spots, or other "imperfections" in your environment bother you.

7.   Your *balance system* gets unbalanced. You feel dizzy, unsteady, light-headed, or faint.

Over time, changes in thoughts and behaviors can also occur. Someone who has repetitive panic attacks associated with panic disorder, for instance, will think she is losing control, and will try to control her environment and the activities of those around her with rules about who drives the car, how long she can be away from home, and how many people she feels safe to be around. Crowds, public transit, and elevators may make her uncomfortable, but she may allow herself to be in these environments if accompanied by a loved one. Over time, she may come to believe that so many elements in the environment can trigger an attack that she doesn't leave her home, a type of panic disorder called agoraphobia.

Phobias also cause panic: the belief that something that most people would consider harmless is terrifying. Phobias can be about something in the environment (i.e., snake, blood) or a usual human activity (i.e., speaking, being in closed-in spaces).

Obsessive-compulsive disorder (OCD) is an anxiety disorder that causes obsessive repetitive thoughts and compulsive behaviors. A repetitive thought replays in the woman's head like a gerbil on a wheel. Somehow, the woman begins to believe that if she performs some action (such as washing her hands, or placing things in a certain order) or mentally prays, counts, or repeats certain words, she will protect herself and others.

Control fanatic, a milder form of obsessionality and compulsivity: To reduce their anxiety, some women are preoccupied with creating an environment around them of perfection, orderliness, and control. The operative word is *control.* They become so preoccupied with controlling the details, rules, schedules in their lives *and* the lives of everyone around them, that their lack of flexibility and vulnerability creates pain and distance in their relationships. This type of anxiety, obsessionality, and compulsivity is much more common in women than the OCD seen in Jack Nicholson's obsessive cleaning ritual in *As Good As It Gets.* Although we may "ooh" and "aah" at their manicured French gardens or their impeccably organized laundry rooms, these women live silently painful lives because their loved ones rarely can tolerate such control or live up to their standards of perfectionism.

Generalized anxiety disorder is a condition in which a person's thoughts are consumed with worry. The excessive worry and emotional anxiety causes "rug burns" in the brain and body. It takes a lot of energy to worry. Over time, general anxiety disorder leads to fatigue, restlessness, muscle tension, pain in muscles and joints, and insomnia.

Anxiety disorder due to a health condition, medicine, or substance abuse. Illnesses change brain and body chemistry to a significant degree that disrupts the fear circuits. Changes in body chemistry, infection, cancer, or inflammation can stimulate brain-body fear circuits and create anxious, nervous feelings and a "sense of foreboding."

In the depression–disease domino effect, mood disorders precipitate illness in the body, and illness in the body causes depression, mania, and irritability. Unrelenting anxiety creates some of these same biochemical changes. Chronic anxiety can also neurochemically disrupt moods and cause secondary problems. If your mood or anxiety stays imbalanced for sustained periods of time, your health is at risk. And, if you have a health problem, say, heart arrhythmia, palpitations, lung disorders like asthma and emphysema, inappropriate treatment may cause an anxiety disorder.

Anxiety problems can also be precipitated by *digestive disorders* like gastroesophageal reflux disease (GERD), irritable bowel syndrome, Crohn's disease; *dermatologic disorders* like hives and psoriasis; *ear problems* like dizziness and vertigo; and *hormonal* imbalances like thyroid disorders and premenstrual and perimenopausal changes in estrogen and progesterone. So it makes no sense to say that nervousness and anxiety reside in the brain. Panic, anxiety, rumination, obsessions, and compulsions—all the feelings, thoughts, and behaviors associated with hyperactive brain circuits—affect your health.

Use of alcohol, stimulants like caffeine, ephedra, amphetamines, and other drugs can also cause anxiety. Stimulants may push an already "hyperactive brain fear circuit" over the edge into panic and edginess. Anyone with a history of panic attacks, phobias, obsessive-compulsive disorder, or generalized tendency toward anxiety is probably better staying away from caffeinated beverages, cold remedies, and diet aids that contain caffeine or other stimulants.

Some medicines for attention deficit disorder, anxiety, and depression may put you into a panicked and apprehensive state. Ritalin, Cylert, and other ADD meds commonly make many individuals tense and edgy, especially at higher doses. Prozac, Effexor, and some of the more "stimulating" antidepressants (see Chapter 4) may also trigger panic and other symptoms. If you have a tendency to be moody and irritable, certain sleep medicines and antiallergy agents can cause anxiety and confusion. Benadryl, Ativan, Xanax, and other anticholinergic medicines lower the neurotransmitter acetylcholine, and so may unleash panic, distress, and a sense of being overwhelmed. People with Alzheimer's or other memory disorders may also get anxious and unhinged on these same medicines.

Anxiety and Addiction

Women who struggle with anxiety are more likely to drink, smoke, overeat, or engage in some other type of behavior to counter their anxiety and turn off the insistent intuitive voice that is telling them something is wrong. Nearly half of these women suffer from obesity, and go from diet to diet, even trying plastic surgery, stomach stapling, and gastric bypass surgery. Yet none of these weight loss methods can have a lasting effect unless a woman addresses her addictive use of food. If she doesn't learn how to manage nervousness and anxiety, the pounds will creep back on no matter what she puts in her mouth or does to her body.

Anxiety, Attention Deficit Disorder, Addiction, and Drama

Women with ADD may be especially prone to complex combinations of anxiety, depression, and moodiness. Since stimulants like Ritalin can frequently help, women with ADD and anxiety are more likely to become dependent not just upon alcohol and other addictive substances, but also on stimulants, both chemical (like cocaine) and environmental (like drama). In most women who suffer from chronic anxiety, stimulants increase fearfulness and panic. But stimulants can help some women with ADD to improve their attentional problems, and some of these women tend to create drama in their lives because it somehow feels comforting.

Anxiety is like finding ants in your house. At first, you may have only one or two, but if you don't find out what they're after, they multiply and attract others, until the next thing you know you're overrun. One day, for instance, I found two big ants in my kitchen near the antique red gumball machine I stock with peanut M&M's. One was eating a small M&M fragment that was sitting on the counter nearby. Another ant had somehow crawled into the gumball machine and was sitting on an M&M munching away. For the longest time, I watched the huge ant on the counter with his feet tucked behind him eating that piece of chocolate. It was fascinating. I thought that there was no harm in letting two ants eat the M&M's. I figured I could share. The next morning, as I was lying in bed slowly waking up, I wondered, "What if those two ants told their friends about the gumball machine with the M&M's?" I went into the kitchen to start the morning coffee and couldn't believe my eyes. The gumball machine that had previously contained a single ant was now filled with hundreds. They had stripped off the coatings of the multicolored candies, leaving white, chalk-like lumps. Apparently, there *is* harm in allowing two ants to stay in your kitchen.

As with ants, one worry can turn into two, multiplying until we are so filled with dread, jumpiness, and distress that we feel as if we have "ants on the brain." Do not try to overlook even one source of anxiety—find the real cause—or your brain circuits will get so preoccupied by worries that you'll have trouble focusing your attention on life around you. All the circuits will be busy.

For women whose brain's fear circuits fire inappropriately when there is no clear and present danger, it is possible to insulate their wiring better so they don't misfire so readily, with a variety of therapies. We'll get into those in detail in Chapter 7.

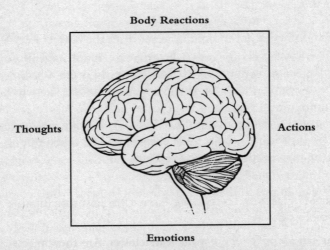

Body Reactions
Thoughts   Actions
Emotions

(Figure 9. Mood and Fear: Drawing of brain with body reactions, thoughts, actions, and emotions.)

Learn Your Feminine Brain's Unique Language for Fear

I hope that these pages have helped you begin to see how your unique feminine brain is wired for fear and anxiety. By looking at your thought patterns and examining your actions and behavior, you can figure out when and how frequently you experience anxiety. And by examining your body's symptoms and health patterns, you can spot if you have overactive or underactive circuits for anxiety.

There are seven basic areas, or emotional fear centers, in our lives in which we experience fear. They include:

- *First Emotional Fear Center: Safety and Security in the World:* Safety and security in a family, an organization of some kind, and the world in general.
- *Second Emotional Fear Center: Relationships and Finances:* Safety and security about relationships with a significant other, or feeling confident with money.
- *Third Emotional Fear Center: Responsibility and Work:* Safety and security about handling responsibility or in work or a career.
- *Fourth Emotional Fear Center: Emotional Expression and Nurturance:* Safety and security about expressing a variety of feelings, including fear, anger, sadness, love, and joy; feeling safe when someone tries to nurture you or feeling confident taking care of others.
- *Fifth Emotional Fear Center: Communication, Will, and Timing:* Safety and security when you try to communicate what you believe to someone at the right time and with the correct intensity.
- *Sixth Emotional Fear Center: Perception, Thought, and Morality:* Security in allowing yourself and others to have a variety of ways of seeing things in the world, and having a variety of opinions.
- *Seventh Emotional Fear Center: Life Purpose, Mortality, and the Spiritual World:* Security about your purpose in life; finding peace in a spiritual world that has good and evil.

WHAT ARE MY *FEELINGS* TELLING ME ABOUT MY FEMININE BRAIN'S WIRING FOR FEAR?

See if you can identify where your fears cluster. Are they in some areas more than others? The following self-test may help.

First Emotional Fear Center: Safety and Security
- ❏ I am afraid of being alone.
- ❏ I am anxious when a loved one is in pain or is going through a difficult stage of life.
- ❏ I am afraid of change.
- ❏ I am afraid of illness.
- ❏ I am afraid of heights, closed spaces. I am afraid to trust people.
- ❏ I am afraid of being helpless.

Second Emotional Fear Center: Relationships and Finances
- ❏ I am afraid of intimacy.
- ❏ I am afraid of ending a relationship.
- ❏ I am afraid of losing money or failing financially.
- ❏ I am afraid of beginning a relationship.
- ❏ I am afraid of having sex.
- ❏ I am afraid of having children, being pregnant.
- ❏ I am afraid of being controlled in a relationship.

Third Emotional Fear Center: Responsibility and Work
- ❏ I am afraid of making a decision.
- ❏ I am afraid of changing a job.
- ❏ I am afraid of commitment or responsibility.
- ❏ I am afraid of competition.
- ❏ I am afraid of being judged or criticized.
- ❏ I am afraid of losing control of my environment.

Fourth Emotional Fear Center: Emotional Expression and Nurturance
- ❏ I am afraid of getting angry in front of another person.
- ❏ I am afraid of having anyone take care of me.
- ❏ I am anxious when someone is angry.
- ❏ I am afraid of accepting help.

Fifth Emotional Fear Center: Communication, Will, and Timing
- ❏ I am afraid of speaking publicly.
- ❏ I am afraid of asserting my opinion.
- ❏ I am afraid of saying "no" when someone asks me to do something.
- ❏ I get anxious when I have to wait.

Sixth Emotional Fear Center: Perception, Thought, and Morality
- ❏ I am afraid when someone disagrees with me.
- ❏ I get anxious if I don't know every detail of a situation.
- ❏ I get nervous if I see a flaw or imperfection in something or someone else does.
- ❏ I get nervous in a situation that is unclear or has ambiguity.
- ❏ I get nervous in a situation that is not rational.
- ❏ I get anxious if I or someone else breaks a rule.
- ❏ I am afraid to take risks.

Seventh Emotional Fear Center: Life Purpose, Mortality, and the Spiritual World
- ❏ I am afraid of aging.
- ❏ I am afraid of dying.
- ❏ I am afraid of God.
- ❏ I am afraid of evil.

WHAT ARE MY *THOUGHTS* TELLING ME ABOUT MY FEMININE BRAIN'S WIRING FOR FEAR?

As in the preceding section on feelings, certain thoughts are associated with fear and tend to cluster in the seven basic emotional areas. Do many of these thoughts percolate in your mind?

First Emotional Fear Center: Safety and Security in the World
- ❏ Others' motives are usually suspect.
- ❏ I must always be on guard in families or groups of people. I am frequently a scapegoat.
- ❏ I must be in charge of the group. I must make order if things get chaotic.
- ❏ I don't have the ability to support myself and be alone in the world.
- ❏ I am going to lose someone I love.
- ❏ If someone I know or love is making a mistake, I must do something to change him or her.
- ❏ I am helpless.
- ❏ I am going to get hurt or harmed.
- ❏ I am going to die soon.

Second Emotional Fear Center: Relationships and Finances
- ❏ I usually get rejected, abandoned, and betrayed in my love relationships.
- ❏ No matter what I do, how well I plan, I always manage to have financial disasters.
- ❏ I'm going to lose something valuable.
- ❏ If I don't have the upper hand in a relationship, I could get hurt.

Third Emotional Fear Center: Responsibility and Work
- ❏ People frequently criticize me and disapprove of my work performance.
- ❏ If people know the real me, they will reject me.
- ❏ I can't risk making decisions because I'm afraid of failure.
- ❏ What other people think of me doesn't matter.
- ❏ We live in the jungle; only the strong survive.
- ❏ I can get away with things. I don't need to worry about bad consequences.
- ❏ No matter how hard I try, I am never good enough.
- ❏ If I try my best and succeed, I will lose the love of some people who are close to me.

Fourth Emotional Fear Center: Emotional Expression and Nurturance
- ❏ I can't tolerate unpleasant feelings.
- ❏ I can't get enough help and assistance.
- ❏ If I'm not needed or depended upon in a relationship, I may be left or abandoned.

Fifth Emotional Fear Center: Communication, Will, and Timing
- ❏ When I say something, I get easily embarrassed or misunderstood.

Sixth Emotional Fear Center: Perception, Thought, Morality
- ❏ If I ignore a problem, it will go away.
- ❏ I should only focus on the bright side of a situation and put a blind eye to its difficult side.
- ❏ If I'm not right, I will lose control.

Seventh Emotional Fear Center: Life Purpose, Mortality, and the Spiritual World
- ❏ God has it in for me.
- ❏ My life destiny is to have pain and to struggle.

WHAT IS MY *BEHAVIOR* TELLING ME ABOUT MY FEMININE BRAIN'S WIRING FOR FEAR AND ANXIETY?

Do you or someone near you notice you act in the following ways? Many of these patterns of behavior are similar to those of moody and irritable people (see "What does my behavior tell me about my brain's wiring for mood and moodiness?" in Chapter 4).

- ❑ I avoid crowds.
- ❑ If I'm home alone, I'm usually on the phone or on the Web.
- ❑ I avoid putting on a dinner party, or doing anything in which I could fail or disappoint others.
- ❑ I have to be in control and in charge of my environment. If things aren't in a precise order, I get edgy. I check my Daytimer or schedule repeatedly since this makes me feel that everything is in order. If we're going somewhere, I need to drive.
- ❑ There are many foods I won't order in restaurants because you just don't know how much you can trust restaurants these days.
- ❑ I avoid buffets, or other areas where multiple people have access or contact with your food.
- ❑ I avoid public bathrooms if I can. I'd rather try to "hold it" until I get home.
- ❑ I usually am "medicated" with pills, alcohol, or sugar when I fly, because I hate it so much.
- ❑ I avoid escalators and elevators if I can.
- ❑ I put off things like taxes until the last minute.
- ❑ I never order or buy things on the Internet. No matter what they say, it's not safe.
- ❑ I rarely go to a concert or other event in one of those big civic center auditoriums. Being in a crowd of thousands of people is not my idea of fun.
- ❑ I don't usually go to horror movies.
- ❑ I usually walk very quickly when I am anxious. Sometimes I pace.
- ❑ When I'm nervous, I talk a lot about things that seem irrelevant.
- ❑ When I'm nervous, my hands or feet shake.
- ❑ Sometimes when I am anxious, I can't speak or move.

People with mood disorders often act the same way as people with anxiety. Do you find yourself acting in the following ways?

❏ I crave and frequently eat carbohydrates in the form of pasta, rice, bread, and sweets, or I maintain tight control over my carbohydrate intake.
❏ I am sensitive to noise, papers rustling, babies crying, smells; I can easily get nauseated or gag. Lint, cat hair, spots, and imperfection make me anxious and irritable.
❏ I shop and look through catalogues to relax.

What Is My *Health* Telling Me about My Feminine Brain's Wiring for Fear and Anxiety?

Your physical health is affected by your brain's fear circuits, and health problems can also precipitate anxiety and fear because of the *anxiety-disease domino effect.*

These symptoms or illnesses can be organized into seven different types of health problems:

1. The bones, joints, muscles, and immune system
   ❏ Do you frequently get jittery and shaky?
   ❏ Do you suffer from hair loss or hirsutism (excess hair growth)?
   ❏ Do you frequently get skin problems like rashes or hives?
   ❏ After you have been frightened or stressed, do you get a cold or do your allergies worsen within twenty-four to forty-eight hours?
2. Reproductive organs, including uterus, ovaries, cervix, and vagina
   ❏ Do you have irregular periods after an especially stressful or upsetting time?
   ❏ Do you frequently have hot flashes and/or cold chills?
3. The digestive system
   ❏ Do you have urinary frequency, going to the bathroom eight or nine times a day?
   ❏ Do you have frequent crampy abdominal pain?
   ❏ Do you frequently have digestive distress in the form of diarrhea or constipation? Abdominal bloating or distension?
   ❏ Do you easily get nauseated, vomit, or gag? Do you have a hard time swallowing pills?
4. The chest area, including heart, lungs, and breast
   ❏ Do you have a problem with arrhythmia or heart palpitations?

❏ Do you get episodes of shortness of breath, heartburn, or chest pressure?

5. The neck region (cervical vertebrae, thyroid, teeth, mouth, gums)

❏ Do you have Graves' disease (hyperthyroidism) or Hashimoto's disease (hypothyroidism)?

❏ If you have thyroid disease, is it hard for you to get a stable dose of thyroid replacement to treat your symptoms?

❏ Do you frequently feel a lump in your throat?

6. The brain, eyes, ears, and nose region

❏ Do you have frequent episodes of dizziness?

❏ Do you have problems remembering what you've read?

❏ Do you frequently notice your attention wandering? Are you easily distractible?

❏ Do you have trouble falling asleep or staying asleep?

7. Life-threatening health problems

❏ Heart disease

❏ Depression and its life-threatening illness (see Chapter 4, "Blue Moon")

As you went through the above list of *feelings, thoughts, actions,* and *health reactions* associated with the feminine brain's fear circuits, did you find yourself checking many of the items? You may have anxiety and hyperactive/underactive fear circuits. In the next chapter, you will learn how to work with fear and how it appears in your feelings, thoughts, behavior, and physical reactions. By doing this, you will learn to decipher the intuitive messages behind your fear and anxiety to feel better emotionally and physically.

SEVEN

In the Still of the Night: Tune Up Your Levels of Anxiety and Calm

One person's excitement is another person's anxiety, so in this chapter I'll help you figure out how to balance your brain's circuits so you have appropriate levels of awareness or anxiety, along with healthy levels of calm and serenity.

Before you can treat anxiety and its related disorders, you need to know your brain's "setpoint" for peace and serenity. A *lower threshold* for distress may give you special intuitive and creative gifts, but may also make you prone to phobias, panic attacks, and resulting illnesses. A *higher threshold* for distress may give you special gifts and skills that may help you excel in athletics and competitive careers, but make you less aware of others' feelings.

Consider the following questions.

What Is Normal Anxiety for You and What Is Pathological?

My idea of peace and serenity is cycling at 100 rpm, listening to fast disco music while reading medical journals. My friend Mildred prefers writing against a background of Baroque music or soothing vocals to feel relaxed. Working in that environment makes me very sleepy. It takes less environmental stimulus for Mildred to experience anxiety or excitement, but much more environmental energy and stimulus for me to feel energized and peaceful.

A mutual friend, Norma, has an even lower threshold for anxiety and the smallest changes in her environment can provoke uneasiness and stress. She maintains calm by keeping a very stable daily schedule, arriving at her office precisely at 7:00 a.m. On Saturday mornings at 9:00 a.m. she pays her bills and vacuums the house. Not surprisingly, Norma's family is prone to anxiety disorders. Many of her sisters and brothers have phobias or panic attacks and suffer from many of the health problems associated with hyperactive brain fear circuits, including irritable bowel syndrome and diverticulitis.

The "Stressometer" Scale: Assessing How Your Brain Handles Risk and Stress

Does taking a risk, being in a challenging situation, make you feel anxious? Or are you slightly energized—so you thrive on challenge and risk?

Where do you find your brain style on the *Stressometer Scale?* (Figure 12)? Is it:

1. Anxiety-prone, hypersensitive to stress?
2. Relatively anxiety-free, craving risk and stress?
3. Balanced: accepting risk and managing stress in a healthy way?

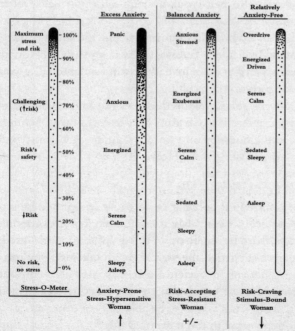

Figure 12. The Stressometer: How easily do you get anxious? How much risk are you comfortable with?

How do you feel during times of maximum stress, no stress, or stress levels in between?

Women who are prone to *anxiety* tend to feel calm only when they feel very safe and have little risk to their health or other areas of their lives. Risk and challenge make them anxious.

But our lives do change and personal growth involves taking risks. Individuals who suffer from anxiety tend to avoid taking personal risks at home, in money matters, or in their work. This kind of "avoidant" behavior tends to prevent them from accomplishing what they want in life.

In contrast, women who are relatively anxiety-free, who are Type A, risk-craving, and stimulus-bound, tend to thrive in stressful, stimulating circumstances. The anxiety "intuitive warning system" seems to be disengaged and these women learn to thrive and feel rewarded with increasing challenge. But they also tend to go into overdrive and fall apart when they stop working or competing. They often enjoy vibrant health during the early years of overworking, but develop later illnesses, especially coronary artery disease and addiction. If they retire, they get depressed and sick.

Women with balanced anxiety do become anxious, but only during periods of maximum stress.

Your sleep habits can also help you determine the normal level of calmness and excitability for your brain and body. No matter how noisy my surroundings are, I can always fall asleep. In fact, unless I am in a highly stimulating environment, I fall asleep because of my narcolepsy. Alice, with her anxiety-prone brain, requires absolute darkness and quiet to fall asleep. She suffers from lifelong insomnia.

If you are *anxiety-prone, stress hypersensitive,* you can buffer your brain and body. Later in this chapter, you will learn how to fortify your fear circuits so you can use the emotional and intuitive guidance behind your anxiety to meet day-to-day challenges. However, if you have a *relatively anxiety-free, risk-craving, stimulus-bound* brain, you can learn to slow down your brain circuits and listen to their warning signals. Your brain will require unique solutions to help it become more aware of fear and its underlying intuition. And even if you have a *balanced anxiety, risk-accepting, stress-resistant* brain style, there is something in this chapter for you. During certain periods of hormonal change, illness, or catastrophic loss, your anxiety-resistant brain may become not-so-resistant. You may need some of the nutritional, pharmacological, behavioral, or other tools in this chapter to get you through a crisis—and you may be able to help other anxiety-prone brain types around you with the same methods.

Additional Factors to Consider

The solutions that will help you successfully manage your anxiety depend upon whether or not:

- You medicate your anxiety with food, drink, or activity
- A similar anxiety disorder runs in the family
- Your anxiety coexists with a difficult-to-treat medical problem
- Your anxiety has been resistant to many treatments already
- Your anxiety is aggravated by a problem with depression
- You are sensitive to drugs in general and usually develop side effects whenever you use them
- You have a frightening or stressful situation in your life that would make anyone anxious

Let's examine how these factors can complicate how you treat your anxiety problem and clarify which solutions are more likely to work.

Do you medicate your fear and anxiety? Do you use the following habits to deal with fear, rejection, criticism, or failure?

a.   Drink alcohol
b.   Gamble
c.   Smoke cigarettes
d.   Meditate
e.   Enter online chat rooms
f.   Smoke marijuana or take other illegal drugs
g.   Take Valium, Ativan, Xanax, or some other benzodiazepine-related medicine
h.   Take Valerian or kava kava
i.   Overeat, binge eat, catalogue shop, surf the Web, or use compulsive behavior to calm you down, help you sleep, or make you feel more in control
j.   Compulsively exercise
k.   Cling to unhealthy relationships

If you regularly drink alcohol, smoke, or engage in some other activity on this list, you may be trying unconsciously to change or chemically alter your brain's fear circuits by numbing them. Alcohol, known as "liquid courage," is an antianxiety agent and hits many of the brain receptors that classic antianxiety drugs do—Valium, Ativan, Xanax and other benzodiazepines. When you take any of these substances daily, you may not even know you have problems with anxiety because they numb or eliminate it. You can figure out if your fear circuits have been medicated in this way by stopping any of these substances or behaviors entirely for twenty-four to forty-eight hours. If you start to have the prototypical feelings, thoughts, behavior, or body health reactions associated with fear, you know you have problems with anxiety. If you feel apprehensive, tense, begin to worry, move around nervously, begin to sweat, get cold chills or hot flashes, develop shortness of breath, become jittery, shaky, have heart palpitations, diarrhea, constipation, or other typical reactions (see Emotional Feng Shui chart in Chapter 3), then your brain's fear circuits have gotten used to being "dumbed down." As a doctor, I have yet to meet a patient whose mental and physical health wasn't negatively affected by an addiction of one sort or another. Medications may give you temporary emotional relief, but numbing fear and anxiety circuits "dumbs" you down, removing a significant but often painful part of our feminine intelligence.

Anxiety isn't pleasant, so it may make some sense to medicate it away, but disconnecting your brain's fear circuits is akin to taking the battery out of your fire alarm. You lose the uneasiness that comes with being an "environmental emotional barometer," but you also disconnect from a key source of intuition, leaving you blind or seemingly unconcerned about risky or dangerous situations in your career, relationships, or world. You may feel better, but you don't want to become like Alfred E. Newman, *Mad* magazine's "What, me worry?" guy. Being cool or indifferent in the face of risk or danger may make you feel socially more in control, but you lose 20 percent of your brain's emotional intuition circuits. If your doctor prescribed a medicine that she told you would remove 20 percent of your vision or hearing, you'd think twice before taking it. However, because this form of feminine insight is painful (or "dysphoric") to experience, women turn to alcohol, cigarettes, or overeating to "dumb it down." But there are other ways to keep the suffering to a minimum and still maintain access to the critical intelligence that your anxiety provides. We'll get to these in a few pages.

When You Numb Yourself, You Dumb Yourself

If you compulsively consume something or have to be consumed by some activity like gambling or sex to escape fear and anxiety, or to feel "more alive," by definition you have an addiction. Addictive eating, gambling, smoking, drinking, and sex have the same biochemical effect on the brain's area for reward. They change your brain's setpoint for anxiety or stress, tricking you into feeling more peaceful, tranquil, and courageous. These activities numb your brain's anxiety circuits in a way similar to Valium, Xanax, and other benzodiazepine antianxiety drugs, by releasing the same neurochemicals: GABA, opiates, and serotonin.

So whether you eat it, smoke it, drink it, do it over and over again, or take it in the form of a pill prescribed by your doctor, addiction disconnects your anxiety and fear circuits, makes you numb, and ultimately disconnects critical circuits for intelligence and intuition. You won't see problems that are coming your way, especially associated health problems (see chart on p. 222, "Addictions That Reduce Anxiety"). Eventually, your health, relationships, jobs, and finances will suffer because you don't have your wits about you. Most of your brain circuits will have been altered neurochemically.

Addicted to Love: The Intoxication of Being a Savior

One of the most anxiety-provoking situations for anyone is watching someone you love suffer. Yet everyone has to go through painful times and all of us must to some degree watch each other come to grips with them. One of the most intoxicating highs, however, is saving people from the "jaws of death" in their life, and we can quickly become addicted to that behavior.

Do you remember the first time someone called you a "lifesaver" or said they couldn't "live without you"? You may have felt exhilaration, a swelling in your chest, powerful, or "high as a kite." Being a rescuer releases the same antianxiety, antidepressant, antipain neurotransmitters that addictive behavior releases in your brain. It's no wonder that many women develop what I call *altruism addiction,* the addiction to being a savior. There's a downside to this addiction, of course. Ultimately, you will tend to attract only people who will be dependent on you. Simply said, saviors need people to save, and these people tend to be alcoholics and drug addicts, and are usually irresponsible with finances and have rocky job histories. Saviors tend to marry people who are dependent, and saviors are dependent on other people being dependent upon them, that is, *codependent.* Ultimately altruism addiction can hurt your health in the same way as alcoholism and drug addiction. Your life tends to spiral out of control because it is linked to someone else who is perennially out of control.

Addictions That Reduce Anxiety

Addiction	Emotional Disorders It Masks	Physical Illness It Creates	Cross-Addictions	Brain Receptors

Eating Disorders
  Obesity
  Binge eating
  Bulimia
  Anorexia nervosa
	Anxiety
	Panic attacks
	Depression
	Irritability/anger
	PMS
	Perimenopausal moodiness
		Heart disease
		Stroke
		Breast cancer and other cancers
		Osteoporosis
		Joint problems
		Reflux and other digestive problems
		Sleep apnea
			Exercise addiction, e.g., running addiction
			Addiction to antianxiety (Xanax, etc.) drugs and pain meds (Oxycodone, fuorinol, etc.)
				Serotonin
				Opiates

Alcohol	Anxiety • Panic attacks • Insomnia Posttraumatic stress disorder Depression • Bipolar disorder • Attention deficit disorder Perimenopausal insomnia and moodiness, irritability, and anger	Obesity High cholesterol Liver disease Heart disease Dementia Osteoporosis Breast cancer and other cancers Ulcers and other digestive problems	Gambling Sex addiction Addiction to antianxiety sleep meds (Xanax, Valium, etc.)	Opiates GABA/benzodiazepines Serotonin Dopamine
Smoking Tobacco	Anxiety/insomnia Depression Irritability/anger Attention deficit disorder	Heart disease • Lung cancer and other types of cancers Digestive problems Emphysema/COPD Skin problems Infertility Miscarriage Other reproductive problems	Eating disorders Gambling Alcoholism Caffeine addiction (coffee)	GABA/benzodiazepines Acetylcholine Opiates Dopamine/norepinephrine
Marijuana	Anxiety	Emphysema • Lung disease • Long-term attention deficit Problems with initiation and motivation Memory disorder Low hormone levels and infertility	Smoking tobacco Alcoholism ? "gateway drug" to other illicit drug addictions	Serotonin Acetylcholine Norepinephrine Dopamine Opiates
Pain Medicines (opiates) Oxycodone	Anxiety Panic PTSD Irritability/anger	Acquired attention deficit Learning problem	Antianxiety medicines (Xanax, Valium, etc.)	Opiates

Addiction	Emotional Disorders It Masks	Physical Illness It Creates	Cross-Addictions	Brain Receptors
Fuorinol Others	Moodiness/ depression		Alcoholism	
Altruism Addiction (codependence)	Anxiety Depression PTSD	Obesity Digestive problems	Eating disorderss	Opiates

DOES ANXIETY RUN IN YOUR FAMILY?

Scientists have discovered that a tendency to anxiety is inherited. Anxiety problems in general, whether panic, phobia, posttraumatic stress disorder, or obsessive-compulsive disorder, tend to run in families. If depression or other mood disorders also run in the family, you may have an increased susceptibility to anxiety as well, which for some women only becomes evident during perimenopause. The medicines or other solutions that successfully treat your relatives' anxiety will probably be successful for you.

DO YOU HAVE AN ILLNESS THAT STANDARD MEDICAL TREATMENT CAN'T TREAT SUCCESSFULLY?

Every physical illness has genetic, environmental, and dietary influences. Some illnesses are caused by viruses, bacteria, or physical trauma, but also have an emotional and behavioral component that exacerbates symptoms or makes them more difficult to treat. Because the brain's fear and mood circuits have connections to every organ in the body, anxiety and depression have a cumulative effect on your health, increasing your chances of developing heart, lung, digestive, endocrine, hormonal, immune, and reproductive illnesses.

Many people don't want to consider that their medical illness may be precipitated or exacerbated by their feelings. They think you're telling them that they're not really sick, that it's "all in their head." But illness occurs *simultaneously* in the brain and the body. If you just treat the body's physical symptoms, the biochemical imbalance that can re-create the illness will still exist in the brain. You may get a temporary remission of physical symptoms, but almost certainly the illness will recur, because soon enough, the signal will make its way again through the anxiety-disease domino effect. People with untreated or poorly treated anxiety disorders suffer from increased risk of other illnesses and spend millions of dollars a year on lab tests, specialists, medicines, and hospitalization for illnesses that could have been prevented. Just treating the body's illness and not addressing the anxiety or mood problem is like continually bailing water out of a boat without patching up a hole in the hull; your health isn't likely to improve.

HAVE YOU RECEIVED A MEDICAL TREATMENT FOR ANXIETY ONLY TO FIND OUT THAT IT STOPPED WORKING?

Most pharmacological, herbal, or nutritional supplements don't provide permanent protection against anxiety or "fix" the imbalance in the feminine brain's fear circuits. This may be because anxiety is a critical part of your intuition and survival instincts. You simply can't medicate it away. Even if you found a medicine to deaden your feelings of apprehension and nervousness, another part of your four-sided emotional brain would "break through" the drug treatment and express itself. Anxiety-associated thoughts, behaviors, or health problems would eventually rear their ugly heads, requiring you to take more medicine or switch medicines.

There are more successful antidepressants available than there are nonaddictive antianxiety agents. The most effective anxiolytic medicines on the market are highly addictive—usually you will need higher and higher dosages in order to neutralize your anxiety over time. Yet even at a higher dose, after a number of years of being on the medicine, your anxiety will return slowly and insidiously. And if you stop taking it gradually, not only will the anxiety recur, it will seem to occur at higher levels than before. The few nonaddictive antianxiety drugs available (see p. 226) are not especially effective for more severe forms of fear, nervousness, and panic.

HAVE YOU RECEIVED MEDICAL TREATMENT FOR DEPRESSION, BUT NOT GOTTEN RELIEF?

Anxiety and depression frequently coexist in women, making treatment of either like a shell game: The ball is hidden under one of three shells that the magician constantly moves around. You just can't locate depression and anxiety exactly in the feminine brain; you need to treat both. If you are receiving pharmacological treatment for depression, and the medicine isn't working, you might want to consider whether you also suffer from anxiety. Alternatively, if you suffer from anxiety problems, and a variety of treatments haven't worked, you may consider looking into treatments for depression.

Medicines That Treat Depression Cause Side Effects of Anxiety

Some medicines or supplements successfully treat depression but have anxiety as a side effect. Some anxiety medicines like Xanax can make women irritable, edgy, jumpy, nervous, and moody. Anxiety can be caused by health problems, or can be the side effect of a drug. It is not uncommon for a woman to complain to her doctor that she feels "nervous" or overwhelmed after taking Synthroid, Advil, Tagamet, Benadryl, or other treatments for a medical problem. Unfortunately, the doctor may dismiss her report, assuming she was "nervous" to begin with. She may accept that her doctor is "blowing off her complaint," and do the same, ignoring her anxiety. Or she may stop the medicine without telling the doctor. Either route is dangerous. Discontinuing a medicine because it makes you anxious leaves your original illness untreated, and unresolved anxiety increases your susceptibility to other illnesses.

Some doctors medicate nervousness and jumpiness by prescribing antianxiety drugs that are highly addictive. By the time an anxiety patient hits her fifties, sixties, or seventies, the list of medicines she takes can become very long indeed, which is simply not good for her. And 30 to 40 percent of the meds on her list could be treating side effects caused by other drugs she's taking! As a doctor, the first thing I look at in every visit is the entire list of medicines that my patient is on to see if she really needs them all *and* if some are actually making her sicker.

Is a Frightening Situation in Your Personal Life or at Work Threatening Your Emotional Health?

Some women try medicine after medicine, therapy after therapy, in the hope of getting relief from their panic, uneasiness, and anxiety. However, if they insist on staying in a marriage with a physically abusive husband or don't want to leave an excessively stressful job in which they are in "over their head," no amount of medicine, herbs, nutritional supplements, or psychotherapy will stop their anxiety. The anxiety is part of the brain's intuition telling them that their lives or health are in danger.

Have You Started Having Severe Nervousness and Panic Attacks During a Health Crisis or Menopause?

You may have spent your entire life cool as a cucumber, only to begin to feel nervous or anxious during an emotional, physical, or hormonal change. You may have had your first attack of anxiety or panic when you were pregnant, postpartum, perimenopausal, infertile, or menopausal. Many of the reproductive and relationship brain circuits are anatomically intertwined with the emotional fear circuits. As a result, women may notice that problems that they once tolerated now make them feel hopeless, angry, overwhelmed, or a nervous wreck. At midlife, you have to do a thorough housecleaning of your life: get rid of what's not working. You can use medicinal, nutritional, and herbal solutions in this chapter to help you. You can also use the exercises in Chapter 8 to rewire thought patterns that increase your suffering and cultivate the intuitive guidance behind your nervousness.

Emotional "Chemotherapy" for Anxiety: The Big Gun Treatments

Antianxiety medicines and herbs temporarily dampen your anxiety, giving you a fleeting opportunity to hear the intuitive warnings underlying your nervousness. These medicines can never permanently solve your problems with anxiety, however. Over time, the medicine will stop working and your nervousness will get worse.

Ativan, Valium, Xanax, and other "big guns" are highly addictive antianxiety medicines—the psychiatric equivalent of chemotherapy and radiation for cancer. Chemotherapy and radiation are reserved for life-threatening cancers, because the longer you take them, the greater your chance of having life-threatening side effects.

Although Xanax, Valium, Ativan, and other addictive antianxiety medicines and herbal supplements don't normally cause cellular organ damage to your body, they can disable key parts of your feminine intelligence. So, how do you know when you should go to a doctor to try some of these medicines? You may need to consider medication if anxiety has distorted your life by causing you to: overeat; drink two or more alcoholic beverages a day; smoke (nicotine or marijuana); stay in a relationship that someone thinks you should leave; stay in a dead-end job; aggravate your health to a degree that standard treatments are ineffective in treating your physical disorders; become depressed and ashamed; avoid career advancement, relationships, socialization, and general emotional growth.

ANTIANXIETY DRUGS (ANXIOLYTICS)

Benzodiazepines: Medicines like Valium (diazepam), Xanax (alprazolam), Ativan (lorazepam), and Klonopin (clonazepam) are frequently used to dampen anxiety, worry, and nervous behavior (see table below). They do this by binding to a receptor in the brain called the benzodiazepine receptor. It is unfortunate the neuroscientists named the natural brain mechanism that calms us down after a group of medicines that are made in a lab. However, we already have a neurotransmitter in our brain that can bind to this receptor and calm us down, and it's called GABA (*gamma-aminobutyric acid*). By taking benzodiazepines from a pharmacy, you supplement your own inborn capacity to calm yourself down. But you can augment your feminine brain's own inner GABA stores so that you can "eat in" rather than always be "ordering out." (Please see "The Healing Power of Repetition," p. 245, and "Meditation, Prayer, and Yoga," p. 244.) Medicines that affect the activity of GABA improve:

Fearful Emotions
- Anxiety
- Nervousness, tension, uneasiness
- Phobias including social phobia, agoraphobia
- Panic
- Dread, fright, terror
- Apprehension, edginess, being overwhelmed

Fearful Thought Patterns
- Chronic worry
- Chronic self-doubt, social phobia
- Ruminations; an inner gerbil wheel playing a situation over and over again in your head
- Chronic self-examination, looking for flaws, mistakes, failures, self-criticism, the "inner Nazi"
- Repetitive thoughts about potential rejection, criticism, and disapproval by others
- Awaiting future pain, illness, and loss of control
- Believing that now or in the future, someone you love will fail, be hurt, or be harmed

Anxious and Fearful Behavior
- Hypervigilance: jumpiness, shakiness, easily startled
- Restlessness: constantly moving in a hurried fashion; can't slow down
- Compulsiveness: a constant urge to put things in perfect order; putting things in "line," making lists, checking to see if things are locked, or that the gas is off; repetitively washing and cleaning

things beyond what most people would think is necessary cleanliness
- Be "frozen," immobile, not wanting to move; hiding from and avoiding work, duties, and people in general

Some Health Conditions That Are Aggravated by Anxiety and Fear
- Panic attacks
- Hormonal: hot flashes, cold chills, difficulty maintaining stable estrogen, progesterone, and thyroid hormonal levels, hairlessness or hirsutism
- Neurologic: dizziness, tremor, spasms, acute or chronic pain, shaking, trembling, choking, seizures, difficulty swallowing, weakness, and insomnia
- Heart: palpitations, arrhythmia, chest pain
- Lungs: shortness of breath, asthma, allergies
- Digestive: heartburn, reflux, diarrhea, constipation, irritable bowel syndrome, and other inflammatory bowel disorders
- Gynecological: irregular menstrual cycles, vaginal yeast imbalances
- Dermatological: psoriasis, eczema, hives, rashes
- Immunologic: allergies

Cognitive/Learning Problems and Emotional Disorders
- Inattention, memory difficulties
- Depression, moodiness, irritability, and addictions of all kinds

Benzodiazepines like Ativan and Xanax have been used to help relax muscle spasms in people with neck and lower back injuries, prevent seizures in people who have epilepsy, and also help some individuals wean or detox off alcohol when they are addicted. These medicines are also used to treat the anxiety that occurs as a result of physical illnesses like Graves' disease and other hypothyroid disorders, as well as the anxiety associated with Ménière's disease and other illnesses that cause dizziness.

Benzodiazepines are only a temporary "quick fix" for *excessive* fear, worry, panic, insomnia and other symptoms of *severe* anxiety. Although benzodiazepines are widely considered effective and safe, many doctors are wary about giving them to patients who suffer from anxiety because addiction and dependence can occur in only six months. If your parents had an addiction to alcohol or were at least "moderate to heavy" social drinkers, your tendency to become addicted to these antianxiety medicines is even higher.

Even the fast-acting benzodiazepines like Xanax and Valium are very addictive. I heard a neurologist say at a medical meeting that the people

Antianxiety Medicine Primer: Benzodiazepines

Medication	Generic Name	Uses	Advantage	Dose Range (per day)	Side Effects (for all benzodiazepines)
Xanax	Alprazolam	Panic disorder Generalized anxiety Social phobia Insomnia (short-term use only)	Fast-acting Rapid onset Highly potent Works for short period of time	2–10 mg	1. Highly addictive, causes physical and emotional dependence. 2. Rebound anxiety: When drug starts to wear off, anxiety comes back with a vengeance. 3. Other withdrawal symptoms: When drug starts to wear off, heightened anxiety occurs including tremor, shakiness, muscle twitching, sweating, insomnia, heart racing, high blood pressure, faintness, and seizures. 4. Buildup of tolerance: Need more and more of medicine over time to get the same effect. 5. Can impair motor skills thus impairing capacity to drive safely. 6. Can impair attention and memory, especially in older people. 7. Can make depression worse in some women. 8. Can cause sleepiness. 9. Women who have experienced physical, emotional and sexual trauma may experience confusion, rage, agitation, and disorientation. 10. Serious interactions with other medicines, including alcohol, estrogens, certain antibiotics, and heart drugs. 11. Do not use during pregnancy.
Valium	Diazepam	Panic disorder Generalized anxiety Social phobia Insomnia Muscle relaxant Good for some pain syndromes Pre-anesthesia; before surgery Insomnia (short-term use only)	Fast-acting Rapid onset Low potency Works for longer period of time	5–40 mg	
Ativan	Lorazepam	Panic disorder Generalized anxiety Social phobia Insomnia (short-term use only)	Highly potent Works for short period of time	3–16 mg	
Klonopin	Clonazepam	Panic disorder Generalized anxiety Social phobia Obsessive-compulsive disorder Epilepsy	Longer acting Slower onset Highly potent Works for longer period of time	1–5 mg	

Sources: Data from C Salzman, et al (1983). Long vs. short half-life benzodiazepines in the elderly. *Arch Gen Psychiatry,* 40:293; WC Demant (1992). The proper use of sleeping pills in the primary care setting. *J Clin Psychiatry,* 53 (supp 12):50; EH Uhlenhuth, et al (1988). The risks vs. benefits of long-term benzodiazepine use. *Psychopharmacol,* 8:161; PP Roy-Byrne, et al (1989). Relapse and rebound following discontinuation of benzodiazepine treatment of panic attacks: Alprazolam vs. diazepam. *Am J Psychiatry,* 146:860.

who've successfully been able to discontinue Xanax meet every year at a conference in Chicago held in a telephone booth. I'm not fond of benzodiazepines as a medicine because they are so addictive. Women seem to have to increase their dose over time to get the same desired effect, and when the effects start to wear off, their anxiety, worry, insomnia, or panic comes back with a vengeance (an effect called withdrawal). Other symptoms of withdrawal include tremors, shakiness, sweating, and heart palpitations. Taking benzodiazepines can impair your judgment, motor coordination, memory, and emotional control and impair your driving as severely as drinking alcohol, since your reaction time can become sluggish.

Before taking benzodiazepines, you may have only one problem—anxiety. However, *after* taking these medicines, you may end up with two serious problems—anxiety *and* addiction. In addition to disrupting attention and memory, especially in older women, benzodiazepines like Xanax and Valium can cause paradoxical rage, agitation, confusion, and disorientation in women who have suffered physical, emotional, or sexual trauma. These medicines can make depression worse and even more difficult to treat.

If you want to stop taking Xanax, Valium, or another of these medicines, don't stop "cold turkey." Stopping these medicines abruptly can result in serious heart palpitations, blood pressure problems, and even life-threatening seizures. If you want to stop, have your doctor help you set up a schedule for gradually reducing your dose.

BENZODIAZEPINE-LIKE NUTRITIONAL SUPPLEMENTS: VALERIAN AND KAVA KAVA

Instead of pharmaceuticals, you can use dietary and nutritional supplements to augment your brain's innate GABA and its calming activity.

Although valerian root and kava kava have both been used widely to treat anxiety disorders, neither herb is any more effective than the above benzodiazepine medicines in the long-term treatment of anxiety, panic, worry, and obsessionality, or any other symptom of excessive fear. Why? Both valerian root and kava kava work basically by the same mechanism as Xanax, Valium, and other benzodiazepines. Ultimately, over time, you may build up tolerance to these herbs just as you would to prescription drugs.

Valerian (Valeriana officinalis) is useful only for the short-term treatment of anxiety and insomnia. You should not take valerian for longer than fourteen days (400 mg/night). If you take it for longer than two weeks, your brain and body get physiologically dependent upon it, and you can experience very uncomfortable withdrawal symptoms, such as heightened anxiety, tremor, shakiness, muscle twitching, sweating, heart palpitations, faintness, and even more severe insomnia. Valerian root is frequently combined with either hops or St. John's wort to treat symptoms of anxiety. Like Xanax and Valium, it also relaxes muscles and relieves some of the health problems of chronic nervousness and worry. By relaxing muscles that go into spasm when the brain's fear circuits go into overdrive, valerian can soothe abdominal crampy pain and lower back, neck, and other chronic pain disorders that are exacerbated by anxiety.

Valerian increases GABA activity in the brain, thus quelling fear and anxiety. In fact, if valerian is used in combination with Xanax, Valium, or Ativan, it amplifies their effect and can result in excessive sedation.

Kava kava (Piper methysticum) (70 mg 3/day) is another nutritional herbal supplement that has antianxiety activity and can improve insomnia. Like valerian, it is recommended for only short-term (one to eight weeks) treatment of anxiety and associated problems. It is not a safe, long-term solution for treating anxiety. Like valerian, kava may work on the GABA receptor as well as other areas in the brain. As a result, if you use kava over time, tolerance develops. Although kava won't impair attention and memory, it does impair muscle control, so you shouldn't use it if you plan to drive. In fact, DUI (driving under the influence) citations have been issued to some individuals who used kava.

Kava can cause gastrointestinal complaints, headache, and dizziness. Chronic use can cause severe side effects. A skin condition with dry flaking skin (kava dermopathy), liver problems with a disturbance in cholesterol metabolism, renal problems (blood in the urine), blood disorders (low platelets and lymphocytes), and other more serious problems can occur. For some women, kava can worsen depression and even increase the tendency toward suicide. Since kava calms the brain down, combining it with other calming, sedating benzodiazepines can be very dangerous, causing excessive sedation and, in rare cases, coma.

Chamomile (German chamomile) (3 g in 1/2 cup water 3x/day). Chamomile has been used to treat anxiety, insomnia, and associated disorders. Although it has mild benzodiazepine effects that may explain how it quells nervousness, fear, and insomnia, it has other biochemical properties that make it effective for health reactions that are aggravated by excessive anxiety, such as allergic and autoimmune skin conditions like hives, eczema, and psoriasis. Chamomile may improve these skin disorders

Antianxiety Medicinal and Herbal Primer

Valerian Root *(Valeriana officinalis; 400 mg/night up to 14 days)*

Uses	Advantage	Side Effects
Short-term use only (less than 2 weeks) Insomnia General anxiety Depression Muscle relaxant Epilepsy Chronic pain disorder Irritable bowel syndrome	"Over-the-counter" use: Don't need a doctor's prescription Can be used in combination with hawthorne for nutritional supplementary treatment of hypertension	1. **Withdrawal syndrome** if used for longer than 14 days: heightened anxiety, tremor, shakiness, muscle twitching, sweating, heightened insomnia, heart racing, faintness. 2. Headache 3. Morning drowsiness, sleepiness 4. Impaired attention 5. Can impair motor skills, thus impairing capacity to drive 6. Hepatotoxicity (liver toxicity in rare allergic individuals) 7. Avoid other sedating herbs and medicines: calendula, Siberian ginseng, chamomile, goldenseal, gota kola, St. John's wort, skullcap, and others; alcohol, benzodiazepines

Sources: See the backmatter notes for sources for this and the next two charts.

Kava Kava *(Piper methysticum; 70–100 mg)*

Uses	Advantage	Side Effects
(Short-term use only) Anxiety Insomnia Muscle relaxant Panic disorder with agoraphobia	"Over-the-counter" use: Don't need a doctor's prescription	1. **Tolerance:** need more and more, higher and higher doses to get same effect 2. Digestive complaints 3. Headache 4. Dizziness 5. Dangerous liver problems 6. Blood disorders 7. Kidney disorders (blood in urine) 8. Skin rash and flaking (kava dermopathy) 9. Avoid using with sedating herbs or medicines (see above)

Chamomile *(German chamomile, Matricaria recutita; 3g in a tea 3x/day)*

Uses	Advantage	Side Effects
Insomnia Anxiety Skin conditions, rashes Inflammatory digestive tract disorders: diarrhea	Can simultaneously treat **emotions** (anxiety) and **health problems** (skin disorders, diarrhea, and other inflammatory digestive disorders) associated with excessive fear and stress.	1. Sedating 2. Vomiting at high doses only 3. Severe allergy in certain individuals 4. Can cause excessive sedation if combined with alcohol, benzodiazepines Xanax, Valium, and others, including Siberian ginseng, hops, kava kava, valerian, skullcap, and others 5. Can cause bleeding if combined with other herbs/nutritional supplements that promote bleeding (see Blood Thinner table in Chapter 4)

Passionflower *(Passiflora incarnata; 2 g in tea 3x/day)*		
Uses	Advantage	Side Effects
Nervousness	Long-term treatment	1. In rare, susceptible allergic
Anxiety		individuals inflamed blood vessels
Restless behavior	Can simultaneously	(vasculitis) and altered
Insomnia	treat:	consciousness
Relaxes muscle spasms in some	Emotions	2. Sedation. Do not combine
pain disorders	(nervousness)	with other sedating herb
Heart palpitations associated	Health reactions	supplements in medicines or in
with anxiety	(digestive cardiac	alcohol.
Digestive disorders aggravated	pain, etc.)	3. Do not combine with
by anxiety: diarrhea,	Behavior	herbs/medicines that are
constipation, ulcers	(restlessness)	"anticoagulants" or "blood
Raises pain threshold in pain	associated with	thinners" (see chart in Ch. 5,
disorders	anxiety disorders	p. 162)

because it has an active ingredient that blocks the inflammatory cascade associated with chronic anxiety (anxiety–disease domino effect). It prevents the histamine release associated with hives, eczema, and psoriasis.

At midlife, many women get hives, eczema, insomnia, and other health conditions that are initiated or aggravated by stress and anxiety. Progesterone, our natural antianxiety hormone, begins to drop as women approach menopause, so they may be at greater risk for anxiety and their bodies more susceptible to anxiety-related skin problems and insomnia. Chamomile may be one solution for both the emotional and physical aspects of anxiety.

Taking chamomile tea can help with insomnia by helping make you feel sedated, but if you combine it with other sedatives including valerian, kava kava, Xanax, or Ativan, you may become excessively drowsy and have a hard time waking up on time in the morning.

Passionflower (Passiflora incarnata; 2g in 1/2 cup water 3x/day). Like other antianxiety herbs, passionflower helps calm nervousness and anxiety by binding to benzodiazepine/GABA receptors in the brain. Some of its other chemical constituents help treat the physical reactions associated with hyperactive fear circuits, reducing anxiety-associated restless behavior (including the restlessness in attention deficit disorder), relieving insomnia, relaxing muscle spasms, and raising the pain threshold for patients with chronic pain disorders. It also improves heart palpitations and digestive disorders that are aggravated by nervousness and stress, including diarrhea, constipation, and ulcers. Passionflower is a sedative, so you have to be careful of combining it with other sedating herbs or medicines. Side effects are rare. Some susceptible individuals, however, may have severe health reactions.

Interestingly, although passionflower has benzodiazepine-like activity, its other ingredients seem to prevent it from impairing attention, memory, or motor skills. More important, it does not cause the usual tolerance problems, addiction, or physical dependence. No one knows why this is true. Because passionflower is non-habit-forming, it may be considered as an herbal nutritional supplement available to treat anxiety for longer periods of time. In addition, passionflower may help mood control. Women with anxiety and depression may find passionflower helps both problems simultaneously.

OTHER MEDICINES TO IMPROVE ANXIETY

In the rest of this chapter, I outline nonaddictive solutions to your anxiety. Ultimately, your health and longevity depend on your ability to tune up your feminine brain's fear circuits.

• *BuSpar.* Books usually list medicines under the heading of "other" when the medicine usually doesn't work or if it needs to be taken with other, more potent medicines. BuSpar is usually used in conjunction with antidepressants in the treatment of anxiety. However, this medicine rarely provides immediate relief from anxiety and panic. Some patients have found some mild relief after taking the medicine for two weeks, but many feel no effect. However, on the plus side, BuSpar isn't addictive and it doesn't make you sleepy or give you problems paying attention or remembering things, problems that frequently accompany the use of Xanax, Valium, or other benzodiazepines. So, if your anxiety is severe, you may want to consider it.

• *Beta-blockers. Inderal* (propranolol) is a beta-blocker that may reduce some of the physical health symptoms associated with panic and anxiety such as heart palpitations and hot flashes, but unless it's combined with several other antianxiety treatments, it isn't very helpful.

• *SSRIs (Selective Serotonin Reuptake Inhibitors).* Although we usually think that Prozac, Zoloft, Paxil, and other SSRIs are antidepressants, these drugs can also be useful to quell the anxiety associated with PMS, perimenopause, panic attacks, obsessive-compulsive disorder, and other disorders (see Chapter 5). However, SSRIs like Prozac and others are notorious for their inability to work after one or two years. It appears that the brain "reroutes" its circuits to make these medicines ineffective. They might buy you a year or two of relief, however, during which time you can get to the source of your discomfort.

Other antidepressants like Effexor, Serzone, tricyclic antidepressants, and MAO inhibitors may also be helpful for women with anxiety and panic, especially if they also suffer from depression.

Nonaddictive, Herbal Nutritional Supplements for Anxiety

• *Lemon Balm* (*Melissa officinalis;* 395 mg/day or 1.5–4.5 g/day in 1/2 cup hot water for tea). Lemon balm is used to stop anxiety and also relieve insomnia. An herbal nutritional supplement, it relaxes the smooth muscle that lines the walls of the digestive tract, thus relieving many gastrointestinal disorders associated with anxiety, including abdominal distension and gaseousness. Lemon balm has unique antiviral and antibacterial properties that help treat both emotional and physical symptoms of stress-induced herpes breakouts. It also helps some women with other chronic viral or bacterial syndromes like chronic fatigue/fibromyalgia (Epstein-Barr virus) and Lyme disease because it can simultaneously treat the viral and anxiety syndromes. No one knows exactly how lemon balm works, but it's not reported to cause you to develop tolerance or be addictive, and it has no known side effects. You do, however, have to be careful combining this herb with other sedating herbs and medicines, since you could become excessively drowsy or obtunded. Lemon balm may interfere with thyroid replacement therapy.

• *Catnip* (*Nepeta cataria;* 760 mg 3x/day). Catnip isn't just for cats; it's an herbal nutritional supplement that can help humans feel less anxious. Although it creates an initial euphoric effect in cats, the active ingredient causes calmness in people and puts them to sleep. It is also helpful for individuals who suffer migraine headaches and digestive disorders. Few side effects are associated with catnip, although there have been reported cases of, yes, catnip abuse, with excessive ingestion leading to euphoria.

Actually, I myself am addicted to buying catnip for my cats. Watching them go through their frenzied catnip euphoria and then fall asleep is very calming for me.

• *Hops* (*Humulus lupulus;* 0.5–1 g/day). People may drink for reasons other than the high from alcohol. Beer's other key ingredient, hops, has a potent antianxiety effect and has been used to treat nervousness, insomnia, and irritability. Alcohol or any other central nervous system sedative combined with hops is very sedating and, in excess, can impair the alertness required to operate machinery or do other skilled tasks. Herbal combinations of hops and valerian root have been shown to be an equal and effective substitute for Xanax, Valium, and other benzodi-azepine sleeping pills.

• *Gingko biloba* (200 mg/day). Gingko biloba improves attention and memory and may also improve anxiety, because it affects GABA/benzo-diazepine receptors like Xanax, Valium, or Ativan, but isn't addictive and doesn't build up tolerance. For women with complicated combinations of anxiety and attention deficit disorder, gingko biloba is a unique, ef-fective, nonaddictive alternative to medicine. However, you have to be careful about taking this supplement. It is a "blood thinner" and can cause bleeding if combined with other blood thinner medicines or herbs.

• *Asian ginseng* (*Panax ginseng*), *Siberian ginseng* (*Eleutherococcus sentico-coccus*), and *Vietnamese ginseng* (*Panax vietnamensis*). Ginseng is a family of herbs that helps buffer your body from stress. Ginseng is used by many people to sharpen their attention and memory skills. If used consistently for at least a couple of weeks, it can lower anxiety levels. Ginseng also treats insomnia and may support the immune system during periods of anxiety and stress. Similar to benzodiazepine medications, ginseng de-creases anxiety levels by binding to GABA/benzodiazepine levels. It does have a very mild addictive potential, so you should take it only for temporary relief of anxiety.

Nonaddictive Antianxiety Medicines and Herbal Nutritional Supplements

There are two basic routes through which a medicine or nutritional sup-plement can dampen anxiety: (1) by turning down the volume of the fear circuits, and (2) by adjusting the activity of the four other emotional cir-cuits, improving mood, anger, love, and joy.

Addictive medicines like Xanax, Valium, valerian, or kava kava only target through one brain receptor, the benzodiazepine receptor. But be-cause the feminine brain is not compartmentalized and many women suf-fer from complex combinations of anxiety with depression and ADD, they may be helped better by nonaddictive antianxiety medicines and nutri-tional supplements since these compounds target multiple brain receptors and pathways. The following are suggestions for treating depression, anx-iety, and attention problems simultaneously.

Nonaddictive Antianxiety Medicines and Nutritional Herbal Supplements

Medicine or Nutritional Supplement	Generic Name	Anxiety Disorder Treated	Advantage	Dose Range	Side Effects
Beta-blockers: Inderal and others	Propranolol	Performance anxiety (stage fright) Social phobia Generalized anxiety Panic attacks	Not addictive Reduces heart rate and palpitations associated with panic	Varies	Dizziness Low blood pressure Asthma Shortness of breath Depression Sexual dysfunction
BuSpar	Buspirone	Generalized anxiety Does not help more severe anxiety disorders • Only a small number of people are helped by this medicine	Not addictive Not sedating No cognitive side effects	15–60 mg/day	Dizziness Digestive distress
Lemon balm	Melissa officinalis	Generalized anxiety Insomnia Physical Health Problems: Digestive disorders Antiviral Antibacterial	Not addictive	395 mg/day or 1.5–4.5g tea in 1/2 cup water	Sedation: Do not combine with other sedatives May interfere with thyroid hormone supplement
Catnip	Nepeta cataria	Generalized anxiety Insomnia		760 mg 3x/day	Euphoria
Hops	Humulus lupulus	Generalized anxiety Nervousness Irritability Insomnia	Used in herbal combination with valerian root		Excessive sedation if combined with alcohol (i.e., beer)
Gingko biloba		Attention deficit disorder • Mild memory disorders	Not addictive	200 mg/day	Excessive bleeding if combined with other blood thinners
Ginseng Asian ginseng Siberian ginseng Vietnamese ginseng	Panax ginseng Eleuther-ococcus senti-cococcus Panax Vietnam-ensis	Increases stress tolerance Insomnia Physical health problems: Supports immune system during stressful events	? only mildly addictive	Varies	Mildly addictive Can be overstimulating for some

See also Chapter 4, "New Moon," tables with SSRIs, tricyclic antidepressants, MAO inhibitors.

TRADITIONAL CHINESE MEDICINE

As part of a complete treatment plan, Traditional Chinese Medicine and its nonaddictive herbal treatments can balance your fear circuits and lower anxiety, panic, worry, and all the other associated disorders. In addition to lowering anxious emotions, the herbs also treat physical reactions that usually occur with anxiety. Western medicine doesn't usually help both body and mind. When I went to medical school, you went to a psychiatrist for anxiety treatment and looked for a dermatologist to address your rash. If you had asthma and panic attacks, you'd see both a pulmonologist and a psychiatrist.

In Traditional Chinese Medicine, a licensed, fully trained practitioner determines the physiological imbalance that set the scene for your emotional and physical problems. Just as there are five basic emotions (fear, anger, sadness, love, and joy), Traditional Chinese Medicine identifies five basic elements—earth, wood, air, water, and fire—that need to be in harmony for emotional and physical health. Each element has a corresponding meridian—energy pathway—associated with it. The Traditional Chinese Medicine doctor identifies the disharmonies that have resulted in anxiety, panic, worry, and associated physical illness and treats you with a mixture of herbs and acupuncture treatments that balance the function of these elements and pathways. In Chinese medicine, anxiety and nervousness basically are the result of (a) an imbalance in the wood element that disrupts the spleen and stomach meridians, and (b) an imbalance in the fire element that disrupts the heart and small intestine meridians.

Typical Traditional Chinese Medicine Anxiety–Disease Treatments	
Physical Health Problem Associated with Anxiety	Chinese Herbal Supplement
constipation	Sm. Biota
night sweats	Zizyphi spinosa
skin problems	Cinnabaris
asthma	Lumbricus
eye problems	Cornu antelopis/Concha
headache	haliotidis
hypertension	Uncariae
insomnia	Magnetitium
GERD (reflux)/ulcers	Os draconis
	Concha ostrea

Source: See Mao Shing Ni (1991). *Chinese Herbology Made Easy.* Los Angeles, CA, Shrine College Tao, *Traditional Chinese Healing.*

Several Chinese herbs treat perimenopausal anxiety and other symptoms:

- *Corydalis tuber* treats nervousness, agitation, insomnia, and headache.
- *Coptidis rhizoma* treats nervousness, anxiety, palpitations, hot flashes, depression, and poor memory.
- *Magnolia cortex* promotes relaxation, decreases anxiety, and treats insomnia. It also treats stress ulcers.

Many of these herbs have been used safely for thousands of years. Scientists have found that they affect neurotransmitter receptors, just as the nonaddictive drugs and herbs that treat anxiety do. Like any medicine, herbs can have complex side effects, so herbal treatment is best used under the guidance of a licensed, board-certified acupuncturist and Chinese herbalist in your area (see Resource Guide).

Hormonal Supplementation for Anxiety

Anxiety and panic can be triggered by inappropriately low progesterone levels compared with body estrogen stores, especially in women during premenstrual time (PMS), perimenopause, and menopause. These lower progesterone levels may also enhance your intuition, letting you know that something is "off" in your life and needs your attention. A traumatic, life-changing event such as divorce can also change your hormonal levels, causing you to have excessive estrogen levels in proportion to progesterone.

Progesterone is an antianxiety hormone that binds to the same receptor as benzodiazepines, valerian, and other herbs. It lowers panic and anxiety, reduces insomnia, and stabilizes mood.

Bioidentical progesterone is available in multiple forms. Do not confuse bioidentical progesterone with Provera, a synthetically derived hormone that doesn't appropriately fit into the brain's antianxiety *benzodiazepine/GABA receptors*. You can buy bioidentical progesterone in a 3 percent cream, over the counter at your local health food store (i.e., without a prescription). This may be a high enough dose for some women, who notice an improvement in their anxiety after taking only 1/4 teaspoon three times a day.

For other women with more severe anxiety, the 3 percent cream isn't enough. They may want to try Prometrium (oral progesterone capsules). This oral form of progesterone can be taken at 100 or 200 milligrams a day.

Over time, however, oral progesterone tends to stop working. The liver creates enzymes that metabolize it or "chew it up," rendering it inactive in the brain and the body. For these women, *progesterone solution,* a very concentrated form, can be prescribed by their doctor. One to three drops per day can be very effective for the more severe levels of anxiety. Finally, for the most severe forms of anxiety and panic (and in some women with epilepsy), intramuscular injections of *progesterone, 500 milligrams a week,* can be lifesaving.

Progesterone helps repair the outer coating of the nerves, called myelin. As a result, it may be helpful in treating chronic pain disorders whose origins are in peripheral nerve damage. It has also been shown to be helpful in the recovery from traumatic brain injury. Progesterone has very limited side effects, although it is sedating. In a few women, it may cause depression. If you have a history of breast cancer or other hormonally-related cancer, you need to talk to your doctor before considering this and other hormonal therapy.

Please don't get progesterone confused with another hormone called *pregnenolone.* Pregnenolone is a precursor to progesterone. At low doses, it has antianxiety effects, but if it builds up in the body, it actually promotes anxiety. If you are prone to moodiness, irritability, and severe anxiety, you're better off staying away from this hormone.

If you have severe anxiety, panic, and fatigue, you do not want to consider taking DHEA. DHEA may make you feel less tired, but it causes anxiety in susceptible women.

If you have a hormonally precipitated anxiety disorder, progesterone is only one part of a total treatment plan. You also need to rewire your brain in therapy.

Psychotherapy—Rewiring Your Brain

Many types of psychotherapy can, in the short term, help you figure out the intuitive information behind your anxiety. The three basic approaches, psychoanalytic, behavioral, and cognitive, are described fully in Chapter 8, "I've Got a Feeling." The traditional psychoanalytic "talk" therapies help you find out what in your past has given you problems with nervousness, phobias, obsessionality, compulsivity, panic, or insomnia, but I hear many women complain that they know *why* they're anxious, they just don't know *how to stop* being nervous and get on with their lives. Cognitive behavioral therapy *can* rewire your thoughts (cognitive) and actions (behavioral) so that you are less likely to perceive your environment, relationships, or work as distressing. This therapy helps you listen to the intuition behind your fear and gives you the skills to respond effectively so that you know you can handle fear.

You may wonder, "Is it really possible to rewire your brain?" or "Aren't these problems hardwired in your brain?" Cognitive behavioral therapy actually changes how your brain fires. In a study on individuals with obsessive-compulsive disorder (OCD), when patients received only medicine, their brains normalized only slightly on a PET scan. When they received cognitive behavioral therapy for their obsessive thoughts and rituals, their brains once again normalized slightly on a PET scan. However, when the individuals took medicines *and also* engaged in this therapy, their brains approached normal firing patterns.

Cognitive Behavioral Therapy Stops Nervous Thinking

Cognitive behavioral therapy is especially helpful if your intuition speaks to you through anxiety. This treatment was initially used to reduce anxiety through thoughts and behavior. In some women, the first signs that something distressing is going on shows up in their thoughts, where they may

- Think about rejection and criticism
- Think about failure now, in the past, and in the future
- Think about being helpless and losing control

If you have anxiety, you usually don't know what is generating these nervous thoughts and symptoms in your body, so you try to ignore them. But if you let these thoughts and symptoms "fester" without responding appropriately, they pick up steam and momentum, and create "rug burns" in your brain and body. The anxiety-disease domino effect is activated and soon you feel panic and pain. Cognitive behavioral therapy teaches you how to identify the prompting events, or thoughts, when you first start to have them, and teaches you how to respond effectively so you can stop this chain reaction.

Cognitive behavioral therapy can be especially helpful for women who experience intuitive warnings about loved ones through their own anxious behavior, in the movements of their hands and feet, in their speech, or in their health. They may talk very fast, not talk at all, talk very loudly, talk very faintly, walk very fast, walk slowly or not move at all, move their hands, tap their fingers, roll their thumbs in a gerbil wheel motion, adjust clothing, fumble papers, adjust the location of items nearby, look up, look away, or stare.

My friends can always tell when I'm intuitively picking up something because I seem nervous. Like the "restless" cows and horses in the pasture before a big storm, my feet will fidget. At dinner I might play with the candle at the table, even trying to light a sugar cube or Sweet-'n-Low packet with the flame. Once, when a sugar cube ignited and dropped onto the tablecloth, a friend took me to the ladies' room and began to interrogate me. "Okay, what's going on with people at this dinner party? You always act this way when you feel something bad is about to happen." I found out later that two people at the table were having an affair, unbeknownst (rationally) to me or their partners, who were also there.

Many women aren't aware that they are anxious when they're acting anxious, but cognitive behavior therapy can teach them how to identify what's making them fearful, help them respond appropriately, and also soothe their nervousness.

DIALECTIVE BEHAVIORAL THERAPY (DBT)

DBT is a special form of cognitive behavioral therapy for women and men who have suffered emotional, physical, and sexual abuse. It helps regulate anxiety and panic, and enables them to regain a sense of safety.

Edie's story illustrates how cognitive behavioral therapy can help someone stop a panic attack.

A Party Phobia

Edie, twenty-eight, was a very successful businesswoman, and no one would ever guess that she had problems with anxiety. Yet in school she had always had trouble doing oral presentations in front of the teachers and the class. Before she would speak, she would feel so nauseated that she would frequently throw up, but would push herself through the panic. When she went off to college, she supported herself selling real estate on the side. Edie was such a go-getter, no one ever guessed that she was afraid of social gatherings. The day before a party she would ruminate over and over again about going. The night before the event, she couldn't sleep. The day of the event, she would be exhausted and a nervous wreck and would begin to eat, craving any carbohydrate available. She felt tension in her chest, and when it was time to go to the party, she would be sweating, tense, and short of breath. Family members would tell her not to go if she was going to get so sick, but Edie didn't want to be a social failure, and wanted to see her friends, and perhaps meet the "man of her dreams."

When Edie got to a party where everyone was drinking, she would immediately have a drink. After that, though, she would fill her glass with water. Edie really didn't like alcohol much because she had had an alcoholic grandfather who was in and out of rehab. However, as the evening progressed, Edie got more tense. She couldn't seem to focus on conversations, since everyone and everything seemed superficial and boring. So Edie would retreat to the side of the room and watch others talking animatedly. Then she would begin to feel waves of sadness. She would see her friends with their boyfriends: Compared to them, she felt like a loser. Eventually, Edie would go home, and for the next few days be sad, dejected, and exhausted . . . until the next party. Then her party phobia would repeat itself.

Edie told me that she had always been a little on the nervous side but had been able to contain it by being very organized at work and in school. She could feel more in control if she practiced her sales pitch or her talk over and over again, but couldn't apply those anxiety management skills to going to a party or finding a boyfriend. So I had Edie bring her attention to the days before the party. Edie began to recall the thoughts going through her mind:

> "When I go to parties, I never find anyone to talk to."
> "When I go to parties, all my friends end up finding boyfriends and I never meet anyone."
> "I am a failure socially because I can't get a boyfriend."

These torturing thoughts would go around and around in her head until she was sick to her stomach.

Since Edie's thoughts seemed to lead to anxiety and panic, we needed to see what truth they held. Edie told me she never lied to herself so her thoughts were always true. In fact, though, her thoughts conflicted and therefore couldn't all be true. Edie's thoughts were tricking her brain into thinking there was real danger, pain, and threat in social situations.

For example: Edie says that when she goes to her friends' parties, she never finds anyone interesting to talk to. On the other hand, Edie feels sad when she sees her friends leave with boyfriends they have met at the party. Why would she feel bad to see her friends leave with boys that she found boring and uninteresting? And if she wanted to meet an interesting guy, why would she expect to find one at these parties that she always declared to be superficial and boring? Edie realized that her thoughts before parties were promoting and exaggerating her natural tendency toward anxiety and panic. So Edie separated going to parties from her desire to meet a boyfriend. She decided to go to parties to see her friends and merely to get out of the house. Edie would choose other venues to meet boyfriends.

Before the next party, she would watch her thoughts. If she started to ruminate, she would sit down and review her new intentions of going to the party; she would just see her friends and "get out of the house." When she started to get bored, she would leave.

Does Edie still have a tendency toward having panic attacks? Absolutely. Edie's brain is wired with anxiety-prone, stress-hypersensitive fear circuits. Her emotional porousness gives her a form of intuition that makes her a genius at business, but it makes social situations agony. However, with cognitive behavioral therapy and a list of other mind–body solutions, Edie has learned to understand the messages behind her anxiety and panic, while simultaneously keeping the associated pain and suffering to a minimum.

Cognitive behavioral therapy, dialectic behavioral therapy, and other types of therapies that are helpful for anxiety and depression are discussed more fully in Chapter 8.

Treatments for Depression, Irritability, and Moodiness That Also Treat Anxiety and Panic

The mechanism behind how the treatments summarized below work to balance feminine emotions is more fully discussed in Chapter 4.

EXERCISE

Regular exercise of all kinds (45–60 minutes a day, at least five days a week) releases opiates, "reward" hormones that can counteract anxiety, fear, and panic, as well as the pain that tends to coexist with anxiety disorders. As long as you choose something that challenges you and doesn't overly exhaust you, running, biking, and walking can, over time, decrease your tendency toward panic anxiety and insomnia.

MASSAGE

Many studies have shown massage to be effective in treating anxiety and associated drug addictions. It increases levels of serotonin, the same neurotransmitter affected by many antianxiety medicines. Massage also provides relief for pain disorders, low back pain, asthma, and other related health problems. Massage releases endorphins that relieve pain and make you feel capable of addressing stressful situations in your life. However, if you have a history of posttraumatic stress disorder, or you have survived physical, emotional, or sexual abuse, you may not feel comfortable receiving a massage, so consult a therapist, psychiatrist, or other doctor before seeking this and other "touch" therapies for anxiety.

Meditation, Prayer, and Yoga

Research studies have shown that *transcendental meditation (TM), the relaxation response, and mindfulness meditation* are particularly helpful for the treatment of anxiety and its related disorders, including heart palpitations, angina, chronic lower back pain, and insomnia. This intentional practice may lower anxiety levels by lowering elevated norepinephrine levels that are present in the anxiety-disease domino effect.

Meditation may help you have more control over your thoughts, like cognitive behavioral therapy (CBT). In fact, one type of CBT, dialectic behavioral therapy, actually uses mindfulness exercises based on meditation to help you monitor your thoughts and correct "wrong thinking" that leads to panic, anxiety, and ultimately, depression.

Prayer has been shown to have a profound effect on the immune system and the inflammatory response. I am not aware of any scientific studies that indicate that prayer reduces stress, anxiety, and panic, but if you were to do a population study on what people do when they're panicked, distressed, and/or hysterical, you'd find that a significant number, probably greater than 50 percent, pray. People pray because it works for them. The act of repetitively saying a prayer like the "Hail Mary" or some other verse or chant may have an hypnotic effect (see below). I do not consider the act of prayer to be a "stereotypical rhythmic act," as some psychologists do. If you believe that there is a power greater than you, somehow appealing to that power in a time of need feels comforting. If you have increased anxiety levels because you are an intuitive emotional barometer, prayer can be an important solution to your nervousness.

Yoga is a form of meditation with poses, breathing exercises, and deep relaxation that has a profound capacity to improve anxiety, obsessive-compulsive disorder, and panic. It has also been shown to be immensely helpful in treating many related health conditions including asthma, heroin addiction, hypertension, and menopausal health complaints. Practiced from twenty minutes to two hours a day, yoga teaches you to observe your thoughts and body reactions. You can learn to sense the first signs that your body's fear circuits are firing and find out why they are signaling danger. Yoga gives you the mental control to find out if your thoughts are driving your anxiety, and lets you apply what you've learned in psychotherapy to change those thoughts.

If you have a history of physical or sexual abuse, you have to be careful with this therapy. Some authorities have documented that some women with PTSD have experienced body sensation flashbacks and memories of their trauma while doing certain yoga postures.

THE HEALING POWER OF REPETITION

Any rhythmic repetitive movement is hypnotic, sedating, and reduces anxiety. Whether you bite your nails, twiddle your thumbs, tap your toe, rock, or drum your fingers on the table, this activity releases the neurotransmitter GABA into your brain and subtly induces relaxation and calmness. Mothers know this instinctively, and rock their babies to soothe them or get them to sleep. It's very easy to fall asleep with the rhythmic rise and fall of the waves on a boat or to the swaying of a train. Repetitive movements such as rhythmic rocking may be nature's Valium, a way to release an inner benzodiazepine that naturally reduces anxiety, stress, and induces sleep.

When autistic individuals get anxious or nervous, they frequently can't talk about their feelings, but soothe their anxiety by rocking. The more intense their anxiety, the more intense the rocking. People who have more language, social, and motor skills at their disposal engage in repetitive tasks or "hobbies"—knitting, needlework, woodworking—to relax and reduce anxiety and stress.

In fact, in every major psychiatric treatment center, an occupational therapy team will engage patients in crafts to improve their anxiety and mood. No matter what you're doing, whether it's painting by numbers or knitting, any activity in which your brain can go on autopilot can be calming.

To relax, do you:

- ❏ Collect things: stamps, figurines, Department 56 houses that light up, Hummel figures, shells?
- ❏ Have a stationery-product fetish: Do you tend to collect pens, 3-M Post-its, and other products that can be found at Office Max or Staples?

❏ Go through catalogues like J Crew, Domestications, Hold Everything, or Pottery Barn, and earmark what you would like to buy?

❏ Go to household gadget stores and research different ways you can better organize your closets, your kitchen, and your office?

❏ Doodle; play with liquid markers, paints, and other artistic materials?

❏ Do hobbies or crafts like stamping, crocheting, needlepoint, candle making, sewing, crossword or jigsaw puzzles, scrapbooks?

❏ Refinish old furniture, fix something that's broken in your house?

In the privacy of our homes, when no one else is around, we all have rituals that lower anxiety and stress in our lives. In the day immediately following the World Trade Center and Pentagon attacks, I felt compelled to go to a local crafts store and buy a lot of Department 56 Village houses. With fourteen houses, I built a village in my bayview window. This is no ordinary village. It is a virtual utopia with tree-lined streets, a waterfront, and paths with miniature people walking peacefully in a park. This miniature city has no chance of being attacked by terrorists. When people visit and see my little village, they say they want to live there. The phone repairmen ask if they can bring their wives to see it lit up at night. Every day, when I look across the room, there, glistening in the sun, is a peaceful utopian society, my model for serenity and exuberance.

You now have an abundance of tools with which to manage anxiety levels in your life. Whether you have nervous thoughts, obsessive worrying and rumination, panic attacks, phobias, or insomnia, you can use these solutions to tame your feminine brain's fear circuits.

EIGHT

I've Got a Feeling:
Monitor Your Intuition to Manage Moods
and Anxiety

I have struggled for years with the physical problems of being emotionally porous. I have to admit that I haven't yet truly mastered managing the moodiness and anxiety that comes to me. For instance, I can't go into an animal shelter without feeling the emotional and physical deprivation of all the caged creatures. I have attempted to put up mental insulation and still be caring by making animal shelters and rescue leagues my number one charity. I know a very passionate woman who has suffered lifelong depression but who is famous for going into these animal shelters and adopting all the pets.

As a neuropsychiatrist, I have had to learn to put up mental insulation between my patients and me. When I was a psychiatry resident, and daily oversaw a group of schizophrenic patients, it took me about a month to figure out that I got irritable, edgy, and anxious after checking in on them because I was hearing *their* auditory hallucinations in my head. Back then, being emotionally and intuitively porous seemed to be a prerequisite for being anywhere near the field of psychiatry, and the physical and emotional fallout occurred in different ways. One by one, nursing staff dropped out. Although no one admitted to hearing the patients' inner voices, everyone went a little nuts if they were on call for too long or did too many double shifts.

To prevent myself from losing my mind, once I graduated from residency as a full-fledged psychiatrist, I decided not to follow any patient for too long. It seemed the more often I saw a patient, and the longer I saw them, the more likely I would start to get "intuitive email" about them when I was home, during what was supposed to be private time. For example, I'd wake up with a bad feeling in the pit of my stomach about Thelma, a patient, only to find minutes later a message on my fax machine that she was in the emergency room after another violent episode. During my exercise routine, my mind would drift to another patient's inability to keep a job. I would get more and more irritable, until it seemed like all my patients emotionally inhabited both my mind and my house.

Many psychotherapists, nurses, doctors, and mothers would attest to the same kind of intuitions. We can be so plugged in to caring for others that they seem to live in our minds and bodies. Some days, we are moody, anxious, burned-out, and numb, and have no idea what has caused our mood.

Nearly 70 percent of nurses, psychotherapists, and social workers are afflicted with healer burnout or the stigmata of "overcaring." The historical stigmata of the Christian saints who feel others' pain have been converted to more modern types in the form of obesity, diabetes, hypertension, chronic fatigue/fibromyalgia, depression, and "burnout" as just a few examples. Mental health workers and group home personnel have the highest rates of these modern-day stigmata or diseases of emotional and physical overwork.

Women with emotionally or physically handicapped children also frequently suffer from depression and chronic physical illness because they spend their whole life mothering children who, for one reason or another, can't leave the nest. These women have to "think" or "feel" for their children in a variety of life situations because the children seem to lack the mental and emotional capacity to respond appropriately for themselves. These "perennial" mothers have learned to avert disaster by intuitively knowing when their children are in distress. To shut off their intuition, and separate from their children would be a Sophie's Choice. Their identity is so shaped by terminal motherhood that allowing their child to carry his own suffering and let other "trained personnel" intervene would feel like amputating a limb.

Chances are, you aren't a saint. It's hard to be one these days given the overly strict Vatican criteria. It is possible, however, to become a modern-day martyr if you are *too* intuitively keyed in to the suffering of others. So what do you do if you are emotionally and intuitively overextended?

An Eleven-Step Program for Managing Mood and Anxiety Problems Using Emotional Intuition

The following program combines many of the principles found in cognitive and dialectic behavioral therapy, twelve-step codependence recovery process, posttraumatic stress disorder treatment, and visualization and affirmation work.

Traditionally, people have tried to treat mood and anxiety disorders by rationally examining the generation of mood in a stepwise, forward progression through the brain; that is, an emotion generates a mood, which generates a thought pattern, which eventually generates specific physical reactions. But intuition examines feelings in a stepwise backward progression through the same brain-body pathway; that is, a physical symptom connects to a thought pattern, which generates an emotion, a signal from your intuitive guidance system.

STEP 1: LOCALIZE THE PHYSICAL SYMPTOMS ASSOCIATED WITH YOUR FEELINGS

Where in the body is the symptom? The physical region (one of the seven emotional centers) that signals distress frequently symbolizes the area of your life that you need to examine. Positive emotions like love and joy usually don't cause symptoms, but actually promote relief or ease in these body areas.

First Emotional Center: Bones, joints, blood, the immune system (families, organizations)

Second Emotional Center: Reproductive or pelvic organs and lower back (relationship, creativity)

Third Emotional Center: Digestive tract, change in weight, problems with addiction (self-esteem, responsibility, work)

Fourth Emotional Center: Heart, breasts, or lungs (emotional expression, partnership, nurturance)

Fifth Emotional Center: Neck, jaw, mouth, shoulders or thyroid gland (communication, will, timing)

Sixth Emotional Center: Ears, eyes, head, and brain (perception, thought, morality)

Seventh Emotional Center: Exacerbation of life threatening illness (purpose in life)

The location of the symptom usually symbolizes the issue that is precipitating the mood, sadness, anger, irritability, or nervousness. For example, getting an uncomfortable feeling in your stomach may indicate a problem with some area of responsibility or work. The next two steps will help you find out what you are thinking and feeling about that issue, so you can pinpoint what is precipitating your mood change or nervousness.

STEP 2: LOCALIZE THE THOUGHT PATTERN ASSOCIATED WITH THE MOOD OR ANXIETY [PLEASE REFER TO EMOTIONAL FENG SHUI CHART, CHAPTER 3]

What words—or, if you are musically oriented, what song lyrics—keep going around and around in your head?

First Emotional Center Thoughts:
- I need people to help me or I feel weak and vulnerable. (Fear)
- People tend to try to control me and make demands. (Anger)
- I feel rejected by family and friends. (Sadness)

Second Emotional Center Thoughts:
- I usually get rejected, abandoned, and betrayed in relationships. (Fear)
- Even when I fall in love with someone, I find a lot wrong with them after a while. (Anger)
- No matter what I do, I always manage to have financial disasters. (Sadness)

Third Emotional Center Thoughts:
- I have trouble making decisions. (Fear)
- A lot of people get opportunities I will never get. (Anger)
- I blame myself for things that go wrong around me. (Sadness)

Fourth Emotional Center Thoughts:
- I can't tolerate pain and unpleasant feelings. (Fear)
- If I don't have the upper hand in the relationship, it doesn't feel just. (Anger)
- Since they left me, my life is stuck in a rut. (Sadness)

Fifth Emotional Center Thoughts:
- If I say how I feel, I lose love and respect. (Fear)
- If I'm not right, I will lose control. (Anger)
- If I speak my mind, it doesn't change anything, so why bother? (Sadness)

Sixth Emotional Center Thoughts:
- If I ignore a problem, it will go away. (Fear)
- I frequently find faults in myself; I'm not trying hard enough. (Anger)

- Things come easier to others; my mind is always in the clouds. (Sadness)

Seventh Emotional Center Thoughts:
- I am afraid of death. (Fear)
- Things should have been different in my life. (Anger)
- God has it in for me; the universe doesn't hear my voice. (Sadness)

If your mood and anxiety are disrupting your ability to think, pay attention, learn, and remember, then see Chapters 9 and 10 in this book to find out how intuition is speaking to you.

Step 3: Localize the Prompting Event

What is the emotion telling you? Is there something different in your life? Or in the life of a loved one? Suppose that the feeling is not merely caused by a thought—it's not simply "in your head." Could it be warning that something has indeed changed? If you have the physical symptom, thought pattern, and typical trigger of an emotion, chances are you are experiencing that emotion whether you are conscious of it or not. As the saying goes, "if it looks like a duck, quacks like a duck, it is a duck." There is an exception to the "Duck Rule," however: You may be "empathically feeling" for someone else. If you are intuitively plugged in to a loved one's life, you may be "feeling for them." Sharing emotions intuitively isn't unique. Twins experience each other's love, joy, pain and sorrow; mothers can sense when a child is in distress. What are your emotions telling you?

EMOTION	PRECIPITATE
Sadness	Things turning out not the way you want or expect
	Loss of love/acceptance or a significant relationship
	Being in contact with someone who is sad
Anger	Things turning out not the way you want or expect
	Losing authority, respect, or power
	Having you or someone you love experience emotional and physical pain
Fear	Entering into an unfamiliar situation
	Being alone, or in the dark
	Being threatened or hurt
	Sensing someone you love is being threatened or hurt
Love	Someone treats you favorably
	Someone gives you what you want or need, raises your status, your self-esteem
	Wanting closeness
	Sharing a special experience with a pet, a piece of land, or having a great workout

Joy	Getting what you want or have worked for
	Being accepted by others
	Achieving a goal

Sources: Adapted, modified, and amended from: A Damasio (1999). *The Feeling of What Happens: Body and Emotion in the Making of Consciousness.* New York, Harcourt Brace; J Panksepp (1998). *Affective Neuroscience: The Foundations of Human and Animal Emotions.* New York, Oxford University Press; M Lewis and JM Haviland-Jones (2000). *Handbook of Emotions,* 2nd ed. New York, Guilford Press; MM Linehan (1993). *Skills Training Manual for Treating Borderline Personality Disorder.* New York, Guilford Press, pp. 139–152.

STEP 4: FIND THE PERSON FOR WHICH THE EMOTION AND ITS ASSOCIATED MESSAGE IS INTENDED

As if you were starring in a good forensics show on TV, you now have to be the detective and find the "body." Is the mood and its related thought and symptoms about your life or another's? Take a fearless inventory, a ruthless survey of your life. First, look in a mirror and ask yourself, "Are these feelings and their message meant for me or someone else?" If you guess that it's about someone else, does that realization, even for a second or two, make your physical symptoms somewhat better? Does it feel, even for a moment, like a weight has been taken off your shoulders? If your body and thoughts respond positively to that theory, then chances are it is about someone else. However, like any other source of information that comes from right-brain intuition, it is critical to find left-brain facts to support your theory. Call up an honest friend or a skilled psychotherapist to double check if your intuition is true or if you're fooling yourself.

Intuitive Buffers: Grounding Techniques

If your moodiness and physical distress are an intuitive warning about someone else's life, you can use grounding techniques to improve your mood and reduce your physical distress. These techniques, in a way, call back the part of your energy that is merging with the other's pain, the essence of what we call empathy. Localize your body and mind on the ground, on planet Earth, where you're standing. You can now perceive that the person for whom you are carrying emotional and physical pain is not you. Your body is standing away from him or her, preferably a good distance away. By holding onto something solid on the Earth, your mind cannot travel as easily to intuitively visit someone else in distress.

Here are some other grounding techniques:

- Stand on cold tile.
- Wash your face with cold water or hold ice in your hand.

- Go for a run, do intense exercise, preferably outside in nature so that you can key in to how your feet are touching the ground and how the wind feels against your skin.
- Listen to loud music and move your body to the beat. Syncopated rhythms are great because they challenge and attract your attention.

Grounding techniques' buffering will usually improve your mood immediately and give you simultaneous relief from physical symptoms. Once you are on an even keel, you may see a way to help others in a more balanced way.

STEP 5: PINPOINT WHAT YOUR MOOD AND INTUITION ARE ASKING YOU TO CHANGE

The word "emotion" comes from a Latin root meaning to change, to move. An emotion is an intuitive signal that something has to change. Once you're ready to heed its message and see the beneficial results of your actions, your mood and anxiety are likely to improve. What needs to change? Frequently, the emotional center in which you experienced a physical symptom or felt a thought will indicate the area that you have to change.

- *First Emotional Center:* A change is needed in your family, the organization in which you work, or within some other key group in your life.
- *Second Emotional Center:* A change is needed within a core partnership in your life, whether it's a primary love relationship or a business partnership, or a change may be required in how you give birth to your own creativity or handle your finances.
- *Third Emotional Center:* A change is needed in your work identity or how you handle responsibility in your life.
- *Fourth Emotional Center:* A change is needed in how you nurture others, or how you express emotion and passion in life.
- *Fifth Emotional Center:* A change is needed in how you assert yourself and have a balanced voice in the world.
- *Sixth Emotional Center:* A change is needed in how you view the world. You may need to see an issue from someone else's point of view, or adopt a more flexible point of view.
- *Seventh Emotional Center:* A change is required in what you see is your purpose in life, i.e., why are you here?

An Intuitive Reading

Mary-Helene, age thirty-nine, called me for a reading.

The physical symptoms: Mary-Helene had two months of lower back pain (Second Emotional Center) and foot pain from plantar fasciitis (First Emotional Center). She was tired of taking Percocet and Demerol pain shots. She wanted to know how she'd do if she had "disc replacement" surgery in her lower back.

Unless Mary-Helene figured out what emotional patterns were associated with her pain disorders, she probably wouldn't have a good recovery from her surgery. Mary-Helene's sadness and fear began four months earlier, when her husband left her for another woman, causing her to feel rejected, abandoned, and betrayed. Her husband had been the primary breadwinner in the family so their separation made her feel terrified of impending financial disaster. Having always been in a relationship with a man, Mary-Helene felt frightened, weak, and vulnerable living alone for the first time.

Mary-Helene was depressed and deeply anxious about being alone. She realized that her physical pain and moods were letting her know she needed to process the grief about her impending divorce, and find emotional and financial support from loved ones and family until she gained the skills to support herself financially. Mary-Helene worked with a counselor who helped her "rewire" her anxious thoughts and a physician who specialized in pain disorders, who helped wean her off her pain meds. For about a year and a half, Mary-Helene used some medicinal mood and anxiety medicines to "splint" her brain chemistry until she could rebuild her confidence and stabilize her finances. She also learned yoga and Pilates, which eased her back pain and anxiety. And slowly, the pain went away.

STEP 6: IDENTIFY EMOTION AND INTUITION CENSORS

Now we need to address that fact that most people's emotional intuition gets stuck between Step 4 (Whose emotion is it?) and Step 5 (What is supposed to change?). Why? Because our brain's frontal lobe can act like a censor, blocking emotions and intuitions. Of course, if we always acted by gut intuition, our society and relationships would be chaotic; sometimes we have to set aside intense emotions and act. When rushing into a burning building, a firefighter sets aside fear in order to get the job done. During the most tension-filled times when a mother wants to run screaming from a marriage, she pulls herself together for the sake of the kids. However, censoring emotions and intuition is only healthy when it's done for a short time. In the long run, it turns into mood problems. Eventually, the emotions leak around the censor and turn into depression, anxiety, and emotional volatility. Soon, you may find yourself breaking down over "little things" in "emotional incontinence," more popularly known as "losing it."

For example, your boss, during a long, exhausting day, may talk sharply to you. Afraid you may be fired, you look down, suck in your emotions, and censor your feelings so that you can survive the rest of the day. However, when you get home and see the dirty dishes in the sink, you may burst into tears, surprising and embarrassing yourself. Depending on your family and personal history, it's possible that you might have no idea why you are crying.

What thought patterns or intuitive censors make it hard for you to read the message behind your moods and panic? Many emotional censors utilize shame, a social emotion that sometimes muzzles our feelings and behavior so that we can function appropriately. However, sometimes shame inappropriately causes us to "stuff" an emotion because we think that expressing it will cause us to lose a loved one, lose status in society, fail at a goal, or appear weak, vulnerable, and inferior in front of others. If you repeatedly have shame about your emotions and intuition and stifle them, you may suffer years of panic, anxiety, depression, and moodiness.

Other censors involve pessimism, a reduced sense of the possibilities for your life. Many of these negative thought patterns come from past experiences, yet you can learn new skills and sprout new brain pathways. You can identify and neutralize pessimistic emotion censors in order to see and realize your true potential.

Do you have any of these censors of emotion and intuition floating around in your brain?

- I can't change a relationship. Who would love me? People usually find me unattractive and unappealing. I would be alone.
- I can't change my job. It's safe where I am now because I have benefits. I don't have a choice; no matter what I do, I seem to end up having financial disasters.
- If people really knew me, they wouldn't respect me. So I must do whatever I can to go along with what other people want.
- If I am angry or sad, people won't love me or like me. If I am always happy and loving, people will always be there for me.

- They can't do it without me. If I don't step in and do something, something bad will happen.
- If I don't do it, it won't get done.
- Things should be different. This is unfair.
- I don't seem to have a special quality or mission in my life.
- A lot of people get opportunities that I never will, so it's best to stay with the job I have.
- I can't change my point of view because if I admit I am wrong, I will look foolish and feel vulnerable.
- When I speak my mind, nothing ever changes anyway, so why bother?
- God has it in for me. The universe doesn't seem to hear my voice.

Identify your censoring thoughts and start seeing and thinking how you can change them to positive, supportive thoughts that will enhance your mood and your life.

Poor Self-Esteem: Unhealthy Thoughts About Yourself

One of the biggest impediments to successfully treating your depression is having low self-esteem. In a nutshell, self-esteem is what you think about yourself. In your frontal lobe circuits, self-esteem is encoded by comparing your aspirations with actual achievements. Your self-esteem is low if your aspirations far exceed your actual achievements (i.e., I'm a failure, I'm a loser). Your self-esteem is higher if your actual achievements equal or exceed your hopes and aspirations. Some psychotherapists believe that your sense of self/self-esteem is static, as cemented in your brain as your personality style and temperament. But from what we know about learning and plasticity, we also know that you *can* in part rewire your self-esteem or at least parts of it.

Improving your self-esteem buffers you against anxiety and depression. Higher self-esteem protects you against anxiety because if you feel that you have success and mastery in many areas in your life, you won't become paralyzed with anxiety in the face of stress and adversity. Low optimism and self-esteem actually predispose you to depression in many phases of your life, including the postpartum period. Low self-esteem affects your body's health as well, especially the organ systems that have an intimate relationship with mood, and it suppresses the immune system, especially natural killer cell activity that protects your body from cancer.

For instance, I grew up believing I was fat. Actually, I was described as "solid." I could never be described as svelte. Even when I had my spinal surgery for scoliosis at age twelve and became taller overnight by three inches, I still *felt* fat even though everyone told me that I was thin. I am 5'3" and a size 4/6, but I still feel fat during stressful times and premenstrually. I know during most other times that I am not fat, but if my mood is low, this inappropriate, inaccurate thought pattern gets played on my mental CD self-esteem player, causing my mood to plummet even further.

The seat of self-esteem, the frontal lobe (the dorsalated prefrontal cortex) has lower blood flow and function in people who suffer from depression. These physical changes are reversed with successful treatment including but not limited to antidepressants and cognitive behavioral therapy. By improving your perception of your actual academic, social, and financial success, your brain areas for self-esteem become more active and your mood elevates.

If you feel like a failure in many areas of your life, you are more prone to mood disorders and depression. We all of us have areas in which our self-esteem is fragile and vulnerable, and others in which we feel more powerful and self-confident. To improve your mood during stressful and not-so-stressful times, you need to assess all *seven self-esteem centers in your life.*

• *First Self-Esteem Center: Families and Organizations.* Do you feel good about your ability to fit into families and organizations? Can you engage in diplomacy and be politically savvy? Do you know when to depend on your family and when to pull away and be independent? Having good self-esteem about the quality of your relationships with family members and other affiliations promotes the health of your mood, bones, joints, and immune system.

• *Second Self-Esteem Center: Relationships and Money.* Do you feel good about your capacity to have a relationship with a significant other? Do you feel attractive to your partners? Are you able to have a relationship with a significant other in which (a) each of you gives as much as you get; (b) each of you makes yourself equally available sexually and emotionally; and (c) both of you have approximately the same money, power, and status?

How do you feel about your capacity to attract money, wealth, and property? Can you pay your bills in a timely fashion and manage debts? Do you always have to earn the money you receive, or have you created multiple wealth streams that bring you money passively?

Having good self-esteem about your relationships with significant others and having a healthy relationship with money affects the health of your lower back and reproductive organs, including your uterus, ovaries, and cervix.

• *Third Self-Esteem Center: Work and Responsibility.* Do you like your daily work and use all of your gifts, talents, and skills in it? Do you get enough recognition and monetary compensation? To be happy, do you have to be in a competitive environment and usually be on top? Do you lack confidence when you are working in a competitive environment? How do you feel about your physical appearance, weight, and fitness? Do you feel good about your ability to assume responsibility and meet deadlines in a timely fashion? Or to be happy, do you continuously have to carry burden and responsibility for others? The health of your digestive tract and having a healthy weight are very much influenced by having good self-esteem about your personal appearance, your work, and your capacity to be responsible and meet your obligations in life.

• *Fourth Self-Esteem Center: Emotional Expression and Nurturance.* Can you feel fear, anger, sadness, love, and joy fully and express them skillfully in a variety of relationships? Are you able to have balanced relationships in which you both receive and give love and nurturance appropriately? The health of your heart, breasts, and lungs is in part dependent on your capacity to feel an emotion fully and release it. In addition, the health of the organs in your chest region is affected by your capacity to experience true partnerships in which both members get as much emotional support and nurturance as they give.

• *Fifth Self-Esteem Center: Communications, Will, Timing.* Do you know how to say the right thing to the right person at the right time with the right amount of intensity? Can you patiently wait during traffic jams, or other times when your personal schedule has been disrupted? Can you tolerate easily someone who has a differing opinion? The health of the thyroid, throat, and neck area is dependent in part upon expressing yourself and listening to others, pushing forward to fulfill your needs or waiting for things to come to you, imposing your will on others or allowing others to impose their will upon you.

• *Sixth Self-Esteem Center: Intellect and Intuition.* How do you feel about your intellectual development, intuitive capacity, and academic achievement? Can you take your intellectual and intuitive style and find a place for it in a vocational setting? Do you believe people understand and appreciate your point of view? Do you think you're usually right? If you do not have good self-esteem about your intuitive and intellectual gifts, the health of the very organs of perception that make knowledge, wisdom, and thought may be affected.

• *Seventh Self-Esteem Center: Faith and Purpose in Life.* Do you have a purpose in life, a reason for being on the Earth? Do you have a balanced capacity to find faith, an inner sense of spiritual security when times get rough? The inability to feel good about your purpose in life in the first place can increase your chance of developing a life-threatening illness.

If you think you have problems in more than one self-esteem center, ask a trusted friend to rate you on your strengths and weaknesses. If you are much more negative about your successes and less able to see how you actually have achieved some of your goals and aspirations, you probably have a form of pessimism, an "inner Nazi," that is self-deprecating and constantly erodes your self-esteem. Your mind may not be a safe neighborhood to visit, especially at night. As a result, you may be particularly prone to depression and chronic sadness. In addition, if you have low self-esteem in a specific center, you may be more susceptible to illnesses related to mood disorders.

Once you have assessed your self-esteem, clarified your self-concept, how do you repair and restructure the thought patterns and behavioral weaknesses that drag your mood down? Cognitive behavioral therapy, especially its assertiveness training sessions, can teach you diplomacy and interpersonal effectiveness skills in families, business organizations, and relationships. Visualizations, affirmations, and hypnotherapy can help you identify and replace thought patterns that hold you back financially, academically, and vocationally (Please see Resource Guide for my *Mind-Body Makeover Oracle Cards*). Treatment for codependence and relationship addiction can help you identify and correct thought and behavior patterns that predispose you to relationships in which you give much more than you get back, or are a compulsive martyr or rescuer. Seeing a neuropsychologist for an evaluation of your attention, memory, and learning style can help you understand your intellectual gifts and find a vocational niche; working with a psychotherapist or spiritual counselor may help you unearth your purpose in life and your own faith and spirituality.

STEP 7: CREATE A BUSINESS PLAN FOR ACCOMPLISHING YOUR GOAL

When you have pinpointed your goal—what you want to change in your life—it's critical to create a profit/loss sheet that will describe what would actually happen if you were to succeed.

On a piece of paper, draw a vertical line from top to bottom. Label the left-hand column "(+) GAIN" in black; label the right side of the paper "(-) LOSS" in red.

For example, if you got a new job:

(+) GAIN	(-) LOSS
More money	Contact with old friends at work
More status	Time—new job is a longer commute
Get a better boss	May intimidate my partner because he will make less money than me
More self-respect	Less time with my kids because I won't be home when they get home
(+) personal and	from school
intellectual growth	Sense of security. Anything new is scary; I might fail

If your plan is lopsided such that gains exceed losses, something is wrong with your plan. Why? Because if you recognize far more pluses in changing, you would have already done it. There is something you're not admitting to yourself and you may need to think again or even do some special cognitive behavioral therapy analysis to pinpoint what is blocking you from moving forward.

If your plan is lopsided such that losses exceed gains, you need to identify whether or not you need to change your perception or gain more skills.

In some depressed people, chemical imbalances make it hard to see positive possibilities. They may have occasional fleeting dreams about what they want, but the pilot light for going after their passion has gone out. If you have a significant problem with your weight, sleep, or any of the other symptoms of depression, you may need medication and nutritional supplementation under the supervision of a trained physician before you can proceed with more clarity.

Alternatively, you may not have the skills to accomplish your goals. Could you gain training or get help knocking off the problems in the loss column one by one? Using the above example, is it possible to maintain relationships with people from your old job? Could you take advantage of a car pool or mass transit to allow you to more effectively use your commuting time? Do your kids really want you to be home when they get home from school or are there after-school programs in which they are eager to become involved? Usually you can reconceptualize the items in the loss category.

Nonetheless, eventually you may hit a wall, a core limiting issue that prevents you from moving forward—perhaps taking a new job will intimidate a partner. In other cases, you may have a core belief or thought that has created a roadblock.

Changes always involve losses and gains. Some losses we are not willing to tolerate, and others we can learn to see as labor pains. If there is an item in the loss category that you can't live without, then come to peace with this fact and skip to Step 9: Radical Acceptance. However, if you aren't willing to live with the limitation that you have just revealed, move forward to Step 8.

STEP 8: GET A COACH = CHANGE YOUR THOUGHTS = REWIRE YOUR SELF-ESTEEM

You can choose to rewire your thoughts alone, with affirmations (see Resource Guide), imagery, and journal work, or you can choose to get help from a coach, a psychotherapist, or other skilled support person who will help you achieve your goals.

Alone or with help, you will

- Rewire new thought patterns into your brain to replace the old ones and thought censors that have blocked your growth
- Acquire the skills you need to accomplish your goal on a deadline, with a schedule
- Recognize and celebrate the goal once you succeed

Changing your thought patterns is akin to doing a "partial brain transplant." The wiring in your brain physically changes.

Coaches and cognitive behavioral therapists are trained to take a negative thought pattern (a censor) and replace it with a more healthy way of thinking. Getting a coach or psychotherapist will also force you to make a commitment to succeed and create a schedule in which you make progress toward your goal.

If you need education, financial resources, or other elements to complete your goal, your coach will keep you on track and steer you in the right direction. Once you've succeeded, and your coach helps you celebrate, your brain and body learns what you are capable of achieving. The stepwise process of succeeding at a goal releases opiates that will elevate your mood and reduce anxiety. Once you've seen what you're capable of accomplishing, more intuitive possibilities will come to you.

Imagery can help you change your thought patterns and has been used successfully to treat depression and other mood disorders. Imagery is, in a way, the opposite of normal, everyday perception, with your eyes and ears.

Normal Everyday Perception
(Feed–Forward Feminine Brain Pathways)

1. You *see* or *hear* something in the world.
2. If it's relevant, you pay *attention* to it.
3. What you see and hear is processed, you make associations, compare it to past experiences, i.e., you *think* about it.
4. You determine how you *feel* about what you see; you attach an *emotion* to it (fear, anger, sadness, love, joy).
5. Your brain and body lay down *memories* about what you see and hear.
6. The emotions and thoughts about what you have seen affect your *behavior* and set the scene for changes in health.

Imagery is generated in your mind's eye.

Imagery
(Feed–Back Feminine Brain Pathways)

6. You become aware of your *body actions, responses,* and *health re-actions,* which . . .
5. Evoke *memories,* which . . .
4. Generate *emotions,* which . . .
3. Stimulate *thoughts,* which . . .
2. Direct your *attention* to an
1. Image, and *insight*

You can use imagery to "rewire" your feminine brain circuits for self-esteem, thoughts, emotions, and mood. You generate an image that gives you insight into how your emotions, thoughts, behavior, and health are interconnected. In a way, imagery is like a quick-and-dirty, technology-free PET scan, a way to find out how your mood circuits are organized and how they ultimately affect your behavior and health, your capacity for achieving goals, engaging in relationships, and fitting into a family or society. And once you get insight into how your mood circuits are wired, you can modify what is getting in the way of your health (with cognitive behavioral therapy, for instance).

Guided imagery has been shown to help patients change their immune cell competence and the activity of the disease in their body. Patients with metastatic breast, lung, lymphoma, endometrial, bladder, and cervical cancers used imagery in addition to chemotherapy, surgery, and radiation to help their immune system get rid of the cancer. The treatment gave patients a sense of well-being and made them feel more in control. It improved mood and morale, and engaging in their imagery treatment two times a day improved the responsiveness of their immune systems, elevated immunoglobulin levels, and improved the capacity of their natural killer cells to destroy cancer cells.

Imaging and Changing Emotions

A cognitive behavioral therapy called dialectic behavioral therapy (DBT), uses imaging of the four components of your mood to rewire your brain: emotion, thought, action, and physical symptoms. Using a psychological and behavioral version of Zen spiritual meditation practice, DBT teaches how to nonjudgmentally (a) *observe;* then (b) *describe;* and finally consciously (c) *participate* in your emotional and physical state. Its mindfulness imagery trains you to experience an emotion in a stepwise fashion, one hemisphere at a time. First, observing your experience without describing or labeling it involves generally trying to stay in the right brain. Then, describing your emotional and physical state takes your observation into the left brain to put it in words.

The final step uses both hemispheres. You enter into the experience, are involved "in the moment," or "at one with the experience." You observe, describe, and experience your actions (what it feels like to sit in a chair), your physical state of health (the state of your stomach, joints, and other body organs), thoughts, and feelings.

As you use imagery to improve mood you imagine a relaxing scene, a secret room, and look to see how it is decorated. You learn to go into the idealized "safe room" whenever you feel threatened. You close the door on anything that can be hurtful, and imagine everything going well in this utopian fantasy inner world. You can also imagine "hurtful emotions draining out of you like water out of a pipe."

Mental Aspirin: Affirmations and Imagery

People have used aspirin-like natural substances such as willow bark for centuries, not knowing how they worked but knowing that they reduced pain and fever. Now, aspirin is used to prevent heart attacks, lower the incidence of colon cancer, and alleviate other serious health conditions. Although we now have more scientific information on the mechanism of aspirin, it really doesn't affect why people use it. People use aspirin simply because it works.

Affirmations are like mental aspirin. Somehow, they work. Although they may not have been studied with double-blind, deaf, mute randomized clinical studies, millions (including myself) use them simply because they are effective.

In 1976, Louise Hay wrote *Heal Your Body,* known by millions as the "Little Blue Book," which brought the practice of visualization to millions of people worldwide. In her later book, *You Can Heal Your Life,* she provides visualizations called affirmations, which transform emotional and thought patterns, ultimately leading to improved health. Her work is deceptively simple yet potent, like aspirin. You can also try my affirmation system, Dr. Mona Lisa's *Mind-Body Makeover Oracle Cards,* to rewire thought patterns that adversely affect the health of your brain and body. This card deck helps you identify and replace thoughts that can trigger depression and anxiety; negatively affect self-esteem, work, and relationships; and increase your risk for illness in every organ of your body.

Belleruth Naparstek has produced a whole library of imagery audio-tapes for mental, emotional, and physical illness that hundreds of hospitals across the United States use. From improving depression (called Releasing Grief) to increasing love (called Empathy for Another), they include exercises to develop healthier boundaries in relationships and improve self-esteem and mood. The effectiveness of many of her imagery exercises have been studied scientifically and proven effective (see Resource Guide).

Although you can begin the process of rewiring your thought patterns with affirmations and visualizations, it's very difficult to perform surgery on yourself and rewire your thinking on your own. Why? When a foreign organ is transplanted into your body, since it's not your own native tissue, your body tends to reject it. Medicine has devised methods of getting around this problem, but when you try to imagine, formulate, and change what you think you can achieve, your thought censors will try to reject the potential goal to protect you from possible failure, rejection, or loss. That's why you want a coach or psychotherapist in your corner. A psychotherapist can also work with you in cognitive behavior therapy, which is a particularly effective way to retrain the New Feminine Brain.

STEP 9: RADICAL ACCEPTANCE

Decide who or what you can and cannot change.

Suppose that you've figured out the intuitive message behind your physical symptoms, thoughts, and moods, and gained awareness of whether the message warns that a change is necessary. If you then decide that you can't change your job, relationship, or situation at this moment, then the only way to move forward in your life is to accept your present circumstance, and find peace and solace in other areas of your life. Continuing to struggle with the reality of the problem adds insult to injury, suffering on top of pain. Here are some thought patterns that can be causing you problems:

- I'll always be miserable like this. I'll never find happiness. (Permanence and Fatalism)
- Things should be different. (Righteous Indignation)
- Ruminating about the problem over again. (The Instant Replay)

To counter these negative thoughts, you can hold these statements in your mind:

"I love myself just the way I am and there are many things in my life that I want to change."
"This too shall pass."
"I trust that everything happens to me in the perfect time and perfect way."

I have never met anyone who had no pain and suffering in her life. Bad things happen; sometimes life on Planet Earth, from our human point of view, is not fair or just. And I'm sure you've met those nauseating, sanctimonious individuals who tell you, "There's a good reason why this disaster happened." Such statements, though they may be accurate from the perspective of a higher divinity whose mind and intentions we cannot read, are seldom helpful if you are in the midst of feeling the visceral grief that occurs with disaster.

In 2000, I had to have three spinal surgeries in four days. My doctor described the process as "kamikaze surgery." Because I was to have my spine fused from the middle of my neck to the tail end of my spine, the procedure was akin to being sawed in half.

Lying in the hospital with an epidural needle in my back and a morphine pump in my arm for pain control, I was miserable. However, the painkillers were not the most comforting help that I received. All of my doctors and friends told me the surgery was necessary so I wouldn't have further spinal deterioration, but they also commiserated, "This is bad. No one should ever have this happen to them." Their love, acceptance, and expectation of the positive outcome helped me eliminate my mental suffering and deal with the physical pain.

Harold Kushner, a rabbi who wrote *When Bad Things Happen to Good People,* gives many ways of handling the spiritual and human pain involved in accepting the unacceptable. Allowing yourself to live with injustice, even temporarily, does not mean that you deserve pain and agony.

As Chris Northrup, who is also a surgeon, once told me, "All bleeding eventually stops." That's gallows humor that illustrates the fact that nothing is permanent. Tolerating the pain of the present moment does not mean that you don't expect future relief. Having faith and hope that circumstances will eventually be different as you gain more skills involves radically accepting the present. Spiritual traditions can be very helpful in achieving this level of faith in the midst of misfortune. Faith becomes a way of life, "not in the sense of an insurance policy against misfortune, but as a tool for overcoming fear, emptiness, loneliness, and cynicism."

STEP 10: IDENTIFY APPROPRIATE "REHAB" CANDIDATES; DIFFERENTIATE THOSE PEOPLE IN YOUR LIFE THAT YOU CAN HELP FROM THOSE YOU CAN'T

Suppose you have determined that your moodiness and physical symptoms are intuitive signals that someone you love and care for is in distress (Step 4). What do you do then? We all get intuitively farsighted about ourselves, although we can still see what someone else needs to do. I think this farsightedness gets worse with age. However, the question remains, how do you donate your intuitive insights to someone else, *and* how do you help facilitate them changing?

First of all, you can't change anyone. The anxiety we experience when we see a loved one head toward obvious disaster compels us to open our mouth and do something. You can point out what your intuition is saying in a skillful way with the correct amount of intensity. However, if the other person doesn't see it your way, you have to do what I call "The Windshield Wiper" maneuver: Wipe away the situation from your mind the way a windshield wiper would wipe away debris that had landed on your windshield. You have to recognize that that person has a higher power, and that his future is created daily by them both. You cannot let yourself become a constant rescuer or codependent—overly enmeshed and in an excessively dependent relationship.

There is a story that makes the rounds at twelve-step meetings for codependents. At one meeting, Mary stood up and told how her husband always came home drunk and passed out in the front yard. Mary had suffered from depression and insomnia for years because she was always waiting for the next time her husband would embarrass himself and her. Whenever Mary found her husband passed out, she'd drag him inside and put him to bed. In the middle of Mary's story, Mabel, a devout Christian, got up and said, "Lady, you need to stop being your husband's higher power." So Mary, who came from a very different spiritual background, answered, "I don't believe in a higher power." Not losing a beat, Mabel shouted back, "Well, can you at least believe you ain't it? Lady, you need to leave him where Jesus 'flang' him."

No matter what your spiritual beliefs, know that even when you get intuitive information about someone, you ultimately can never be a higher power for anyone. I've changed the famous phrase, "You can lead a horse to water, but you can't make him drink," to meet the needs of the moody, porous, overcaring intuitive population, "You can lead a horse to water, but you can't give him an IV." When people hear me say this, they say, "That doesn't make sense, you can give a horse an IV," at which time, like Mabel, I reply, "Yes, but what would be the point? You'd have to put that horse on life support, and you'd be that support. Eventually, you'd end up getting drained dry."

When your mood plummets and you get a bad feeling that something's happening with a loved one, call him or her up. Diplomatically obtain left-brain data to find out if your intuition was accurate. And if it is, gently state your perspective once . . . maybe twice. Then let it go. And when your intuitive warning signals of moodiness and physical symptoms of distress keep going off, do the radical acceptance exercise in Step 9.

If your loved one insists on going forward with a course of imminent danger, at this point you have to identify him or her as "NOT A REHAB CANDIDATE," someone that you cannot help.

What do you do if you find out your partner, husband, daughter, son, mother, father, patient, or (fill in the blank) is not a "rehab" candidate? Please read Step 11.

STEP 11: ONE LIFE TO LIVE

One of my favorite soap operas from my teenage years was *One Life to Live,* because I liked the philosophical concept behind its title. We are all given one life to live. We can't truly help anyone else in making the "right" choices, because we are all "issued" our own life to take risks, make mistakes, and fall in love with the wrong people.

I once did a reading on a woman, Nora, who had diabetes. She was having problems with depression, panic attacks, and headaches. She also wanted to get pregnant. My immediate reaction was, "What, are you nuts? Don't you know what can happen to someone who has severe diabetes and gets pregnant?" Instead, a little switch went on in my mind and I saw a clip from the movie *Steel Magnolias*. Sally Field, the mother, is trying to convince her diabetic daughter, played by Julia Roberts, not to have a baby. To Nora's utter surprise, I began to recite Julia Roberts's lines (in a Southern accent, I must admit), "Mama, I'd rather have a few moments of something wonderful than a lifetime of nothing special." In fact, Nora had seen the movie and it made a tremendous impact on her desire to have a child despite the fact that it could take years off her life.

I told Nora, "If, one, you know all the left-brain rational reasons why you shouldn't have a baby, and, two, your right brain and body intuition are screaming at you to get pregnant, and three, you still really want to get pregnant . . . Do it. It's your life to live. This is what you need to do. Your loved ones will still love you, and they will have to deal with their feelings about it."

PART THREE

*The New Feminine Brain Way of Thinking,
Learning, and Paying Attention*

NINE

I Can See for Miles and Miles: Attention and Perception, Impulsiveness and Compulsiveness

I am the poster child for the New Feminine Brain's adult form of attention deficit disorder with hyperactivity. When I was a resident, my physical hyperactivity was so great the medical students who followed me on call were always told to wear running shoes. I simply can't sit still. I fidget; I squirm; get up to get highlighters, stickies, file cards, and magazines. I walk fast, talk fast, think fast . . . everything fast. It's physically painful for me to slow down. When I give a public talk, I scotch-tape numerous signs on the floor of the stage that read "Talk Slowly." These help me, but still people's written comments include, "Dr. Schulz has so much to say. Why does she have to speak so fast?"

A friend of mine, Naomi Judd, describes my speech pattern as "sixty miles an hour with gusts up to one hundred." She asked me how I could have attention deficit disorder when I could sit for twelve hours at a time and help her work on her book. I said, "Look, I have a strong emotional attachment to getting this done, which pumps up my attention circuits. I don't want you to get in trouble with your editor, so fear is also a great motivator that . . . Oh my God . . . Why is Larry [her husband] running across your back pasture?" My response demonstrates my extreme distractibility.

I have the more masculinized brain form of ADD. I was good at math and science and not big on reading. I played with blocks while my sister read *Little House on the Prairie.* I am addicted to sugar, which I control with

273

the help of a gumball machine that dispenses peanut M&M's but only takes pennies. To get an M&M's dose, I have to hunt for a penny, which is agony for me. It's my "portion control device" so I don't get insulin resistance eating too much sugar.

Intuition and attention are both core functions of the right brain and have a unique relationship. When your attention wanders, and you enter a dreamlike state of consciousness, you have enhanced access to your intuition. Meditation, a process in which we intentionally alter our level of consciousness, may help open you intuitively. Even people with disordered attention, ADD (attention deficit disorder), or ADHD (attention deficit disorder with hyperactivity) seem to gain access to their intuition when their attention wanders. And the feminine brain seems primed to pick up when a child, partner, or patient is in distress.

Virtual Nurturance: Women's Intuition and ADD

Alice-Marie, thirty-five years old, called me for a reading.

The reading: Alice-Marie had no emotional distance between her and a very troubled loved one, for whom she was anxious and fearful. This family member was either developmentally challenged or handicapped in some way, so Alice-Marie couldn't fix the main problem, but only run interference when other problems occurred. As a result, Alice-Marie was constantly, intuitively monitoring danger in her loved one's life and was distracted from critical issues in her own. Her body's neurological system seemed to be chronically on "red alert," making several of her organ systems feel like they were "fried." Her throat appeared chronically irritated by allergies or upper respiratory infections. Her digestive tract seemed red, either due to food allergies or nervousness, and she was chronically exhausted, sad, and moody.

The facts: Alice-Marie was very worried about her twelve-year-old daughter with Asperger's syndrome, Betty, who was failing many classes in school, had few friends, and was always complaining about stomachaches. Alice-Marie could always tell when her daughter was having a bad day at school because her own nerves would get "on edge," and she couldn't focus at work. Alice-Marie had been diagnosed with ADD and had always had trouble paying attention to the task at hand. When she wasn't paying attention to her own life, her mind wandered into the lives of loved ones, worrying about their problems, and was adept at picking up on their troubles. But her intuition was making her sick. Her intuition came to her through her brain's developmental flaw in attention, but how could she come to peace with her ADD, improve her ability to focus and her physical problems, and heal herself but also maintain access to her intuition?

Distractibility in the Twenty-first Century

Why is paying attention a challenge for women today? The New Feminine Brain has been shaped to be more distractible, impulsive, and compulsive, because a woman has to:

1. *Divide attention* appropriately between the physical needs of her outer world of family and friends, and her own inner emotional needs
2. *Focus attention* on a job or task *without being distracted* by everything else that's going on around her
3. *Focus attention* on what her *intuition* tells her so she can anticipate future opportunities and potential problems

Since the feminine brain traditionally has more connectivity than a man's, usually a woman can divide her attention among different roles, but adding more pressure in any one area may make her drop a ball in this mental juggling act.

In order to succeed in business, for instance, a woman must reel in her attentional circuits so that she isn't so intuitively keyed in to other's feelings and thoughts. One of the major impediments to women advancing to top positions in the workplace is that they care too much what others think. A testosterone-dipped, more compartmentalized brain is better suited to follow the motto "It's not personal, it's just business." Over the last three or four decades, as women's earning power and socioeconomic status have increased, we have sprouted new brain pathways for competing in the workplace and unplugging from the feelings of our opponents, but that has a cost. When women detach from their intuition and empathy, they increase their vulnerability to emotional and physical problems.

But, in the long run, it's about as easy to censor your intuition as it is to stop a woman in labor from delivering her baby. Intuition is so much a part of every brain-body circuit you have that it's impossible ever to truly unplug it. When you try to convince yourself that feelings for your co-workers, competitors, or other businesspeople don't matter, those feelings and thoughts don't go away—they merely go underground into your brain and body. Empathetic feelings and thoughts simmer in your brain until they set off a domino effect, a biochemical chain reaction, that disrupts your mood and ability to pay attention.

Later in this chapter I will talk about ways to use all of your emotional, cognitive, and intuitive abilities in balance.

Subscribing to Too Many Channels

At every life stage, women today have more input and channels of information to pay attention to than at any time in history. No wonder it seems as if everyone has ADD and the world is on Ritalin and Prozac. The New Feminine Brain is sprouting new neurons and synapses—new nerve cells and connections between them—to deal with the challenges of sifting through information. More and more women are being diagnosed as having attention-deficit disorder, and almost none of these cases looks the same.

One woman might tell you in a dreamy monotone, "The psychiatrist says I have ADD. That's why I always seem to be so out of it, my head in the clouds. Now I know why antidepressants have never worked for me." Another might rattle on nonstop: "Oh, my God, I can't believe I messed up all those forms! I can't believe I lost that report. I don't know where that file is. Oh, by the way, did I tell you my psychiatrist just told me I have ADD?" One talks at twenty words a minute, the other at 150 words a minute.

Then your daughter goes off to college, spends hours researching and preparing, but never seems to be able to finish her term papers or hand in her assignments on time. She phones home to announce, "I just went to Health Services, and they told me that my problem is ADD. I get lost in the details and lose sight of the big picture." Finally, your best friend, who's going through perimenopause, phones in distress because she's forgotten to pick the kids up at school and mail the tax forms. "My brain feels like it's on Novocaine," she wails. "I keep having 'senior moments.' I think it must be late-onset ADD."

How can all these women have attention disorders? The functions involved in paying attention are distributed across the brain. It takes at least five different areas of the brain to focus your perception, distribute your attention, prevent you from being distracted, help you see both the whole picture and the details, then funnel all that awareness into directed, purposeful activity that will give you a feeling of reward. Given all that, it makes sense that the wastebasket diagnosis of ADD would be applied to so many different women: those with their head in the clouds, those who worry too much, those who seem preoccupied, those who can't see the forest for the trees, and those who feel as if their brains are on Novocaine. All these women have challenges in their attention circuits because their brains are trying to keep up with a novel world.

How Attention Works: Your Attention Circuits

Let's look at your responses to the questionnaire in Chapter 3. In each section the responses labeled 5 and 6 relate specifically to attention and perception. Your answers will tell you if you have a balanced proportion of all three components of attention or an imbalance of one component that gives you an "extreme" attention style (see below). Ultimately, to survive as an individual and as a member of society, you have to have a flexible mindset that uses all three of the components of attention:

1. *Focused attention.* The ability to ignore distractions, prioritize what to pay attention to and what to ignore (primarily frontal lobe brain function)
2. *Divided attention.* Your ability to divide attention between the outer world and your inner experience or pay attention equally to both the whole picture and details (primarily right brain parietal function)
3. *Emotional attention.* The ability to pay attention to emotionally charged issues. Empathic attention is a form of emotional attention devoted to the health and welfare of a loved one (primarily temporal lobe–limbic system function)

If you repeatedly chose answer 5 in parts I through V of the questionnaire, you may have problems with all three kinds of attention; and your distractibility, impulsivity, and other symptoms may interfere with learning and memory. On the other hand, if you answered 6 in parts I–V of the questionnaire, you have a balanced attention style that lets you readily focus on something, divide your attention to other elements of your surroundings, and at the same time be emotionally present to yourself and others. (By the way, how do you do it? I'll hire you.)

Consider the first question in the questionnaire:
You have entered a crowded department store. What do you do?

a.   I always have a list and I always follow it.
b.   I have a list, but I lose it and just wing it.

FOCUSED ATTENTION

If you can enter a crowded store without a list, keep "in mind" the things you need to buy, and successfully leave the store with those items and without getting sidetracked, you have *focused attention.* If you enter that store with a written list of items and follow it, leaving the store without getting waylaid, you also have focused attention. A department store tries hard to distract us. Can you keep your attention on the task at hand, or do you need a list to organize you? A shopping list, or any list for that matter, is a "prosthetic frontal lobe"—like the frontal lobe it creates a plan, organizes, and prioritizes what you should focus on first, then second, and so on. It keeps you on track and prevents you from getting distracted by exciting things around you (stimulus-bound) and ultimately acting impulsively. If you make a list then lose it, you have *distractibility*. You lack the focus necessary to hang onto the list. If you answered 5 on the questionnaire and impulsively buy things displayed at the cash register, you have an attentional deficit symptom called "impulsivity," which distracts your focus.

Distraction can take many forms. Some people with attentional problems start things but don't finish them; that's *impersistence*. (Your teachers might have written on your report card: "Lacks perseverance.") Other people get so "glued" to something they are doing that they block out inadvertently other, more critical things. That's called *perseveration*. ("How can she have ADD when she's on the computer for hours on end?") Or maybe you get too easily overwhelmed, your mind gets "clouded," and you can't focus on anything. "If Louise doesn't take a study break every forty minutes, she can't retain anything she's trying to learn." Finally, some people have "selective" areas of inattentiveness called a *field of attentional neglect*. "How come Mary's sock drawer is a masterpiece but her financial records and office work space are a disaster?"

ATTENTION = MEMORY

Much of what people think of as memory is really attention. The frontal lobe organizes what you perceive and attend to, which helps you lay down a memory. When a woman in perimenopause complains that she can't remember a thing, it's probably not a memory issue, but an attentional one: changes in hormone levels in her frontal lobe are causing inattentiveness.

A common example of how we confuse attention and memory is the task of keeping a list on your mental blackboard, for instance, hearing directions. When you ask someone for directions, and he says, "Well, you go down this street, then turn right at the second light, then go past the gas station until you get to . . . ," unless you're exceptional, you've probably already forgotten what he's said so far. Writing down information is another adaptive compensatory strategy people use when their attention is shaky.

Making change or doing other arithmetic computations in your head tests your attention. You have to manipulate figures in your mind, holding them in your attentional circuits' mental scratch pad as you compute. In one of my favorite vignettes from the TV show *Seinfeld,* Jerry goes to pick up a rental car at the airport. The woman at the rental desk tells him, "We have your reservation, but we have no more cars." Then he says, "But I should have a car because I made a reservation." She repeats, "We have your reservation, but we have no more cars," to which he says, "You're not understanding me." "Yes, I am," she insists. Finally, Jerry snaps, "Anyone can *take* a reservation. You have to *hold* the reservation."

The same principle holds true with attention. *Taking* the information—perceiving it, hearing, seeing, feeling it—is one thing; being able to *hold* it in working memory, so you can manipulate it, involves attention. If you can't make change for a dollar, it may not be that you have acalculia—the inability to do math. It's more likely that you have an attentional problem.

DIVIDED ATTENTION

In Question II, which looks at your habits in a restaurant, response 5 relates to divided attention, the capacity to be aware of your own thoughts but keep "in mind" what's going on around you. After the waiter recites the list of salad dressings, can you keep them in mind, on your "scratchboard memory," as you think about what you want to eat? If you can recite the salad dressing list without having the waiter repeat it, you have good *divided attention* (see below), which is very important for *memory.* However, if you answered 5 and you can't keep the items in your mind if you're thinking about something else, you have problems with distractibility and dividing your attention between your internal and external environments.

Speaking of restaurants, are you *stimulus-bound,* or overly responsive to your surroundings? In a restaurant, are you likely to get caught up in what others are ordering, and prefer others' meals to your own? Can you stop yourself from reaching over and taking a tomato out of someone else's salad, or plucking a french fry from the side of his burger? While sitting at a desk, are you driven to scribbling with the pens or doodling on the edge of your papers? Do you find yourself continuously capping and uncapping the pens? While standing in a hallway, is your hand drawn to flipping the light switch for no particular reason? If you can't stop yourself from "using" things, that's an attention challenge called utilization behavior, another form of impulsivity, and is seen in *hyperactivity.*

People with attentional challenges tend to be either hyperorganized or disorganized. A compulsively organized person has carefully programmed her car radio to favorite stations. Her CDs are meticulously alphabetized by artist. At the opposite extreme is the disorganized person who lacks the persistence to program the radio and habitually punches the scan button, and is too distracted to listen to a CD all the way through.

You often need to be able to focus simultaneously on two different areas, say, your feelings and your outer environment. For example, you may become absolutely captivated by an old song on the radio, remembering how you felt the first time you fell in love. As you listen, your attention is divided between the outer and inner worlds. The capacity for internal reverie may be waning in the New Feminine Brain, though, because these days, instead of our brains creating a unique internal imagery to go along with a song, MTV and music videos do it for us. The title of the song "Video Killed the Radio Star" may be true.

Another form of divided attention is the ability to see both the *details* (left-brain, focused attention) and the *whole picture* (right-brain, global attention). Being able to see both the trees and the forest gives a balanced perspective. People with excessive left-brain attention are overly detailed and compulsive, and tend to have trouble finishing projects on time because they can never get it perfect. On the other hand, people with excessive right-brain attention tend to approach any task with broad brush strokes, neglecting most of the details, so the final product is sloppy and slipshod.

Some people were either born without or have lost the ability to divide attention between themselves and their outer environment. Either they are born spacey or they acquire a spacey mind-set through meditation or repeated hallucinogenic drug use. Cyclic changes in hormones may also disconnect a woman's capacity to divide attention between herself and others, making her feel like a space cadet (see below).

You need both your left and right brain to see and pay attention to the world. How you approach a buffet table can offer insight into global (right-brain) and local (left-brain) awareness and how we handle choices in daily life. Someone with balanced attention sees the whole (right-brain) forest as well as the individual (left-brain) trees. She would be able to scan the whole buffet table and plan ahead, then go through the line systematically, making selections. Someone with excessive left-brain attention—a hyper-attentive sort—might take a long time in the salad area at the beginning of the buffet, pay too much attention to the individual vegetables, and never get to the rest of the buffet or find her favorite dishes. Someone with excessive, global, right-brain attention, on the other hand, might take in the whole table at a glance but skip around so much when serving herself that she, too, overlooks her favorite dishes. Any extreme sort of attention presents challenges.

EMOTIONAL ATTENTION

Your feelings are the greatest factor in determining what you pay attention to: whatever makes you angry, sad, fearful, loving, or joyful. Advertising executives create commercials and magazine ads laced with images of sex and other emotionally provocative situations to get our attention.

Nonetheless, too much emotional attention can be a problem. In school, were you frequently more focused on the mood of someone near you than what the teacher was talking about in the front of the room? If one of your parents, children, or partners is in distress, can you focus on your work or remember what you've read? Do you usually know shopkeepers by their first name? Do you write personal emails two or even three times a day or get so lost in a conversation that you forget your surroundings?

Emotional attention is motivated by our passion and sense of caring. To learn and remember well, you need to use this 3-D emotional attention together with *focusing and dividing* attention. Some women can divide their attention easily but others are so keyed into emotions that they can't attend to anything else.

In women, there are three basic extreme attention styles: *bull's-eye focused, transcendent,* and *empathetic* attention.

1. *The "Bull's-eye," Focused Attention Style:* Society rewards us for our capacity to hyperfocus on one thing and block out everything else. The traditional male, compartmentalized brain is better adapted to this sort of focus, while the traditionally hyperconnected feminine brain has a much greater difficulty maintaining it and staying free from distractions. Because our culture values focused attention more than other ways of attending to our environment, if your attention style isn't riveted to a "bull's eye," you're more likely to be diagnosed with attention deficit disorder.

2. *The Transcendent Attention Style:* Most trained, successful athletes have been able to develop this extreme form of attention to perform at their peak. They manipulate their right brain, whose parietal lobe enables them to divide attention equally between their outer environment and inner emotional world. Expert meditators also learn how to "disconnect" these right-brain areas to get an ecstatic focused feeling of "oneness with the world." During this "transcendent" form of attention, time seems to stand still. Golfers who get a hole in one, gymnasts who really "nail" a routine, quarterbacks and receivers in "the Zone" frequently report this single-

minded, timeless feeling. Transcendent attention ignores the rules of time and space. After natural childbirth, when a woman holds her baby for the first time, her brain is biochemically primed to focus on her baby in this blissful state of mind. Childbirth and other dynamic hormonal events facilitate a transcendent mind-set.

3. *The Empathetic Attention Style:* Some women's brains are so keyed in to emotional undercurrents that they can't focus on anything else. For example, it's hard to enjoy a meal or even focus on what you're eating if your dinner companion is looking angry or distressed. Your attentional circuits may get so glued to what is bothering your friend that no circuits are available to pay attention to what you're putting in your mouth.

Diagnosing Attention Disorders

Because many women do not have the classic male "compartmentalized" style of *focused attention,* when they complain to a doctor about their lack of focus, they receive a diagnosis of ADD and get put on Ritalin, Adderall, or some other medicine. Most women do not receive lasting benefit from this, since it cannot "fix" their native style of paying attention, which is underappreciated. Unfortunately, most children are being labeled as having ADD or ADHD by a teacher or parent who identifies symptoms on a checklist, not by objective measures on professional tests. A diagnosis of childhood ADD is based on three main symptoms: inattentiveness, hyperactivity, and/or impulsivity. The primary diagnostic tool is called the Connors Scale. It is an imperfect measure at best: a checklist of items that the child's teacher ticks off, based solely on his or her observation of the child's behavior.

Signs of *inattentiveness* on the Connors Scale are:

- inattention to details
- careless mistakes
- difficulty sustaining attention
- not listening when spoken to
- failing to follow instructions
- difficulty organizing tasks
- avoiding and disliking sustained mental effort
- losing items necessary for tasks
- distracted by extraneous stimuli
- forgetful in daily activities

If the teacher checks six or more of these items, the child receives a diagnosis of ADD. But the Connors Scale doesn't take into account other factors that may contribute to the child's observed behavior. What about the instructor's teaching style? Perhaps the teacher speaks in an emotionless monotone, or fails to make the material lively, relevant, or emotionally compelling. Perhaps the child finds the subject matter dull: He may be bright and inquisitive but bored by the history of the baskets of Mesopotamia or whatever uninteresting material is being presented. If the material is not engaging, the student will not perceive it, pay attention to it, learn it, and remember it. The child might also be very empathetic, intuitive, and preoccupied with other, disturbing issues (problems at home, etc.) that preempt her capacity to attend to what's going on in school.

A child may be diagnosed with ADD on the basis of six or more signs of *hyperactivity* and *impulsivity:*

- fidgeting
- leaving one's seat
- running and climbing
- difficulty being quiet during leisure activities
- motor-driven, always on the go
- talking excessively
- blurting out answers in class
- difficulty with waiting one's turn
- problems with interrupting
- intrusiveness

But here, too, there could be other reasons a child might exhibit this behavior. Perhaps she is emotionally disturbed by stress at home. Children seldom verbalize inner distress; they tend to act it out, becoming agitated, pacing, or getting into fights.

A child might meet the criteria for ADD on the Connors Scale without really having a disorder in attention. A child who's impulsive, blurts out answers, interrupts, and intrudes into others' space simply may not have been taught how to be polite. The problem may not be frontal-lobe inattentiveness but a lack of education in proper social behavior. Before deciding if certain behavior warrants the label ADD, it's important to look at the social environment in which the person was raised.

For example, years ago, while I was in college, I was invited to dinner at the home of a Japanese friend. Throughout the meal no one said a word, and the mother stood at the door to the kitchen and watched us eat. At the other extreme, interruptions and in-your-face boisterousness are the norm in certain cultures, including my own Portuguese family dinners.

As we hit puberty, our frontal lobe grows into its executive task of managing our behavior and inhibiting our impulses. Some girls are genetically less likely to be hyperactive and impulsive. A cluster of genes on the X chromosome actually mediates social behavior by inhibiting the frontal lobe and right brain. The feminine brain structure tends to prevent butting in on conversations, and tends to help women more than men read facial expressions, social cues, and body language. If a pregnant woman has excessive androgens, however, the brain of a female fetus when grown may develop more impulsivity and hyperactivity. With society's changing sexual roles and social expectations, a girl (and ultimately a woman) may be more likely to be accepted if she is hyperactive and impulsive. This behavior may be labeled by others as "driven" or "Type A" and may actually have some social and economic advantage.

A child with ADHD may "grow out" of a lot of the hyperactive symptoms as her frontal lobe matures at puberty and develops circuits to inhibit stimulus-bound behavior, and she may funnel her energy into socially appropriate routes like work and perfectionism. However, some women will tend to internalize that energy and develop symptoms of anxiety, depression, and restlessness. You've probably sat next to someone on a plane who's constantly getting up and down, or asking for a blanket, a pillow, another magazine. Impulsivity may also come out in antisocial behavior and high-risk behavior such as reckless driving. Substance use and abuse is common among adults with ADHD, but it is not clear if the use of alcohol, marijuana, and other drugs is a compensatory strategy for calming down the hyperactivity to facilitate increased focus and productivity.

Attention and Development

A variety of factors mold your brain and determine how you ultimately pay attention. If your mother was stressed when pregnant with you, especially in the first trimester, her elevated androgen levels would have altered how your right and left brain perceive the world. In addition to an increased risk for dyslexia, you're less likely to develop the traditional focused attention. Your atypical attention style is likely to give you exaggerated empathetic and intuitive gifts and possibly creative and artistic skills. If a pregnant woman drinks alcohol, however, all attention pathways in the fetal brain become disordered. Alcohol not only damages the developing corpus callosum, the connection between the right and left brain, but also injures developing white-matter nerve pathways involved in every aspect of attention. Children and adults with fetal alcohol syndrome suffer the most severe forms of attention deficit disorder, with profound hyperactivity so disabling that they have trouble functioning in the world.

Your childhood environment also shapes how you learn and pay attention later in life. From birth to two years, the nursery environment further affects your attentional circuits. Ultimately, we need a balance of left-brain details and right-brain spiritual, emotional, and empathetic enrichment in our environment to develop healthy attention. In early childhood, were you raised in a crowded environment with other siblings and an extended family? How often were you picked up and hugged? Was the TV or radio always on in your house? Did you live on a farm, with wide open spaces, or in a busy, crowded city?

Was your childhood enriched or deprived? An enriched environment simply means one with lots to see, hear, and pay attention to; a deprived environment is one that is sterile and lacks input. Either extreme will affect your attentional circuits. Too much input will overwhelm and not help your development and too little will impoverish it. If the atmosphere you grow up in is chaotic, you'll have higher levels of two stress hormones—norepinephrine and cortisol—that will, over years, affect your attention and memory. A childhood injury to the brain from an accident, fall, or sports may also affect your attention and memory circuits.

Your reproductive history—whether you have a child early or late, or never give birth—also affects the brain areas for attention. The hormones your brain is "dipped into" in utero, in puberty, in pregnancy, postpartum, and through emotional, physical, or sexual trauma—estrogen, progesterone, testosterone, and others—all influence your attentional circuits. Your inner environment—the emotional challenges you've had to face—also influence your attention. Unresolved emotional issues use up your mental reserves and leave you with insufficient "cortical tone" to attend to events in your present life. Your body develops symptoms of illness until you attend to past conflicts and feelings that are holding you back.

Finally, if you are a child of the twenty-first century, opening multiple windows on your computer while watching TV, talking on your cell phone, and downloading email, your new feminine brain may adapt neurochemically and anatomically to this overwhelming input and excessive overstimulation in a way similar to a baby's and child's developing brain. Your attention may become shorter and you may find it difficult to read a long book or report. You may need special effects, quick changes of scenes in a movie to stay interested and alert; a slower, dialogue-driven drama may easily lose its appeal. And your attentional circuits will be molded over time to accommodate an ever more complex, fast-paced environment.

Clearly the influences of the twenty-first century on the New Feminine Brain look nothing like those of the fifteenth century. What arouses our interest and emotions, what seems relevant and worthy of response, is very different from back then. And with so much input coming at us today, something has to be increasingly novel to get and hold our attention.

The New Feminine Brain's Attentional Styles

The following case studies illustrate the most common attentional styles of the feminized brain and the ways in which each type is likely to be challenged.

CASE STUDY 1: SPACE CADET, THE FINAL FRONTIER: TRANSCENDENT ATTENTION

Suzanne, age fifty-seven, was better suited for transcendent meditative states than for the demands of school and a career. Her primary care doctor had diagnosed her with ADD in high school. She had trouble paying attention in school, was always disorganized and late, and became easily overwhelmed when there was a lot of noise and stimulation in her environment. She excelled in English literature, writing, and other left-brain classes, but failed miserably in right-brain "spatial"-type classes such as geometry. She flunked her driver's ed test three times because she couldn't parallel park.

At work, Suzanne was easily overwhelmed by the details of a task and the activity of her co-workers. She had spent years teaching TM (transcendental meditation) in a spiritual community, which helped her focus, as did spending time with her husband, Bill, an accountant, who was everything Suzanne was not—organized, grounded, focused, and driven.

Suzanne had other emotional and physical concerns that aggravated her attention problems:

- Borderline low thyroid function
- Family history of addictions; an alcoholic father and son addicted to marijuana
- Excess weight with constant cravings for sweets, pasta, and bread
- Fibroids, breast cysts, and "excess estrogen"
- Depression and irritability that didn't improve on medicines

When she was depressed or tired, Suzanne had an even harder time paying attention at work. She was also quite upset about her son's drug problem and about his failing many school classes. She consumed sweets because they "pepped" up her attention. As her weight ballooned, so did menstrual problems, breast cysts, and fibroids. A psychiatrist prescribed Adderall, a Ritalin-related medicine for ADD, and her attention and mood improved for about a year, but after several dose adjustments, it stopped working.

Suzanne's brain probably had a developmental problem in her right parietal lobe, an area critical for attention. Her problems with depression, motivation, initiation, and lack of direction were primarily due to her transcendent attention style, but the food and meditation she used to improve her mood probably made her problems worse over time. Studies show that long-term meditation can alter the attentional circuits in the right hemisphere in some susceptible individuals. She also had trouble dividing her attention between her obligations in the world and what was going on in her inner meditative emotional life; extrapersonal space and intrapersonal space became one vague area for her. In *Why God Won't Go Away,* researchers Andrew Newberg and Eugene d'Aquili report that meditation decreases arousal in the right parietal area, the same area for directed attention in extrapersonal space. For meditators, intrapersonal (inside themselves) and extrapersonal space (the external world) feel like one. In Suzanne's case, she may have used meditation to get her out of her left brain and give her some peace, but having done it for years she may have exacerbated her spaciness by rewiring her right parietal lobe.

Suzanne's son had the more masculinized form of attention deficit, ADHD, with hyperactivity. He was easily distracted and his impulsive, stimulus-bound behavior made it difficult for him to focus on, prioritize, and complete tasks. Women who developed in utero in an androgen-excess environment are more likely to have this more masculinized attention style, and one third of them are also likely to be dyslexic.

The Estrogen Connection

Suzanne's attention problems were probably aggravated by her hormones. Even though she was postmenopausal, her excess weight made her body have inappropriately high levels of estrogen, a condition called "estrogen dominance," which, as with some women on the Pill, made her irritable, edgy, depressed, and unable to focus. There seems to be a connection between estrogen and ADD. Estrogen affects mood, attention, and memory by somehow acting on serotonin, norepinephrine, and other neurotransmitter systems. Girls with ADD may have increasingly severe problems with attention at puberty because of changing levels of estrogen and progesterone since it influences serotonin levels in the brain. Estrogen at appropriate levels can treat the mood and attention problems in PMS and menopause, like the serotonin medicines Prozac and Zoloft.

Thyroid disorders (either hypo- or hyperthyroidism) can precipitate changes in attention. Suzanne and her son were both sugar addicts, which is common among people with attentional problems, some of whom develop weight problems as a result.

Boys are more likely to have attention deficit disorder with hyperactivity whereas girls are more likely to have the calmer, dreamy form. Yes, many nontraditional boys do have the inattentive form of ADD, and atypical women can be hyperactive. No one knows why boys tend to be more hyperactive than girls. It could be due to elevated androgen or testosterone levels, since girls and women with higher androgen levels are more likely to demonstrate ADHD. Social pressure may also be a factor, since usually girls who demonstrate hyperactivity are more likely to be shunned.

As Suzanne's son got older, his attention style became more similar to his mother, more dreamlike and distracted. As someone grows older and develops more frontal-lobe control over behavior, hyperactivity seems to disappear. However, since ADD/ADHD is an inborn trait, like blue eyes, curly hair, or left-handedness, drug treatment with Ritalin or getting older doesn't cure these problems or give them "normal" attention.

Both Suzanne and her son had to come to terms with their unique brain style. Suzanne's brain was better adapted for being a therapist or counselor. She could also use her left-brain writing skills in a career, but she would need to hire a surrogate frontal lobe organizer, an editor, who could hold her to a schedule and maintain a logical structure in her writing. Psychotherapy, medicine, and nutritional supplements could help Suzanne pump up her ability to focus (see below).

CASE STUDY 2: "I'VE FALLEN AND I CAN'T GET UP": EMPATHETIC EMOTIONAL ATTENTION

Karen, fifty-two, had a long history of distractibility and problems paying attention in school and later at work. Her résumé is a long list of jobs, each lasting one or two years. Whenever the work environment got tense, Karen got sick with episodes of dizziness, fatigue, a lump in her throat, and chest pain. Over time, these episodes got worse, affected her job performance, and Karen would get fired for making mistakes. Even though she eventually was able to get a job that allowed her to work from home, without the distraction of co-workers and a supervisor, Karen fell behind more and more deadlines. After a minor car accident and concussion, Karen went on disability. No matter what medicine her psychiatrist gave her for attention deficit disorder, she wasn't able to clear the mental fog from her brain.

Karen's empathetic attention style was too vulnerable to environmental interference and distraction, and was easily derailed by the emotions and thoughts of people around her. She had developed this ability to switch her attention because of a chaotic, traumatic childhood. Her mother was institutionalized shortly after Karen's birth, and she was shuttled from foster home to foster home. Shortly after her mother committed suicide, Karen married a man who turned out to be an abusive alcoholic, but because she had few job skills and two kids, Karen stayed in the marriage until her husband abandoned them for another woman. Forced to go to work to support herself and her two kids, she developed depression, fatigue, panic, and mental fog, which worsened her attention.

Karen's circuits for fear, attention, and intuition were shaped by her traumatic childhood, her mother's suicide, and her husband's violent temper. For survival, Karen had learned to focus empathetically on the people around her, and be on constant surveillance for potential anger, betrayal, or abandonment. As a result, she wasn't able to focus on work. Karen had ADD, but not ADHD, since she wasn't hyperactive or impulsive. In fact, she was inhibited, timid, shy, depressed, and anxious. Ritalin wouldn't help her focus. Karen's attention was probably derailed by long-term anxiety and depression, which were "burning up" serotonin and opiates, making it harder for her brain to get and stay focused and organized. Karen's empathetic attention circuits were so consumed by emotional pain and suffering in herself and others that there was no room to pay attention to anything else.

Karen needed to detox and rebuild her brain. She needed psychotherapy combined with medical and nutritional treatment for depression (see Chapter 5) and anxiety (see Chapter 7), which would make more space in her brain so she could pay attention to work and other more rewarding pastimes.

Case Study 3: "Seeing the Trees but Not the Forest": Excess Left-Brain and Insufficient Right-Brain Attention

Joan, forty-seven, is hard-working, but has difficulty focusing her attention in the outside world. She loves people but feels very alone. Despite her efforts to get along with others, her co-workers find her difficult to work with. She always seems to have "tunnel vision," to be in her own world and not plugged into her colleagues' concerns. Joan works in a college admissions office. When I asked her what her job involved, she told me, "I file acceptances and rejections. I have a lot of file folders. I'm very systematic and organized."

Joan's attentional style is obsessive-compulsive: She organizes and plans, but with a hyperfocus that hangs her up in the ordering of details so that she seldom executes the bigger plan. As Joan puts it, "I focus so much that I run out of time and it doesn't get done." Her organizational efforts annoy and alienate fellow employees. "No one else can figure out how to work the plan I set up," she says.

Joan wants to get married and signed up with a dating service to find a mate. But in love, as in work, her obsessive-compulsive attentional style seems to work against her. "It took me a long time to fill out the form; I wanted to make it perfect," she recalls. But her answers seemed devoid of warmth. She spent so much time investigating dating services that she saw how to improve them and she actually created her own, starting a new business that helped others. She sold the business for a profit but unfortunately never made a match herself. Her sadness and sense of failure is poignant. "I just don't understand why I can't have passion in my life," she laments.

Tunnel and Tree Vision: Excessive Focus on Details

Joan is so focused on the trees that she can't find the forest. Joan's left-brain attention to details make her unable attend to right-brain emotional nuance and warmth. In the dating service application, Joan was so attentive to getting every detail perfect that she missed its overall purpose, which was to get a date. If you are driving down a road, it's important to have divided attention: to see not only what's directly ahead but also to be aware of cars, cyclists, and pedestrians in the periphery. Joan's tunnel vision was so focused on her assignments that she wasn't aware of the emotional reactions of people around her. Partnership or team work was also hard for Joan. Unable to change how she organized her work, Joan couldn't understand why she was repeatedly told that her methods were hard to follow. She constantly made lists, and new, increasingly complex organizational strategies. Her inattentiveness was compulsive, not impulsive.

Joan has too much frontal lobe function: excessive organization of everything, every fact, file, is so exaggerated in importance. Her temporal lobe limbic area that is important for emotional states is peripheralized and her inattentiveness to the feelings of people around her caused her repeated rejection and social isolation. Her obsessive-compulsive personality and preoccupation with extreme orderliness and perfectionism made it hard for her to be happy and healthy. Joan eventually developed alcoholism to medicate her despair and isolation.

Medicines are usually not much help for increasing a person like Joan's ability to focus simultaneously on left-brain details and right-brain empathy, but cognitive behavioral therapy and other forms of psychotherapy can be very successful pumping up her empathy.

Attention deficit disorder is supposed to be an inborn problem, but as you can see, it is complicated by environment, experience, and hormonal and immune system disorders.

CASE STUDY 4: HELP! ALL MY HORMONES ARE EVAPORATING!

Deborah is forty-four and wants to know if she could have developed ADD in her forties. She had problems with infertility, but after five years of unsuccessful in vitro fertilization treatments, decided to give up on the process and adopt. Deborah had never had trouble paying attention until she had medical treatment for infertility. Pergonal and other fertility drugs that stimulate the ovaries, and Lupron, and other GnRH agonists used to shrink fibroids, can induce a mental fog that mimics ADD. The surge of hormones caused by infertility medicines and the dramatic reductions seen in fibroid treatments unplug attention circuits in the brain's frontal and temporal lobe. If you subject your brain to rapid shifts in hormones over and over again, as Deborah did, it will make you feel incapable of focusing or sustaining attention. Additionally, Deborah's grief and sadness over her unsuccessful efforts to get pregnant made it hard for her to pay attention to matters outside herself.

Kathleen is another example of how hormones can affect attention. At fifty-two, she is at an important crossroads and having a hard time working as a lawyer. Each case seems to blend into the next and her mind wanders in court. For years, Kathleen has felt that her creativity has been straitjacketed by her career. In her dreams, she sees herself opening a flower shop with friends. Kathleen also has mood changes and an "unbalanced" feeling in her head. In perimenopause, she was trying hormone replacement therapy, but it didn't seem to work. The changes in estrogen and progesterone levels were affecting her brain circuits for attention and retention. That is no coincidence. The attentional circuits in her brain were changing because what she was supposed to pay attention to was changing. Perimenopause basically invites women to reevaluate their relationships and vocation at midlife, and make changes if they're not satisfactory. At various times in our lives—in crises, when someone close to us dies—we are forced to search for new meaning. Our attention may withdraw from the outer world so that we can find out what our inner voice is really saying. It may be tempting to medicate that inattentiveness, especially if we are not in the habit of self-reflection.

For Kathleen, having problems with focusing attention, orienting to her environment, exploring, concentrating, and being vigilant at work was her brain's ways of disconnecting her attention from an outer unsatisfying career (extrapersonal space) and directing it inward to find out her true purpose. She was not able to focus on her job because she was supposed to figure out what's going on in her heart.

Maximize Your Attention Potential

How can you learn to appreciate the genius in your particular attention style and minimize the difficulties it may cause? Which environmental, educational, and career settings are likely to bring out the best in you? Which do you probably want to avoid? What sort of people should you hire, marry, or hang out with to augment the attention areas in which you have challenges? What addictions and other compensatory strategies do you need to stop and what medicines, nutritional supplements, and therapies can you take to sharpen your focus?

RELATIONSHIP THERAPY: BORROW A FRONTAL LOBE

If you are hyperactive, distractible, and stimulus-bound, you may need to "borrow" a frontal "executive" lobe from someone else (or a team of people), to help you resist distraction and organize and plan your work and life in general. You can borrow someone's frontal lobe to augment your own attention in a marriage, friendship, with a roommate, employee, employer, or some other relationship in which you divide up the responsibilities. In Case 1: Space Cadet, the Final Frontier," Suzanne did this by marrying a very competent accountant who helped her get it together. The person with strong frontal-lobe attention could provide the motivation, organization, and planning skills that would help you focus, stay on task, and complete projects on time. Karen (in Case 2: "I've Fallen and I Can't Get Up") depended on her relationships, although not the healthiest, to provide structure, which improved her focus and attention somewhat.

But, like a chemical dependency, excessive dependence on the people around you to pump up your attention circuits is risky. It's best if you can learn to provide some of that function for yourself and get the cognitive therapy retraining that will help you.

CLARIFY, ORGANIZE, AND FILE AWAY INNER EMOTIONAL TURMOIL WITH THE HELP OF A COUNSELOR OR THERAPIST

When you have a lot of turmoil inside, it's hard to pay attention to the details of daily life. Working with a psychotherapist or counselor (see Chapter 8) can clarify and file away emotional turmoil and trauma that are keeping you focused inward. Deep-cleaning of your psyche is especially needed during developmental turning points—postpartum and menopause, meeting a mate, getting married, or changing your career. At such times you may simply need to book time for yourself so you can process all that is going on.

Each of the predominant attentional styles of the New Feminine Brain has its own compensatory behavior:

• *A graphic organizer.* A Daytimer or Filofax can help people with Space Cadet inattentiveness who have problems with organization and planning. The book serves as a "prosthetic" frontal lobe and keeps you organized. It's a prompter, telling you what to do, who to talk to, what to see. You might be a brilliant musician, but if you don't show up for the nine o'clock meeting, you won't get the recording contract.

• *Environmental organizers.* Working in cooperative groups is also helpful. The other members of the group (if you like them) provide stimulation to activate your brain circuits and can also help you organize, plan, and keep you away from distraction. Many people successfully compensate for attentional deficit by using maps and flow charts. Some keep a TV or a radio on to increase environmental stimulation, thus priming their brains' attentional circuits. Other people find background noise more distracting than helpful. Frequently, people with attentional problems find that if they alter the task they are involved in multiple times a day, the continuous feeling of novelty pumps up attention.

• *Carbohydrate cravings.* Women like Suzanne with Space Cadet attentional style often crave and eat sweets and carbohydrates—a form of self-medication. Carbohydrates contain the amino acid tryptophan, which helps the body make serotonin, the neurotransmitter important for attention. Of course, carbohydrates contain a lot of calories and constant intake means weight gain. Too many calories make your fat cells swell, so, to keep your blood sugar stable, the number of insulin receptors on the cells increases. Then your pancreas has to produce more insulin to keep up with the calories you're consuming. Eventually it can't keep up and you develop insulin resistance. That, in turn, can lead to estrogen dominance, which increases the chances of other health problems like menstrual problems, fibroids, and breast cysts.

• *Addiction to alcohol, marijuana, cocaine, and other drugs.* Many people with hyperactivity and ADD use alcohol, marijuana, and other drugs to self-medicate, which releases the brain's natural opiates, inducing feelings of calm and well-being that make it easier to pay attention.

• *Vocational rehab.* Like all the women in the case examples, a lot of people with ADHD or ADD have a history of inconsistent or even poor job performance and difficulty deriving satisfaction from their work. But how much of a poor job performance is due to a "poor-performing job"? Perhaps there is too much distraction or not enough stimulation in the workplace. Maybe there's not enough structure (a supervisor prompting you to complete tasks)? Or perhaps this is the wrong job for you because it doesn't capture your interest enough to pump up your attentional circuits.

Some schools offer peer tutoring and cooperative learning where the students work in groups; four or five children might work together to complete a task. Similarly, some organizations assess employees' strengths and weaknesses, then team them up with people who have strengths they lack.

Distractible and impulsive people do best in creative jobs with a high degree of novelty and stimulation, where there's a different task with a different challenge every hour or so throughout the day. Hairstyling or stock or bond trading or working in an ER would be examples: Dealing with many different clients every day would reduce the chances of boredom. Someone else could take responsibility for the frontal "executive" lobe tasks of organizing and keeping your schedule and the left-brain details of handling the bookkeeping.

For me to pay attention, I have to be in an ever-changing environment full of stimulation, so that my brain's attentional circuits are pumped up. When I first worked in a lab, if I was given a routine task such as doing the same assay over and over, the lack of novelty would increase my chances of making mistakes. I dropped a lot of beakers and had other accidents. My supervisors learned not to put me in a situation where I was doing routine jobs. Instead, I was given things to invent, which I found challenging and stimulating. Eventually, I was given my own lab—with a door to lessen distraction. I'm a bonder, so if I'm working around other people, all somebody has to do is say something like "Hey, how about those Red Sox?" and the next thing you know, I'm not getting anything done. Having my own office with a door closed cuts down on the distractions.

Now I work for ML, Inc.—myself. Even though I do not have enough frontal-lobe "executive" attention, organization, and planning to manage my business on my own, I hire frontal lobes: I have very organized people who take care of administrative tasks that I would make a mess of. But they don't work in my office; that would be too distracting. I also plan different tasks every day—medical intuitive consultations, neuropsych evaluations, working on a newsletter, and working on my books. Each task is challenging and stimulating, and if something begins to get cumbersome, I switch off to another task for a while to maintain my attention, and then come back again when I'm better focused.

Activities like work and sports that give us a sense of reward release natural opiates that sharpen our attention and are chemically related to Ritalin. If you have chronic pain, putting yourself in a vocational setting that gives you a sense of reward releases natural opiates, which can help you focus your attention as well as reduce your pain.

• *Environmental Ritalin: Importing Stimulation.* Many people with attentional challenges thrive in stressful work environments, where the pace is very active—a hospital emergency room, say, or a daily newspaper. The fast pace stimulates the brain stem to produce norepinephrine, which allows you to focus.

Some people need background noise to concentrate. Other people with inattentiveness need a silent, monastery-like environment to focus and stay on task.

I almost always work with the TV on. I have a library of 1,400 movies on tape that I watch regularly. For a movie to work as "background environmental Ritalin," I have to have seen it many times before. If I haven't seen the movie, the novelty will make me pay attention to it and not to the work I need to finish. When Chris Northrup and I work on her newsletter, I can't read unless we have a movie playing. Sometimes we'll rent something at the video store. Chris will ask, "How about this one?" And I might say, "Oh, I haven't seen it. We can't get it or I'll watch it." At that point, people around us look at us in astonishment. Then Chris may say something like, "How about *My Cousin Vinny?*" I'll say, "Oh, great. Let's get that one. I've seen it twelve times." That works for me because while the movie is playing, I'll glance up every once in a while and realize that one of my favorite parts is coming. When it does, I watch it briefly and laugh—get my pump of norepinephrine for stimulation—then go back to work.

• *Focus with a smile.* One of the most effective strategies for improving attention is to laugh or elevate your mood. A positive mood pumps up your attentional circuits so that you're better able to explore your environment, concentrate on what's in front of you, and pay attention longer. Research shows that a positive mood can improve performance in both math and reading.

Attention Boosters

We've talked about some of the ways that the New Feminine Brain compensates for attentional problems, but you may wonder if there are more direct ways to pump up the attentional circuits—with Ritalin and other medications, for example. What are some other things you can do to make the most of what you have?

Ritalin is perhaps the most commonly prescribed drug for the treatment of attention deficits, but it is by no means appropriate for everyone or for every attentional problem. Ritalin (methylphenidate) is a mild brain stimulant. Although no one knows exactly how it works, it allegedly activates the brain stem arousal/attentional system. Don't take it if you're anxious or tense, since it may aggravate those symptoms. Ritalin and other related stimulants reduced the core ADD symptoms but can disturb sleep and appetite (see the ADD chart, below, for other related medications and their side effects). However, Canada recently suspended the use of British-made Adderall, a stimulant, owing to twenty reported deaths. So the jury is still out on the safety of this class of medicines.

Stimulants like Ritalin have been used for ADHD for over thirty years. Ritalin and medications like it are considered by many experts to be among the safest drugs for children, but many others don't agree. They can be abused and addictive, and doctors and parents are concerned about their being overprescribed. Newer, nonaddictive, nonstimulant ADD medicines are coming on the market every day. Strattera (atomoxetine) is being heavily advertised for the treatment of children and adults with ADD/ADHD. I'm not a fan of using any medicine in which long-term usefulness and effectiveness hasn't been established.

Other medicines available for ADD and ADHD are tricyclic antidepressants (see Chapter 5), which are less potent, don't work as well, and also

A Medicine Primer for ADD

Brand Name	Generic Name	Dose	What It's Used For	Don't Use If You Are or You Have	Side Effects
Ritalin	Methylphenydate Ritalin SR = slow release	20–60 mg/day (divided dose)	Mild brain stimulant ADD • ADHD Also narcolepsy	Anxiety • Tension • Agitation Glaucoma • Tourette's syndrome Severe depression • Hypertension Coronary artery disease Hyperthyroidism • Avoid anticoagulants/certain antidepressants, Clonidine	Addictive potential • Beware if you have a history of alcohol or drug addiction • Nervousness • Insomnia Lowered appetite • Palpitations Increased blood pressure • Don't take with other stimulants •Psychotic reaction
Metadate CD	CT Methylphenydate	1 x/day	ADD • ADHD	(Same as Ritalin)	(Same as Ritalin)
Metadate ER	ER Methylphenydate	2–3 x/day	ADD • ADHD	(Same as Ritalin)	(Same as Ritalin)
Concerta	Extended release methylphenydate	18–54 mg/day	ADD • ADHD	(Essentially the same as Ritalin)	(Same as Ritalin)
Dexedrine	Dextroamphetamine	5–60 mg	ADD • ADHD Narcolepsy	(Essentially the same as Ritalin)	(Same as Ritalin) with high abuse potential
Adderall	Amphetamine salt XR variety Extended release	10 mg/day 5–60 mg/day 1 x/day		(Essentially the same as Ritalin)	(Same as Ritalin) with high abuse potential
Desoxyn	Methamphetamine	5 mg–60 mg/day	ADD • ADHD Obesity		(Same as Ritalin) with high abuse potential
Cylert	Pemoline	56.25–112.5 mg/day		(Same as Ritalin) plus associated with liver failure	(Same as Ritalin) with high abuse potential
Nonstimulants: Catapres	Clonidine	0.1 mg–2.4 mg	ADD • ADHD Hypertension	Low blood pressure Kidney disease	Dry mouth, • Drowsiness Dizziness • Lower BP
Strattera	Atomoxetine	40–100 mg	ADD • ADHD	Glaucoma Hypertension Heart arrhythmia	Digestive disturbance Headache Dry mouth

have many side effects. But their advantage is they aren't addictive like stimulants. Clonidine and other antihypertensives have been used as well as an array of nontraditional antidepressants (Wellbutrin, a.k.a. bupropion) and antipsychotic medicines, but no real studies have documented whether they really work.

If you are inattentive, spacey, disorganized, and impulsive, Ritalin and other stimulant medicines may be worth a try, but if you have had problems with addiction, stay away from this class of meds. Likewise, if you have a hormonally or immunologically induced problem with attention, Ritalin is not the best initial approach to clear your brain fog. You need first to find the right medical, hormonal, nutritional, and herbal treatment for your endocrine and immune system dysfunction.

SUPPLEMENTS THAT BOOST ATTENTION

A number of vitamins and nutritional supplements have been found helpful for improving attention. (As with any medication, check with your doctor before taking these supplements. Carefully follow any instructions regarding dosage, and be aware of any warnings about contraindications and possible side effects.)

Taking 120 to 200 milligrams of gingko biloba a day will increase the brain's production of acetylcholine, a neurotransmitter that is important for attention and memory, as well as norepinephrine, dopamine, and serotonin, which are key to the initiation and maintenance of attention. Gingko prevents age-related changes in these neurotransmitters. Since gingko biloba influences multiple neurotransmitters, including GABA (as well as those listed above), it would be particularly effective for someone like Joan ("I have a lot of file folders"), who is obsessive-compulsive and anxiously focused on the details to the exclusion of the big picture.

Like aspirin, gingko is used as a treatment for atherosclerosis, to regulate blood pressure, and to treat heart disease. But gingko biloba should *not* be used if you are prone to bruising or bleeding easily. Gingko biloba prevents or inhibits blood platelets from sticking together to form a clot, so it would be dangerous to take it with other herbs or medicines that have a similar effect on clotting (herbs such as dong quai, feverfew, garlic, ginger, ginseng (Panax), chamomile, or medicines such as heparin, aspirin, and other "blood thinner" medicines). Other herbs that could theoretically increase bleeding if combined with gingko are angelica, anise, arnica, capsicum, clove, fenugreek, horse chestnut, horseradish, licorice, onion, papain, passionflower, red clover, turmeric, and others. If you are concerned about bleeding, or are on a blood thinner, please consult your physician before taking gingko or any of these herbs.

If you are concerned about your fertility, you may want to stay away from gingko, because some animal studies suggest that it may interfere with egg fertilization.

Since gingko biloba influences multiple neurotransmitters, it has other effects that make it especially useful for the New Feminine Brain. If you are inattentive and crave carbohydrates (pasta, rice, bread, and sweets), and suffer from irritability, melancholy, and sadness, gingko may help control those cravings, since it increases serotonin metabolism. If you have an attention problem and a chronic pain disorder, this supplement would also be excellent for you, since serotonin inhibits pain transmission. If you have an attention deficit with apathy and a lack of initiation, gingko biloba's effect on dopamine and norepinephrine will increase your motivation.

Finally, if you're prone to anxiety or panic in addition to inattention, gingko biloba would be especially helpful since its GABA activity could lessen your nervousness.

Omega-3 fatty acids, polyunsaturated fatty acids, including DHA (docosahexaenoic acid), are found in fish oil and some seeds, and are essential for brain functioning. Taking 200 to 300 milligrams a day of omega-3 fatty acids can help improve membrane function in the brain. All the neurons in the brain have fat along their membranes, and if the fat or oil content is not the right composition of DHA, the shape of the membrane changes as well as the configuration of neurotransmitter receptors along its length. Many children with ADHD have been found to have lower omega-3 fatty acid levels in their blood. Ultimately, if the brain cells don't have the proper amount of DHA, attention (and associated neurological functions) will be altered. It is thought that as the fats in our diet are oxidized, these membranes become "leaky."

Pycnogenol, also known as grapeseed extract, is also helpful for improving attention. The recommended dosage is one 40 milligram tablet, three times a day.

Other supplements that are helpful for boosting the attentional circuits are *vitamin B$_6$* (200 mg/day), *folic acid* (400 mcg/day), *vitamin B$_{12}$* (100 mcg/day), and the amino acids *glutamine* (500 mg/day) and *tyrosine* (250 mg/day). They help the brain make the neurotransmitters that stimulate your attention circuits for focus and arousal.

S-adenosyl-methionine (SAMe) is a nutrient and dietary supplement that can be used to treat ADD/ADHD. It has been used by more than a million people in Europe primarily for depression and arthritis since the 1970s.

Distributed through all the body tissues, it's mostly concentrated in the brain and liver.

SAMe is a natural supplement that has been found to be effective for adults with ADD and ADHD, particularly people who have difficulty with impulsivity, in dosages of 400 to 1600 milligrams a day. Some people experience side effects, such as mild headaches, loose bowels, and dry mouth, but for the most part, preliminary studies show that SAMe is very helpful. There are no available studies examining SAMe's effect on the female brain, but in a study of eight adult men with ADHD who were treated with very high doses of SAMe, 800 mg three times a day, six of the eight were helped with their symptoms.

Since it has mild stimulant effects like dopamine and norepinephrine, SAMe might be of particular help to women with attention and motivation problems, ADD, pain, and depression. It is not addictive like Ritalin or other stimulant medicines. SAMe has been shown to help fibromyalgia and osteoarthritis at doses of 400 to 800 milligrams a day. Even though SAMe is expensive, it can be extremely effective. It must be taken at the recommended dosage and on an empty stomach or it won't be absorbed. SAMe has very few side effects and doesn't cause weight gain or insomnia like other meds.

Two distinct types of *ginseng* also can be helpful in boosting the attentional circuits. *Panax ginseng* (Asian ginseng) improves concentration and is an antidepressant. It is also used as a general tonic to stimulate immune function. The principal active ingredients lower blood pressure and act as a brain stimulant, alter carbohydrate and fat metabolism, and stimulate natural killer cells (cells that fight cancer). Preliminary evidence suggests that Panax ginseng improves psychological function in postmenopausal women by increasing DHEA.

You should be careful taking ginseng with other stimulants, including coffee, guarana, and tea, because the stimulant effect may be intensified. Ginseng should not be combined with other herbs or medicines that promote bleeding since ginseng inhibits blood platelets from sticking together. These include angelica, capsicum, chamomile, feverfew, gingko, licorice, and red clover.

Since ginseng is a stimulant, it may cause insomnia and increase heart rate or palpitations. It has been associated with euphoria and abuse. Since it can affect hormone levels, it can be associated with achy breasts and vaginal bleeding. High blood pressure, nervousness, insomnia, increased libido, and hormonal effects may be signs that you're taking too high a dose. Panax ginseng is meant to be used for less than three months.

Siberian ginseng (eleutherococcus) is not the same as Asian ginseng and is used to treat Alzheimer's disease and attention deficit disorder of chronic fatigue syndrome/fibromyalgia. It also helps the immune and cardiovascular systems and has some estrogenic activity. Siberian (like Asian ginseng) is best used for sixty days, then stopped for two or three weeks. Dosages of Siberian ginseng vary depending on if you use the root (0.6–5 g/day) or ethanol extract (2–16 ml 1–3 x/day).

Siberian ginseng's active ingredients affect the brain's pituitary-adrenocortical system. Like Asian ginseng, it prevents or inhibits platelet aggregation, so it shouldn't be taken with other blood-thinning herbs or medicines.

Gotu kola, a supplement also known as centalla asiatica, is used in southeast Asia to relieve mild depression and anxiety. Gotu kola may work like Ritalin to increase arousal in the brain-stem area for attention. Gotu kola reduces fatigue and improves memory and intelligence. Large amounts of gotu kola may elevate blood pressure and cause skin photosensitivity and itching. A typical dose is 600 mg 3 times a day. Avoid gotu kola if you are on sedative drugs, cholesterol-lowering drugs, and diabetes drugs, because it may counteract their action.

Caffeine is one of the most popular forms of self-medication and has been shown to be similar to Ritalin in its effect. It helps with memory by increasing the production of acetylcholine. Low levels of caffeine added to Ritalin improve more symptoms in ADD than Ritalin alone.

Coffee and tea are not the only sources of caffeine. Diet Coke is the New Feminine Brain's coffee substitute since it contains 40 to 60 milligrams of caffeine in a twelve-ounce serving. A five-ounce cup of tea contains 20–100 milligrams of caffeine. And then there's chocolate. A cup of cocoa or a NoDoz tablet contains 100 milligrams.

Ginseng, gotu kola, and caffeine are stimulants, so they may be helpful for the more hyperactive form of ADD, as well as the fog due to chronic fatigue and autoimmune dysfunction.

Meditation is an attention-booster for some people, although it has no effect on others. Some people can learn to change their EEG patterns—their brain wave patterns—by meditating. It makes me fall asleep.

Environmental and Education Strategies

One of the most important ways of sharpening your mind is coming to peace with your unique style of paying attention to the world. Whether you have focused attention, dreamlike transcendent attention, or empathetic attention, you have an innate talent in how you home in on information. Robin Williams's and Ellen DeGeneres's comedic genius has many of the features of attention deficit disorder. In elementary school, someone who acts and thinks like these comedians is given a diagnosis of ADD and Ritalin. Yet Robin Williams has made a career out of his impulsive, hyperactive mind-set, and Ellen DeGeneres charms audiences with her unique, self-deprecating "space cadet" persona.

The feminine brain is uniquely adapted to have a "roving intuitive intelligence" rather than a focused mind-set, so you don't want to straitjacket it. By learning to appreciate and utilize your intuitive way of thinking and paying attention, you will avoid problems with mood, anxiety, and obesity, and stay healthy. You can find a niche for yourself—the right environment at work, with peers, and with your family—where your unique attentional style will best operate.

If you have a problem focusing and paying attention, below are a list of programs to help you derive the genius behind your unique feminine mind-set.

1. Inattention, Spaciness (Transcendent Attention Style)	
Unique Feminine Brain Style Symptoms	Inattentive, "mind in the clouds" • Carbohydrate craving LH>>RH, usually better at English, history than math or science +/- history/family history addiction +/- weight problem, insulin resistance, hyperestrogenism +/- melancholy/sadness Restless, purpose in life • Hormone cycles aggravate attention problems
Solutions/ Adaptive Strategies	*Supplements/Medications:* A good multivitamin with: Pycnogenol 40 mg 3x/day Vitamin B$_6$ 200 mg/day • Folic acid 400 mcg/day Glutamine 500 mg/day • Tyrosine 250 mg/day • SAMe 400–1600 mg/day Siberian ginseng 0.6 g/day • Gotu kola 600 mg 3x/day Gingko biloba 120–240 mg/day • DHA 200–300 mg/day Ritalin/stimulant meds sometimes useful *Diet:* More carbohydrates earlier in the day • Fewer carbohydrates after 3 p.m. *Exercise:* Aerobic 30 minutes a.m. • Walk briskly 30 minutes p.m. *Environment/Vocation:* Peer tutoring/cooperative learning in school environment • Increase supervision/structure in workplace • Stimulating job with novelty Vocational counseling or professional coach for life purpose exploration Minimize meditation until attention circuits are maximized *Other Treatments:* Treat addiction if present • Self-esteem promoting treatments (see Chapter 5) • Treat mood disorders if present (see Chapter 5)

2. Unfocused, Hyperactive (ADHD)

Unique Feminine Brain Style Symptoms	Hyperactive • Impulsive Stimulus-bound Carbohydrate craving RH>>LH usually; frequently better at math/science than English/history/languages
Solutions/ Adaptive Strategies	*Supplements/Medications:* A good multivitamin with: Pycnogenol 40 mg 3x/day Vitamin B_6 200 mg/day • Folic acid 400 mcg/day Vitamin B_{12} 100 mcg/day • Glutamine 500 mg/day • Tyrosine 250 mg/day L-acetyl carnitine 500 mg/day • Gingko biloba 120–240 mg/day Chromium 180 mg/day • SAMe 400–1600 mg/day DHA 100 mg 3x/day • Siberian ginseng 0.6–5 g/day +/- Ritalin or stimulant • No Ritalin if have history of addiction *Diet:* Minimize artificial sugar, aspartame, MSG, food dyes *Exercise:* Active daily exercise program that can be incorporated into work schedule *Environment/Vocation:* Graphic organizers • Organizational elements at work like highlighters, file cards • Environmentally stimulating environment (TV/radio noise) helpful to some. • Career with diversity/novelty *Other Treatments:* Treat addiction if present Self-esteem promoting treatments (see Chapter 4)

3. Empathic Attention: Anxious, Edgy, in Pain, and Overwhelmed

Unique Feminine Brain Style Symptoms	Inattentive • Problems dividing attention between inner emotional world of feelings and outer environmental demands • Distractibility Decreased sustained attention • Prone to anxiety, panic, or phobias Usually history of trauma insomnia +/- history of chronic pain +/- history of concussion or head injury +/- history of chronic use of sleep meds/alcohol/pain meds
Solutions/ Adaptive Strategies	*Supplements/Medications:* A good multivitamin • SAMe 400–1600 mg/day (good also for pain disorders) • Ginkgo biloba 120–240 mg/day (will also treat anxiety and depression) • *No* Ritalin or stimulant meds (will increase anxiety/panic) • DHA 100–300 mg/day *Diet:* No caffeine • No aspartame • Minimize alcohol *Exercise:* Relaxation/visualization and imagery exercises *Environment/Vocation:* Daily work outside of home that is regularly scheduled and that is rewarding

	Other Treatments Treat anxiety/panic (see Chapter 7) • Treat pain and mood disorders (see Chapter 5) • Treat addictions Self-esteem–promoting treatments (Chapter 11)

4. Attention Deficit and Immune System Dysfunction

Unique Feminine Brain Style Symptoms	Inattentive • Distracted • Exhaustion, fatigue Insomnia or hypersomnia • Health that's very stress-responsive At times apathy, low initiative, and low motivation Chronic immune system dysfunction like chronic fatigue, fibromyalgia, lupus, Gulf War syndrome, environmental illness, multiple chemical sensitivities, systemic candidiasis, ulcerative colitis, Crohn's disease, Lyme disease Frequently have pain syndrome
Solutions/ Adaptive Strategies	*Supplements/Medications:* A good multivitamin (See Boxes 1 and 2) • SAMe 400–1600 mg/day DHA 100–300 mg/day • Cat's claw/Samento (see Resources) Ginkgo Biloba (will improve pain and mood) 120–240 mg/day Panax ginseng (see practitioner for appropriate dose) *Diet:* See practitioner for diet that is appropriate for your unique health problems *Exercise:* Have a trainer or physical therapist work on increasing aerobic endurance • Yoga, Pilates *Environment/Vocation:* Avoid quitting work and going on "disability." • Calm, consistent, reliable work that uses your gifts, skills, talents Get vocational coach or professional coach for life purpose exploration Meditation, prayer, art therapy, music therapy *Other Treatments:* Treat depression (see Chapter 5) • Treat pain/immune system dysfunction • Minimize or eradicate pain meds, sleep meds

5. Attention Problems from Hormonal Fallout

Unique Feminine Brain Style Symptoms	Inattention • Problems with sustained attention Complaints of memory loss Melancholy, sadness • Irritability Carbohydrate craving
Solutions/ Adaptive Strategies	*Supplements/Medications:* A good multivitamin • Ginkgo biloba 120–240 mg/day See Chapter 10 for supplements for memory, including possible estrogen and progesterone supplementation, soy supplementation, and also phytoestrogen supplements *Diet:* Carbohydrates balanced with protein in 1:1 ratio at breakfast, lunch Few carbohydrates after 3 p.m. • Smallest meal: dinner

> *Exercise:*
> Aerobic exercise 30 minutes in a.m., 30 minutes in p.m. after dinner
> *Environment/Vocation:*
> Vocational coach to assess best use of skills, talents, and creativity in
> second half of life • Meditation or retreat time to listen closely to
> information that's coming from inner space
> *Other Treatments:*
> Treat melancholy/sadness (see Chapter 5)

My Mind Is Like a Hummingbird

I was diagnosed with ADHD in 1989 and prescribed Ritalin, which for me was (yes, past tense) a wonder drug. Instead of sitting on a chair in the runner's starting position looking like I would bolt any minute, after Ritalin, I could actually lean back in the chair with my muscles relaxed. My face relaxed, my speech got slower, everything seemed slower. I felt like the world had gone from a Mario Andretti sports car to a Conestoga wagon. People noted the new change immediately. I was so quiet, they thought I was mad at them or depressed. Then I got a side effect. My joints got all inflamed, and a rheumatologist told me to get off the medicine. So I had to learn to compensate.

I organized all my work and notes on three-by-five file cards that are organized in Pottery Barn wooden drawers, all alphabetically labeled. Scientific journal papers are arranged in five-inch black binders organized by categories. I have twenty-five wooden file cabinets downstairs with files that serve as a prosthetic frontal lobe for organization and planning. I carry a Daytimer into which I glue my daily schedule. When I read, I always highlight (yellow, orange, pink, or green) to maintain my attention on the line of the written word. I always have a TV on when I read or work to give me the stimulus I need to focus.

Compensatory strategies for managing hyperactivity and impulsivity are much more difficult to develop. To a public place, conference, or theater, I always bring a book, a journal, highlighter pens, and file cards with me to pump up my attentional circuits, and to distract me so I am less likely to fidget or leave my seat. I know it appears rude, but the alternatives would seem even more rude, I'm sure. So that I don't impulsively blurt out something in the middle of someone's talk, I literally hold my hand over my mouth, pressing both lips together. My friends have gotten used to seeing my eyes go off when they are speaking, for they know that my attention span is like a hummingbird's. I even bring a newspaper to distract me when I'm in line at McDonald's, because even a four-minute wait seems like forty minutes.

I take a lot of supplements for my attention. I take SAMe (800 mg a day), which does a world of good. My attention and focus are as superb as they could ever get for me. I take DHA (100 mg 3 times a day; any more than that, I get so calm, I fall asleep). I take an excellent pharmaceutical-grade supplement mega-vitamin (USANA, see Resource Guide) containing B_6, B_{12}, and other nutrients that are supposed to support attention. Magnesium (300 mg/day on an empty stomach) calms down (a little) the hyperactivity. I also take 180 milligrams of chromium, and a small amount of Siberian ginseng. I drink two twelve-ounce cups of coffee at 4:00 p.m. each day. Only once a day do I drink an aspartame-containing drink like Diet Coke. Instead, I drink a diet beverage called Diet Rite, which does not have aspartame, and, frankly, I drink Kool-Aid. Yes, I drink Kool-Aid. This makes people wonder about me, but it really helps. Finally, I take gingko biloba (130 mg a day). I'm careful whenever I have surgery or some other procedure to discontinue all of these supplements, and I share with my physician what I am taking. This is indeed a lot of vitamins, and many local restaurants and friends are familiar with my little Ziploc baggie of supplements.

Am I a perfect person? Hardly. I know that my ADHD can make me appear quite flawed and adolescent at times, but it also gives me intellectual and intuitive gifts and a capacity to produce work that I wouldn't have if I weren't connected to "a little Edison Electric Company" in my brain. My inattentiveness, hyperactivity, and impulsivity can irritate others, so my self-esteem over time has been bruised, but the people who are closest to me love me anyway. Quite frankly, many of them are hyperactive as well.

I meet a lot of kids and adolescents who have the same brain wiring and I try to tell them that they too can use the unique wiring of the brain they have to love, appreciate, and grow in life. Sometimes they do need meds, but sometimes supplements can capture and hold on to that hummingbird in their mind.

If you have a problem with attention—and you now see that the New Feminine Brain is vulnerable to them—I strongly recommend that you maintain good "emotional hygiene." If something is bothering you, if a fight is brewing, if there's conflict beneath the surface of a relationship, bring it out into the open and resolve the matter. Otherwise, you will have dirty linen piling up in your interpersonal space—and it will be harder for you to pay attention.

Discover your unique brain style for attention, learn to accept *how,* as well as *who,* you are—and you'll find your intellectual and intuitive genius.

TEN

What's Too Painful to Remember, We Choose to Forget: Memory, Wisdom, Aging, and Trauma

Girls and women learn differently from boys and men. Yet our unique anatomy for memory increases our chances of having memory problems like Alzheimer's disease and other dementias later in life. In this chapter, you will learn how to minimize your chances for dementia and other memory disorders now and as you get older.

Intuition Comes Through the Memory

Hunches and intuitive flashes can come to you through memories that are stored in your brain and body. To get your attention, your brain may re-play a specific memory clip to communicate symbolically what you need to know. The right brain may signal intuitions through memories of songs, sounds, or vague images of the past. The left brain may signal you symbolically through archetypal images, letters, words, lyrics, and other language–based information. Finally, your body signals you through symptoms of illness that communicate that something in your life is out of balance.

The Anatomy of Memory

What we remember about an event is never the whole truth and nothing but the truth. Rather, it is an approximation of the truth, colored by emotion and past experiences, tempered by age and health. Let's look at how memory works and how your brain lays down memories.

The hippocampus lays down memories you can talk about and the amygdala lays down memories that are stored in your body, memories that you usually don't talk about but act out. The left brain is more important for "verbal memory" and the right brain is critical for "body memory."

When I was twelve years old, I watched a program on TV called *Welcome Back, Kotter,* starring a guy with blue eyes and a crooked smile—John Travolta. Like every other preteen girl in America, I got goose bumps. What I saw, heard, and felt registered in my brain while watching the show, and for the rest of the evening he stayed on my mind, in my *short-term memory.* Later, as I slept, the sight and sound of John Travolta made its way to the memory centers (hippocampus and amygdala), where he was tagged a "very important person" and stored multimodally all over my brain in a network.

Years later, when I was on a ferryboat in Maine, I heard a male voice that was eerily familiar. I gravitated to his side of the boat even though I wasn't conscious why, feeling I remembered this guy from somewhere. Once I saw the distinctive blue eyes and dimpled chin, I screamed, "Oh my God! That's John Travolta!" (This may not be as happy a memory for him as for me.)

Our brain remembers in two different ways:

1. *Body memory areas (the amygdala)* of what's familiar, causing us to act or our health to react to similar situations in the future, and
2. *Verbal memory areas (the hippocampus)* identifying names, recalling facts, and laying down events in the form of symbols.

So, intuition can come to us in right-brain body memories and physical symptoms or through symbols that appear in our waking or dreaming experience.

LEFT-BRAIN MEMORY: SYMBOLS AND FACTS

Verbal memory (a.k.a. left-brain semantic memories) stores facts in words and symbols. Your hippocampus may help you store biographical data like whether you're married and other simple, declarative facts. The information you'd need to play and win the game show *Jeopardy* would all come from verbal memory: What is the capital of Arkansas? Who is the president of France? Who is buried in Grant's Tomb?

RIGHT-BRAIN MEMORY: HABITS AND HEALTH

In contrast, the amygdala or right-brain nonverbal memory captures memory in shapes, images, body health, or habits. Your choice of mates, your likes and dislikes in food, a lot of what you gravitate to or avoid are based on this kind of nonverbal memory. For instance, the right brain is involved when you put together a jigsaw puzzle and remember the shapes of missing pieces. On Monday morning, when you drive to work absentmindedly on "auto-pilot," body memory helps you follow the correct route. Who you choose as a mate, that which you are drawn to love or hate, are in part driven by memories stored in your body. In fact, body memory provides many feelings behind our hunches and intuitions. You might get a wonderful feeling in your heart that the guy you've met is "Mr. Right," not realizing that he has some of the best and worst characteristics of your father. You may feel a terrible sensation in your stomach when you choose the wrong answers on a test. If you don't listen to the first subtle twinges that your body makes to get you to go in the right direction, those sensations can evolve into symptoms and escalate into overt physical illness.

Body Memories Shape Habits and Behavior Unconsciously

In the lab, before an experiment begins, if a complicated machine is involved, we first run fluid through the tubes in its system to "prime the pump." This makes the machine work more smoothly when the real experiment begins. The body uses memory to prime behavior, too.

In priming, information that we see, hear, and feel but don't pay attention to gets stored in our brain and body. Later, this information, without our knowing about it, influences our habits and choices. If the Coke commercial is repeated often enough in the background, like it or not, we're more likely to get and drink one. If enough fashion magazines on the newsstands and stars on TV feature a new length of skirt, we are more likely to gravitate to that style. We have been primed or, rather, our brains have been primed, by what we have seen and stored in our memory banks.

I once asked a friend, Larry, who is in the country music industry, why it is that I can usually tell when a song will be an instant hit when I first hear it on the radio. Larry told me chances are that song has already played several times on the radio in the background while I'm not really paying attention. By the time I actually consciously hear it, my brain and mind have been primed so many times that unless it's really a terrible song, just the familiarity and repetition would increase my recognition and affinity for it.

For most brain functions, we women use both our right and left brains simultaneously. Men tend to use one side of the brain at a time, especially for communication. Because the traditional male brain is more compartmentalized, his body and memory are more likely to be segregated, and he is less inclined to talk about either. Women's two brains communicate more, so women base decisions on a combination of left-brain conscious experience and right-brain body memory and intuition.

The Feminine Brain's Multimodal Learning Style

Because women's brains have more functional connections between individual brain areas, they more readily use body and symbol memory to learn, remember, and benefit from experience. So, for example, in history class, a woman with this type of "ambi-brain," bilateral style wouldn't do well just listening to the teacher rattle off facts about the Pilgrims or the pyramids in Egypt. Just passively going to class and doing the assigned reading won't help her perform well in a class. She is more likely to do well if she copies over her notes, makes charts, has a discussion group with friends, and pays attention to her intuition on the final exam.

The Traditional Male's Unimodal Learning Style

The traditional male would prefer to learn one hemisphere at a time, that is, hearing the left-brain facts first and then engaging in hands-on, practical, experiential learning later. Of course, some atypical men also benefit from a bilateral learning style. They usually, but not always, are left-handed, ambidextrous, and have dyslexia or ADD. Since standard pathways for perception, attention, memory, and language may have a "developmental ding" in them, the men may compensate by using multiple pathways simultaneously to reroute information around their learning disability.

Stress and Trauma Shrink Verbal Memory and Create Body Memory

A little bit of stress, with its release of cortisol, will actually pump up function in the hippocampus and improve attention, learning, and memory. For a limited amount of time, putting right-brain emotional distress into words, and talking with a trusted adviser, purges and actually improves wisdom and intelligence. However, high doses of stress push the cells of the hippocampus over the edge, inhibit memory formation, and make a person feel like she has Alzheimer's disease.

The hippocampus is very vulnerable to stress and stress hormones during development in utero and late in life as well. And lifelong vulnerability to stress in your brain may be influenced by how your brain was conditioned to stress in utero: Severe maternal stress increases a child's chance of having mood and anxiety disorder later in life, but an antidote to this prenatal priming of the brain's circuits may be in gentle infant massage or repeated handling, which seems to decrease this tendency toward anxiety, moodiness, and emotional reactivity.

Stress can cause learning and memory problems, it releases cortisol and norepinephrine, and over time it actually causes nerve endings in the hippocampus to shrink or atrophy.

Stress also creates physical symptoms that can mimic menopausal complaints, including memory loss. The amygdala has lots of connections to the heart, lungs, blood vessels, skin, and body temperature centers, so body memories are expressed through a change in heart rate, cold chills, and hot flashes that resemble menopausal symptoms. Premenopausally the feminine brain has some protection against chronic stress because of its higher estrogen levels, but once they begin to decline in menopause, women become more susceptible to stress's irritating effect on memory. The song's suggestion that anything that's too painful to remember, we just choose to forget is more applicable to the premenopausal brain; after menopause, it is harder to stay in a situation that makes us uncomfortable or reenacts past unhappiness or abuse because intuition, body memories, and failing health are more than ever likely to warn us to make changes.

Nonetheless, women with untreated posttraumatic stress disorder can suffer dramatic problems with memory. Their brains' chronic elevated levels of cortisol and norepinephrine can actually accelerate brain aging, which resembles symptoms of Alzheimer's disease.

Normal Aging and Memory

Felice is seventy-three years old and called me, concerned about her memory. A clinical psychologist, she has a thriving practice, and a wide circle of close friends and colleagues who treat her like Yoda, the wise being in *Star Wars*. Felice divorced her alcoholic husband fifteen years ago, and since then, her life has been busy and productive. She goes to many self-help conferences and symposia, and frequently travels with friends and family. However, in the last year, she got her hearing checked because she was having a hard time picking up on conversations in a crowded room. Although her hearing was perfect, she still felt lost at times in conversations. Frequently, Felice would have a word or someone's name on the tip of her tongue but not be able to get at it. Having always prided herself on her quick, facile mind, she now felt it seemed slower. Yet, tests revealed that her memory was entirely normal for her age and educational level.

Memory Matures as We Age

Generally speaking, our memory improves as we age, but the way we learn and remember events changes as we mature. Nonetheless, a variety of physical and emotional stressors can alter or accelerate age-related changes in our brain. Repetitive emotional trauma, financial crises, broken relationships, health problems such as hypertension and diabetes, brain injury, and exposure to toxins in the environment all take their toll. Ultimately, however, many of these factors that increase cognitive decline in the brain with aging are avoidable or preventable.

A population of older people as a whole has more *variability* in how their brains perform as they get older. Some people's brains slip in learning, memory, and IQ points, and others hold fast to their abilities. Scientists believe now that people whose memories are slipping have the early stages of cumulative brain injury and disease.

In Normal Aging, We Retain Our Brain Power and Mental Faculties

Education, nutrition, and general health changes affect the brain's health. People with more education seem to maintain their capacity for learning and memory, although this may be due to either the fact that they had healthier brains to begin with or that they are more likely to remain lifelong learners.

Normal aging begins in infancy: The brain changes quite a bit from birth to death, through plasticity. As we get older, the cellular and anatomic changes from brain plasticity and sprouting new pathways actually improve our brain and help us develop emotional wisdom and intellectual maturity. Normal aging does not necessarily mean a total decrease in the number of nerve cells, as commonly believed. In normal aging, there is a cumulative *increase* in memory nerve cell endings branchings even beyond the age of seventy. Dementia, senility, and Alzheimer's disease may actually be a breakdown of this ability to "grow."

By continuously putting yourself in novel environments that are emotionally and intellectually challenging (but not *excessively* stressful), you are more likely to maintain brain cell growth. The phrase "Use it or lose it" definitely applies to the brain as we age. Too much challenge and change is stressful, and leads to excess cortisol, norepinephrine, and brain atrophy and memory loss. Too little challenge or not enough change and environmental enrichment leads to atrophy of the brain memory area and probably loss of memory.

Wear and tear vs. Use it or lose it

Adults like Felice who continue learning retain higher brain size and capacity. Lifelong learning may not just involve the 3R's, reading, writing, and arithmetic, which only involve exercising the left brain. Any part of the nervous system, if not emotionally and mentally challenged or "exercised," may shrink or atrophy just as muscles do when we don't exert ourselves. Yet science indicates that our emotional reaction style or "personality" becomes more "crystallized" (i.e., stuck in a rut) in our brain over time. The longer we hold emotional beliefs, the more likely we will ignore or discount experiences that contradict those beliefs.

Newer studies suggest, however, that you can change some of your personality characteristics by learning from past trauma and living in a healthier, enriching environment. In women between the ages of forty-three and fifty-two, occupational experiences—working in improved environments and conditions—were shown to change some personality characteristics that were not thought to change across one's lifetime, like the capacity to be extroverted and conscientiousness. Apparently, changing environments, changing who you relate to, getting rid of what's unhealthy helps keep your right brain's emotional responses fluid and varied.

As We Age, Some Tasks Become Easier, Some Harder

Most abilities stay about the same as we get older, but it can become difficult to do more than one thing at a time. For example, the ability to pay *attention* may stay about the same, but your capacity to divide your attention among many competing things may be more difficult. Dividing your attention requires a kind of rubber-band quality in the mind, a cognitive flexibility that begins to diminish somewhat as we age. The speed with which women think or speak also tends to decrease.

Learning and memory don't change much with age. Reading, writing, and other aspects of language stay relatively the same, but the way the brain stores and organizes information may change. When learning someone's name or some other fact, you may not organize the information into a specific category (called "chunking"), and so you may take longer to remember or retrieve peoples' or object's names.

OLDER BRAINS ARE SLOWER AND ALLOW SELF-REFLECTION AND GREATER PERSPECTIVE

Kids' thoughts move from one idea to another, like Ricochet Rabbit—ping-ping-ping. As we mature, we tend to think and move slower. Normal aging may slow us down so we can think things through and not act as impulsively.

I am about thirty years younger than Felice, and visit her about once every two to three months. Being somewhat hyperactive, when I talk I jump from topic to topic. Felice will sit and listen, and when I finish, there will be a long, pregnant pause. Usually, I sit in intense, anxious anticipation until Felice delivers the most articulate, well-thought-out statement so rich with meaning that I stay silent in utter admiration and respect. The wheels in Felice's mind may roll more slowly, but the engine as a whole moves incredibly efficiently, so she generates the same number of ideas and thoughts.

Recently, from a catalogue, I bought a sign in Greek that says, "I'm still learning—Ancora Imparo," one for me and one for Felice.

Dementias

Knowing and understanding the molecular and cellular foundation of Alzheimer's disease will help you understand why some treatments may decrease your risk for this illness, or slow its progression if you already have it.

Alzheimer's disease is the most common cause of dementia; most cases begin by age sixty-five, although some rarer genetic, more severe forms can occur as early as thirty or forty years of age. People argue about how common this disease really is. Ten percent of people in their sixties have some form of Alzheimer's, and 40 percent of people in their eighties. Only five percent of all patients with Alzheimer's disease have an abnormal form of chromosome 21, 14, or 1. In these early severe cases, the disease begins very early (age thirty to forty). Any diagnosis of Alzheimer's disease is only tentative since the only way to truly diagnose this illness is after the person dies and their brain is examined by a pathologist. While the patient is alive, no test result is "diagnostic." An MRI may show a loss of volume in the hippocampus, a key memory area of the brain. The fluid surrounding the brain and spinal cord (cerebrospinal fluid, or CSF) may have abnormal amounts of neurotoxin, which causes inflammation. Immune cells become activated and produce inflammatory mediators, cytokines, and nitric oxide, causing a domino-like cascade of inflammation, which leads to cell death.

Mrs. Brown was seventy-eight years old and had always lived a very independent life in the Boston area. Then she broke her hip and needed a home health aide to help her prepare some meals, and do light shopping and cleaning. I needed a part-time job until I got into medical school, so helping Mrs. Brown seemed perfect. When I arrived at her apartment, I knew immediately that something was wrong. Her mail was piled outside the door with "disconnection notices" from the gas, telephone, and electric companies. I knocked on the door and, after a very long time, Mrs. Brown opened it. As I introduced myself, warning bells were going off in my head.

Mrs. Brown was half-dressed, partially clad in her slip as she casually waved me into her apartment. There were bags of groceries on the floor in front of the door, containing spoiling milk, eggs, and produce. I could hear a tea kettle whistling in the kitchen. When I called her attention to it, she beckoned me into the kitchen to sit down and have a "chat."

I turned off the stove to silence the kettle and we sat down in the living room. I tried to figure out what was going on. It was clear that Mrs. Brown couldn't remember my name, no matter how many times I repeated it. She'd lose track of what she was saying in mid-sentence, and she had trouble with speech and finding words. Her conversation was rambling, vague, and impoverished. She would say, "Why don't you put the groceries in the . . . in the . . . box in the kitchen. . . . Isn't it a beautiful day?" She repeated these phrases several times within the course of fifteen minutes. "Well, it's that thing you want to . . . well, you uncap it and . . . then you get a new one when you can't write with it." A twenty-four-word phrase instead of using the word "pen."

Mrs. Brown had little insight; she didn't seem to realize how dangerously disorganized her life was. The piled-up mail with overdue bills was scary. The kitchen had several burned-out pans, and the apartment was a general disaster. Because her sense of smell had deteriorated, the rotting produce and groceries went undetected.

It began to get dark and I had to get home. I mentally committed to coming the next day to clean out the refrigerator, which was another disaster. When I started to put lights on, Mrs. Brown began to get panicky, agitated, and started anxiously picking at her sweater. So instead I called an ambulance and took Mrs. Brown to the hospital. I couldn't leave her like that.

The next day I visited her at the hospital. The doctor had diagnosed her with a "tentative" dementia of Alzheimer's type (see box below). When I walked into her hospital room, Mrs. Brown said, "Oh, are you my new social worker?" So I said, "Mrs. Brown, it's me, Mona Lisa? Do you remember me? We were together almost twelve hours yesterday." And she looked at me and said, "Oh yes, dear. Come in. They cleaned my apartment all up. Have a seat . . ."

After looking out the window confused for a few minutes, she turned back to me and said, "You know . . . I knew another Mona Lisa once. She looked just like you. She came to help me out years ago . . . she was a very nice girl." I couldn't believe it. I said, "Mrs. Brown, that was me . . . I'm Mona Lisa." She looked at me closely, scanning my face for any familiarity, and I could see she really didn't recognize me at all. Since she started to look uncomfortable again, I let it pass, and asked, "So, Mrs. Brown, how's the food here?"

Mrs. Brown had dementia, a chronic, progressive decline in intellectual function and social behavior which causes more and more loss of function in relationships, vocation, and society. An individual with dementia gradually loses the capacity to pay attention, learn, or remember, to think abstractly or symbolically, and loses her sense of direction or spatial concentration. In the later stages of the illness, she won't understand the cause of her incapacity.

Characteristics of Alzheimer's Disease
- Poor insight and judgment
- Lack of social propriety and modesty (change from prior personality)
- Apathy and disinterest
- Disoriented to time or location
- Wandering attention
- Speech and language problems: problems finding words; impoverished distractible speech
- Sundowning: confusion when the sun sets
- Loss of smell
- Forgetfulness, problems learning new information

Alzheimer's disease isn't the only cause of memory problems. Many other illnesses can make a person have problems with "mental sharpness" and forgetfulness, including *infectious diseases* like Lyme disease, Epstein-Barr virus, or AIDS; *autoimmune and inflammatory illnesses* like lupus; *nutri-*

tional deficiencies as in anorexia nervosa, vitamin B$_{12}$ deficiency, and alcoholism; *stroke* (cerebrovascular disease) and heart disease; *repeated brain injury* as from boxing, auto racing, and football; and *other brain illnesses,* like Parkinson's disease.

Dementia Is More than Simply Having a Problem with Memory

For a while, in its early stages, Mrs. Brown's dementia may have been missed because she was very bright, had a high school education, and was very clever at hiding her symptoms. She may have had a mild forgetfulness for years that had gone unnoticed because she lived alone and was retired.

But by now when you met Mrs. Brown, you realized that something was terribly wrong with her brain. And memory wasn't the first problem you realized she had. Her lack of insight and judgment and her inability to attend to the day-to-day details of life were the most obvious features of her case. Opening the door to a stranger dressed only in a slip showed that her brain's frontal network, programs for social propriety and modesty, were a little shaky. Changes in judgment and insight were obvious. Even though I found multiple areas of confusion in the apartment that I pointed out to her, Mrs. Brown was unconcerned, apathetic, and indifferent. Even though it was obvious from the apartment's clutter that she had lived there for years, she seemed lost and disoriented and didn't seem to know where things belonged. Most of her activity was restless, disoriented, and confused wandering, searching for things. Only after introducing myself to Mrs. Brown for the third time did I realize that she also had a severe memory problem.

The Heart Disease–Cholesterol–Alzheimer's Disease Connection

There may be some relationship between the tendency to have heart disease and cholesterol problems and Alzheimer's disease. Fat doesn't just go to your thighs and hips, it's also very important for brain function and helps make and repair nerve cell membranes. Apolipoprotein E (ApoE) is an important mediator of cholesterol metabolism in the brain and in the body. If you inherit one type of ApoE, ApoE$_4$, you are at an increased risk of having both Alzheimer's disease later in life and atherosclerotic heart disease. ApoE$_4$ in women seems to have a worse effect on memory than in men. How can one gene increase your risk of having two apparently different diseases? Normal ApoE helps clear low density lipoproteins (LDL) from the blood, reducing one's risk of developing atherosclerotic plaques. Normal ApoE also scavenges lipids, which are used to repair brain cells. If you have the ApoE₄ mutation, then you are more likely to get atherosclerotic heart disease and an accumulation of brain cell injury over time, thus, Alzheimer's disease. Beta amyloid may be secreted in response to the accumulated nerve injury, which increases inflammation, cell damage, and ultimately the nerve cell plaque formation seen in Alzheimer's disease. But if you keep your cholesterol levels low, you reduce your risk of Alzheimer's disease.

In Alzheimer's disease, the brain areas that are involved in memory, attention, behavior, language, and judgment usually have tangles and plaques, the end result of a disruption in cell growth and brain plasticity. Brain-irritating amyloid plaques cause nerve cells to die, leaving behind tangle "ghosts." Nearly everyone over sixty has some tangles, but they are much more numerous in Alzheimer's disease. In Alzheimer's disease, the tangles don't just stay confined to the memory region (hippocampus), they spread to other brain areas that are involved in the symptoms of the disease. In the final stages, tangles eventually spread to the motor areas, leading to incontinence, immobility, and ultimately death from heart arrest or lung infection. Tangles also spread to areas in the brain and brain stem that produce the "battery fluid" of the brain—neurotransmitters like acetylcholine, serotonin, dopamine, and norepinephrine that fuel the brain's memory, attention, and other functions.

Women Have a Greater Risk for Developing Alzheimer's Disease

Recently a friend of mine was very sick, so I volunteered to sit with her and watch movies on her DVD. Usually I tend to watch the same kind of movie, a slapstick comedy (*Tommy Boy* or *Wayne's World*), or a romantic comedy (*Moonstruck* or *My Big Fat Greek Wedding*). Since she was very ill, I let her pick out movies that I would never see, mostly what I call "bonnet" movies, usually set in eighteenth- or nineteenth-century England, with women in ridiculous hats and long skirts and men who wear many layers of clothing. It was a good exercise for me. *Pride and Prejudice* really vacuumed out the synapses in my brain. Listening to a new dialect and accent forced me to pay attention in a new way. Without its usual stimuli of physical slapstick, comedy, and special effects, my brain was forced to dust off some cognitive areas that hadn't seen the light of day in quite a while. By breaking out of my personal movie rut, I exercised and promoted growth in many different brain areas.

One of the movies she chose was *The Buena Vista Social Club,* the wonderful story of a group of musicians in Cuba that was famous in the 1940s and '50s. A producer decided to look up some of the musicians to see if they were still playing. It seemed ridiculous to assume he'd be able to locate them, because all would be in their seventies, eighties, and nineties. And I expected that since they've been living in Castro's Cuba, their health wouldn't be all that great because of the country's poverty and underdeveloped health care system. I also expected that a significant number would be demented. Yet the director found them all in relative good health and interviewed them eating, drinking, and smoking cigars. Even with the stress and trauma of living in Cuba, they seemed not to have a high incidence of dementia.

The movie was incredible. Most of the musicians were still very active in music. Since I'm a neuropsychiatrist, I listened and watched *very* carefully. And all of the musicians remembered much of their musical past as well as recent events and experiences. Many of the musicians were still very socially active. One pianist played for a children's ballet and gymnastics troupe. Many of them taught and were actively involved in passing their gifts to younger people. The director got them all to play together again. Their bodies showed signs of aging, their posture was stooped, and their hands and fingers showed osteoarthritic changes of overuse, from playing musical instruments for decades. Yet despite all the cigars and alcohol consumption, and their nonvegetarian, nonorganic diet, the Buena Vista Social Club musicians were sharp as tacks. They were verbally articulate, answered questions with a wide variety of words in an organized, nontangential way. They were very social; their thoughts were neither slowed nor impoverished. They walked and moved normally without any of the slowing characteristics of many people in their eighties. After the movie was made, the musicians recorded an album, winning a Grammy. They went on a world tour that included a Carnegie Hall performance.

Although women may have an increased incidence of Alzheimer's disease over men due to hormonal issues, we are not all destined to dement. Estrogen plays a role in the frontal lobe's production of acetylcholine, which is central to memory function, and also protects nerve cells from injury and promotes their growth. Menopause with its drop in estrogen may decrease the production of the neurotransmitter acetylcholine, which is essential to memory function, and increase production of the neurotoxin beta-amyloid, which increases nerve cell inflammation and cell death. Although not all studies agree, women who take estrogen replacement may be at a lower risk of Alzheimer's disease. However, not all women who go through menopause and don't take hormone replacement get Alzheimer's disease, so clearly there are other factors.

Interestingly, testosterone may also play a role in memory dysfunction in Alzheimer's disease. In men with Alzheimer's disease, testosterone levels are lower than in men without Alzheimer's disease. No one has studied whether this hormone affects Alzheimer's disease in women. Also, women tend to get Alzheimer's disease earlier than men. In women, significant atrophy is found at average by age fifty, about the time of menopause. Men are more likely to get it in their sixties.

Reversible Memory Problems

Mrs. Brown has five daughters, all of whom are concerned about their memory. Their stories illustrate a variety of reversible memory disorders that are *not* Alzheimer's disease.

Hormonal Chaos and Infertility Cause Memory Problems

Abigail, at thirty-nine the baby of the family, had married late. Finally, when the time was right and she "met the right man," she decided to get pregnant and start a family. She had several surgeries for endometriosis, but wasn't able to get pregnant, so she had three rounds of in-vitro fertilization (IVF). Sadly, after five years, all the IVF, and $75,000, Abigail was not pregnant and her brain felt like "mush." She also felt apathetic, had a low sex drive, and kept forgetting important appointments. Her attention span was nonexistent; when she read a page in a book, she couldn't remember what she had read.

Abigail's brain and body suffered from the aftermath of treatment for infertility. She had been given Lupron, which is also used to treat endometriosis. Unlike her mother, Abigail's pseudodementia was temporary and the short-term use of bioidentical estrogen and progesterone would stabilize her hormone levels. Then her brain areas for memory, attention, and frontal-lobe executive function could come back "on line" and her attention span and forgetfulness would return to normal. Yet you cannot minimize the emotional aftermath of infertility. Women need to examine their grief about not having gotten pregnant and also try to see how the series of treatments affected their relationships with their husbands. Unresolved grief could turn into a major depression that over time could increase the chances of developing memory problems, heart disease, and cerebrovascular disease, which could cause a form of dementia or memory loss, what people used to call before the 1980s "hardening of the arteries and senility."

Immune System Disorders Cause Memory Problems

Betty-Lynn had always had a lot of colds, flus, and allergies. Growing up, Betty-Lynn had fatigue, joint pain, and lethargy for years which she thought was due to Epstein-Barr virus (EBV) and chronic fatigue syndrome. However, after a bout of eye inflammation, "iritis," she was diagnosed with systemic lupus erythematosis (SLE), an autoimmune illness in which the body makes antibodies against many organs. Every once in a while, her lupus will flare up and she'll have to take a round of steroids, or more recently, methotrexate. Now, at forty-six years of age, she has trouble remembering names and constantly has to write notes to herself or she forgets things.

In any illness where there is chronic immune system activation (including rheumatoid arthritis, chronic fatigue/fibromyalgia, Lyme disease, and others), the brain's attention circuits (and ultimately memory) will be a little shaky. When the body's white cells are chronically activated, they release inflammatory mediators, IL_1 and IL_6, that influence brain function, causing a mild delirium, apathy, sleepiness, fatigue, and inattentiveness and make it difficult to lay down memories. Cognitively, the person feels like she's on another planet. Multiple medicines that treat autoimmune illnesses can also influence attention, learning, and memory. Betty-Lynn and other women with autoimmune illnesses may take repeated rounds of steroids in an attempt to put out the fire in their immune systems. However, these medicines are similar to our own body's stress hormones, which tend to disrupt the brain memory area, the hippocampus.

Methotrexate is one of many medicines that can cause memory problems. Used in the severest cases of lupus and certain types of chemotherapy, these medicines may be lifesaving, but unfortunately may injure, sometimes permanently, the white matter pathways of the brain for attention, learning, and memory. Patients with these types of illnesses need to take these side effects into consideration as they plan their treatment programs with their doctors or practitioners.

Perimenopause, Antianxiety Medications, and Other Drugs Can Cause Memory Complaints

Christine, forty-eight and the middle daughter, is just getting off the tail end of a very difficult divorce battle and messy custody fight with her ex-husband. Her periods have always been "as regular as clockwork," but now are "all over the place." For the last year, she has had a period every eight to twelve days, which is getting to her. Her moods are up and down. Christine is trying to finish up her Ph.D. dissertation, but can't seem to "keep all the studies" in her head. She forgets what she is saying in mid-sentence when talking to her adviser or when teaching her students. She has developed intense cravings for carbohydrates and sweets, which some-how make her head feel clearer. Unfortunately, she has also put on twenty pounds. Christine has developed a host of medical problems for which she takes medicines that include Tagamet for heartburn; Benadryl to fall asleep; Xanax for panic attacks and palpitations; and oral contraceptive pills for dysfunctional heavy periods. As her mood plummets further, she gains more weight, and her memory gets worse.

Christine did not have Alzheimer's disease but several other physical and emotional disorders that cause problems with forgetfulness. Mood problems and depression, from the rapidly changing hormone levels of perimenopause, the influx of high levels of synthetic estrogen from the Pill, and the protracted divorce and custody battle could cause a "pseudo-dementia." Memory problems are frequently associated with depression. Rapidly changing hormone levels can induce mood disorders, just as rapidly changing temperatures can make a glass break. And mood affects memory. Depressed people usually complain a lot about their memory problems. They tend to tire easily on memory tests earlier when the ques-tions get more difficult. They can't freely recall information but they will be able to *recognize* the name, location, or phone number if they hear some-one else say it or if they see it written down somewhere on a list. People with "memory loss" complaints associated with depression are more likely to say "I don't remember" when asked to remember something they can't recall. In contrast, someone with Alzheimer's disease will make up an an-swer or distract others in an attempt to cover up the memory problem.

The memory problem may in fact be secondary to a problem with at-tention. When you are upset for a *very* long time (like Christine) in a situ-ation that is inescapably stressful, it wears down the brain's attention circuits, making learning and remembering difficult. Some people may not feel a change in mood, but they'll feel the trauma's effect on memory instead.

Tagamet, Xanax, Benadryl, and other drugs can cause memory prob-lems. Benadryl and Xanax lower acetylcholine, a critical neurotransmitter for attention and memory. Sleep medicines, antiallergy medicines, an-tianxiety medicines, and a variety of other over-the-counter medications all can induce a pseudo-delerious inattentive state that can lead to for-getfulness. Tagamet blocks histamine, another neurotransmitter critical for attention and memory.

Other substances can cause memory problems. Alcohol abuse can ultimately cause dementia. So can severe abuse of amphetamines and cocaine, especially if snorted. Cocaine "freebased" can over time cause tiny strokes. So can abusing inhalants like gasoline, glue, and Wite-Out, or smoking large amounts of marijuana for decades.

Painkillers can induce changes in attention and ultimately make someone believe she has a dementia. Morphine, Demerol, and other painkillers can disrupt the neurochemistry of your brain for laying down new memory. Advil, believe it or not, can also cause some confusion and memory loss in some individuals.

Low levels of vitamins in your diet and poor nutrition can hurt your memory. Not enough vitamin B_6 or B_{12} (which occurs in severe alcoholism, peptic ulcer disease, or poor dietary habits) can cause memory loss. On the other hand, excess supplementation of vitamins A and D can do the same. Excessive dieting and anorexia nervosa cause diffuse brain atrophy and memory problems, which are reversible when your weight normalizes. The neuronal pathways are coated or insulated in fatty myelin. As Margaret Cho says, the first place you lose weight isn't your hips and thighs, but in your head. During your reproductive years, if your body fat is so low that your periods have gone away, chances are there isn't enough fat in your brain to be emotionally and mentally healthy.

Thyroid Problems Can Cause Memory Complaints

Debby, fifty-five years old, had originally been a stockbroker, but when she found out her mother had Alzheimer's disease, she took alot of time away from work so she could became very involved in her treatment and placement in a nursing home. During this time, Debby was also very concerned about her own memory. Her husband had begun to call her a "space cadet," since her mind seemed to always be in the clouds. She had problems with low sex drive, fatigue, and lack of initiation and motivation. She had gained weight and was constipated.

Adequate thyroid hormone levels are critical for normal memory. In fact, there are thyroid receptors in the hippocampus, the key memory area. Debby's symptoms were caused by an elevated TSH. Too little or too much thyroid hormone affects cognition, attention, and memory—and "More is not better." The very stressful state of having too little or too much thyroid hormone causes cortisol and other stress neurotransmitters to be released, changing the brain for an extended period of time. Many patients with hyperthyroidism (Graves' disease) may still have attention, memory, and mood problems even when their thyroid levels are returned to normal. However, after normal thyroid function is maintained for a period of time, these residual memory effects eventually correct themselves.

Tamoxifen and Other "Antiestrogen" Medicines Can Disrupt Memory Function

Edith, fifty years old, had always been a nurturer. A nurse, she volunteered at local soup kitchens in her spare time, and would drop anything to help a friend. Edith was horrified when she found out her mother had Alzheimer's disease. It took several stressful months for Edith to "settle" her mother's financial affairs. During that time, Edith discovered a lump in her left breast that was found to be cancerous. Edith was put on tamoxifen. Soon, her brain began to feel "fuzzy."

Antiestrogen medicines, like tamoxifen, may also affect the mind. The most common adverse effects of tamoxifen include menopausal symptoms like hot flashes, nausea, and vaginal bleeding, but it also has been associated with fatigue, an inability to concentrate, a change in mood (especially depression), irritability, and nervousness. Although tamoxifen may be a key drug in the treatment and prevention of breast cancer, it can cause cognitive and emotional symptoms. It may also affect the immune system function that's inextricably related to mood. In fact, major depression occurs in between 1 and 15 percent of patients on tamoxifen and has been associated with mental slowing, problems with initiation, motivation, fatigue, and problems with sleep, which can make a woman feel like she is dementing.

Tamoxifen and other antiestrogen medicines switch the brain suddenly from its customary cycles to the more stable menopausal brain, condensing a change that's supposed to occur over a decade into a much shorter period of time. This sudden change can make a woman feel her brain is malfunctioning. If this medical treatment is something you need to stay healthy, there are nonhormonal ways to improve your memory (see below). For women without a history of breast cancer, taking bioidentical estrogen temporarily can ease memory complaints and buffer your hormonal transition.

Aging or Evolving: Are You Acting Like an "Old Lady" or a "Wise Woman"?

It is very possible to age gracefully and maintain your mental faculties, but it takes work and a willingness to change, grow, and take risks. Simply put, if you don't use your intellect, you'll lose it. If you continue to learn and challenge yourself, you can age gracefully and lower your risk for dementia. To age gracefully, you have to exercise every area of your brain:

- Attention, learning, and memory of new things
- Reading, writing, and other language skills
- Three-dimensional skills like map reading and navigating a car
- Relationships and social skills
- Physical and mental flexibility and agility
- Self-organization and purpose.

Please look at the paired statements in each of the ten categories listed below. Which of the statements in each set most closely approximates your cognitive style? Are you aging gracefully, or getting old and becoming "over the hill"?

Aging Gracefully • Acquiring Wisdom	Getting Old • Becoming "Over the Hill"
1: Learning and memory	
I read about 1–2 books at least per month.	There are few books in my living room and den.
I've either taken a class recently or bought a how-to book in the past year	I can wait in an airport lobby or doctor's office for more than 30 minutes without reading something.
2. Language	
If I don't know the meaning of a word, I look it up in a dictionary or ask someone what it means.	You'd never want to choose me as a partner in Scrabble.
If there was a movie out that everyone was raving about that had subtitles, I'd go to see it.	I don't know two synonyms for the color "red." I won't see a movie with subtitles no matter how good it is.
3. Spatial "Direction Sense"	
If I had to, I could fly into a strange city, rent a car, and drive around by myself.	I have one route, one way I usually go to the nearest city; if I don't go that way, I get lost.
I could learn to drive in England if I had to.	I couldn't put together a 50-piece puzzle in less than 1 hour.
4. Social/Relationship Skills	
I could go to a party where I know few people and meet one or two that I'd have contact with after I left.	I usually don't socialize or mingle at a party if I don't know anyone.
I call up 1–2 friends a week to go to a movie, etc.	Most of the people I spend time with are related to me.
5. Attention	
I could watch TV in one room if kids were having a party in the next room.	I have trouble hearing at a cocktail party and my hearing is normal.
I can remember the phone number in my head after dialing 411	I can't read if someone is talking.

6. Skilled Movement	
I could learn to drive a car with standard transmission.	I could never learn how to do the hand jive or dance the Macarena.
I could follow the directions in a VCR manual and program the time to record.	Dance classes are out of the question. I avoid technology and hate updating my cell phone and computers.
7. Organization/Planning	
If I were to enter a new supermarket, I'd figure out how it's laid out first rather than go up and down every aisle.	I have to go back to the house frequently to get something I forgot before leaving for work or a short drive in the car.
I'd know if someone had gone through my purse.	When cooking something with a recipe, I frequently find out that I don't have a key ingredient.
8. Idea Density	
I have many projects around the house that are "in progress."	I really can't read an article in the *New York Times* from start to finish.
My living space shows I have a busy mind.	When writing a paper for school, I usually had a hard time meeting the page requirement for length.
9. Cognitive Flexibility	
I could reorganize my sock drawer by two different methods.	I usually don't do well if someone changes the rules on me once I've gotten used to my routine.
I could go to a foreign country, where I don't speak the language, and make my way with a dictionary and a map.	If a cleaning person changes the location of things in my house, I have to put everything back the way I had it.
10. Motor Slowing	
I am usually never the last person to finish eating.	I usually bring up the rear when walking in a group, but I don't have an orthopedic problem.
I can get in and out of a public restroom in less than 5 minutes.	It takes me longer to come up with the answer to a problem than most people.
+/20 positive	-/20 negative

Now, add up the number of endorsed items in the Aging Gracefully column. Then put a (+) sign in front of the number. Then add up the number of endorsed items in the Getting Old, Over the Hill column. Put a (-) in front of the number. Subtract the Over the Hill score from the Aging Gracefully score to see how much you're buffered against aging and Alzheimer's disease. The higher your score, the less likely you are to get Alzheimer's disease.

The more you learn, the more "connections" you build in your brain, and this cognitive reserve somehow protects you from brain aging.

Activities like viewing television, listening to the radio, reading newspapers, magazines, and books, playing cards or checkers, doing crosswords or other puzzles or going to museums all involve language, attention, learn-

ing, memory, visuospatial abilities, organization, planning, social and relationship skills, cognitive flexibility, and motor programming networks in
the brain. Frequently participating in these relatively simple activities is associated with a 50 percent lower risk of getting Alzheimer's disease.

Political Correctness and Ageism

When I worked in the inpatient psychiatry unit, we had older patients on
the floor we called the "senior team" (aged sixty-three and up), who were
treated differently from younger patients. There was an unspoken policy of
political correctness about how you should act with these older patients.
You were supposed to hold your senior patient's arm when you walked
down the hall, treating him as if he were "frail." It made me want to
scream. Whenever residents did this, everyone else looked on and smiled.
To me, it felt like we were infantilizing these patients.

At first, when the patients were depressed, they walked and talked
slowly, and acted "frail" whether or not they had a physical problem like
arthritis. When their depression improved, they talked and walked more
quickly, the weakness and slowness disappeared, and their arthritis improved as well. Many of the age-related changes in physical function that
we have come to believe are "normal" frailty are really ageism. Whenever
I had a patient whose thinking, speaking, and walking was slowed to a
near crawl, I wouldn't slow down and I wouldn't lower my expectations.
It may sound mean, but I would leave them at the nursing station and tell
them I would meet them in the day room. After initially being annoyed,
they would speed up. I wouldn't talk to them any differently than I talked
to any other adult. If they weren't hard of hearing, I would talk at a normal volume and speed. I would never simplify the grammatical construction and I'd never lower my expectation of what they could do
cognitively just because they were older. Gradually, they stopped acting
like frail "old ladies" (or old men). Once released from these stereotypes,
it seems these women were free to expect more and want more in life.
They went from being "old ladies" on the senior team to being "wise
women."

To be old is not to be frail. Frailty is a state of mind that leads to disease in
the brain and the body.

We can all age gracefully, remain mentally and physically agile and
quick. Frailty is not a part of normal aging, it's a disease associated with

heart disease and dementia. Imbedded in our culture is the "old lady" stereotype, that is, that walking slowly (and probably talking slowly) are inevitable parts of aging. In some older people, gait speed and swing time, the amount they pick up their feet, are reduced, and sometimes associated with Parkinson's disease and arthritis. Usually, it's just associated with inactivity and fear of falling, poor physical fitness, a dependent attitude, depression, and a stereotype that they assume when they get older.

A recent study of people between sixty and ninety years old investigated whether or not "age-associated" changes in physical function, especially walking, is influenced by ageism. In one group, the people's brains were primed for ageism. When they watched a computer screen, "old lady" type or ageist words were flashed at speeds that allowed perception without conscious awareness—words like "senile," "dependent," "diseased." The other group's brains were primed with "wise woman" type words: "wise," "astute," "accomplished." The "old lady" group who heard ageist words exhibited no change in walking speed or swing time. In contrast, those who heard the "wise woman" words walked 9 percent faster. Their swing time went up as well.

The authors of the study concluded that if you reinforce "positive stereotypes" by rewiring someone's self-concept from "old lady" to "wise woman," you can increase the efficiency of one function of the brain, that is, walking speed and swing time.

Pump Up Your Memory Circuits
"Ancora Imparo"/"I'm Still Learning"

Memory loss is not a natural consequence of aging. But if you do have trouble remembering things, there are ways to pump up your Feminine Brain's memory circuits.

PUTTING OUT THE FIRE: INFLAMMATION, FRAILTY, AND AGING

Many of the risk factors for accelerated aging and Alzheimer's disease are associated with inflammation in the brain or body.

So many of the anti-inflammatory treatment approaches that lower the risk of heart disease and stroke also lower the risk of developing memory problems and help people age gracefully.

Inflammation in brain and body may even be the basis of frailty, a wasting syndrome. A physiological state of vulnerability that increases one's chance of disease and death, frailty creates a higher risk of falling, fractures, infection, hospitalization, and institutionalization. However, frailty is not caused simply by advanced age.

The various treatments for memory problems (1) slow or prevent oxidative and inflammation damage in brain pathways and blood vessels that nourish the brain with oxygen; (2) bolster neurotransmitter levels that are critical to memory and brain function; and (3) influence plasticity, growth, and repair of the brain.

Antioxidation and Anti-inflammation Medicines and Supplements

Nonsteroidal anti-inflammatory drugs (i.e., NSAIDs) have been shown to delay the onset of Alzheimer's disease. Your chance of developing this disorder is reduced by 50 percent if you use this class of meds, which includes aspirin, Tylenol, and Advil. NSAIDs also decrease cognitive decline, especially in language (i.e., naming), visuospatial processing, and visual memory.

1. *Aspirin* (75–325 mg/day or 1 baby to 1 adult aspirin per day) is a potent inhibitor of an inflammation cascade called the "prostaglandin pathway," as well as a blood cell clotting mechanism called "platelet aggregation." Aspirin decreases your risk of stroke and heart attack. Do not take any other "antiplatelet" or "blood thinner" medicines or herbs, such as Warfarin, gingko biloba, or St. John's wort, which would give you an increased risk for bleeding. In some people, aspirin can cause cognitive side effects, agitation, confusion, and headache. In individuals with a history of digestive problems, aspirin can cause stomach pain, ulcers, nausea, and other gastrointestinal problems. In some people, especially with respiratory problems, aspirin can aggravate shortness of breath and asthma. Other anti-inflammatory agents may have a therapeutic effect on the inflammation and oxidative chain reaction associated with the neurofibrillary tangles and amyloid plaques of Alzheimer's disease.

Deprenyl (selegiline 10 mg/day) and melatonin have a beneficial effect on inflammation. So does vitamin C (500 mg/day).

2. *Indomethacin* (25 mg twice a day), like aspirin, is an NSAID and an inhibitor of the inflammatory prostaglandin cascade. Its mechanism is similar to aspirin's in delaying or preventing the occurrence of Alzheimer's disease. Zinc (100 mg 2x/day), selenium (200 micrograms per day), alpha-tocopherol (100 mg/day), and other types of vitamin E (2000 iu/day) all quell free radicals that cause oxidation that leads to inflammation. High levels of antioxidants correlate with better cognitive and memory performance in older persons.

3. *Zinc* is an antioxidant and stabilizes biological membranes, especially

in the nervous system, protecting the nerve cell membranes against oxidative damage. Older persons are at greater risk of having zinc deficiency, especially if they are heavy alcohol consumers and also take a lot of medicines, including diuretics. Zinc also bolsters immunity by inhibiting virus replication of the common cold, and may also decrease the chance of getting age-related macular degeneration.

4. *Selenium* doesn't just prevent oxidation of cell membranes, but also regulates thyroid hormone metabolism. As you may recall, a thyroid hormone imbalance which can cause an attentional problem (confusional state) can cause memory complaints. Selenium helps convert T_4 (thyroxine) to T_3 (triiodothyronine). T_3 is supposed to be more important for mood and cognitive function than T_4. Selenium functions with d-alpha-tocopherol to prevent oxidative damage of membranes.

5. *Vitamin E* is a collective term for a family of substances that are structurally and functionally related. Abnormally low levels of this vitamin increase the risk of degenerative disorders, including Alzheimer's disease and blood vessel disease (atherosclerosis) and heart disease, that also can set the scene for dementia and stroke. There are two types of vitamin E, *tocopherols* and *tocotrienols.* Both have antioxidant activity. Alpha-tocopherol and alpha-tocotrienol are the most important forms of vitamin E because they have the most potent antioxidant activities. Some studies suggest that alpha-tocotrienol is a more potent free radical scavenger and antioxidant than alpha-tocopherol. Tocotrienols are found in some plant oils, including palm oil, rice bran oil, palm kernel oil, and coconut oil. (But canola, cottonseed, olive, peanut, safflower, soybean, and sunflower oils contain very little tocotrienols.) Tocotrienols, similar to cholesterol-lowering "statin" drugs (e.g., Lovastatin), inhibit cholesterol synthesis. Tocotrienols are available in a nutritional supplement form as "mixed tocotrienols." In addition to lowering the incidence of heart disease and stroke, tocotrienols also lower cholesterol levels, which when elevated increase one's chance toward Alzheimer's disease and dementia.

Tocotrienols have also been shown to have an anti–breast cancer effect. Tocotrienol–rich palm oil has been shown to inhibit the growth of human breast cancer cell lines. Women with a breast cancer history present a special challenge for pumping up brain memory circuits. Estrogen replacement for preservation of memory circuits (see below) is generally considered inappropriate, whether or not their tumors were estrogen positive. In fact, tamoxifen treatment for breast cancer may further lower estrogen binding to brain hippocampal memory circuits. Tocotrienols may be a wonderful supplement option for women who have had breast cancer who are concerned about their memory either because they themselves have memory complaints or they have a positive family history of dementia. This supplement is one of the most potent antioxidants known and may lower a woman's risk of Alzheimer's disease by reducing the inflammation cascade that leads to neurotoxicity and brain cell death. At the same time, tocotrienols may inhibit breast cancer cell growth and lower their chance of recurrence. In fact, some researchers have suggested that tocotrienols be combined with tamoxifen as a breast cancer treatment.

High-dose tocotrienol (200–300 mg/day) should be stopped one month prior to surgery because of its antiplatelet "blood thinner" activity. Beware of combining tocotrienol with other "blood thinning" supplements or medicines that may cause bleeding problems, especially gingko biloba and St. John's wort.

6. *Selegiline* (Eldepryl, Deprenyl) has also been used in Parkinson's disease. Selegiline blocks the breakdown of dopamine, norepinephrine, and serotonin, critical neurotransmitters in the frontal lobe executive function network that are important for memory.

7. *Cholesterol-lowering "statin" drugs* appear to lower the incidence of diseases that have chronic inflammation. Drugs such as Lovastatin and Lipitor reduce the level of low-density lipoproteins (LDL). Long-term treatment with these drugs may prevent heart attack and stroke through effective control of high blood cholesterol, which can clog small arteries, forming plaques, that cause dementia by multiple strokes. In addition to lowering the risk of osteoporosis, statins may also lower the risk for Alzheimer's disease.

However, "statin" drugs can be very toxic to the liver and may interfere with hormone production since hormones are made from cholesterol by the liver. There may be a variety of other ways to lower cholesterol, including exercise, diet, weight loss, stress reduction, and a variety of traditional Chinese herbs (the list of which is beyond the scope of this book).

8. *Coenzyme Q_{10}* (200 mg/day) also seems to lower inflammation and oxidation in the body and the brain since it is cardioprotective, cytoprotective, and neuroprotective. No one really knows for sure how it works, but coenzyme Q_{10} seems to protect cell membrane lipids and cholesterol from being oxidized, thus preventing inflammation. Coenzyme Q_{10} lowers cholesterol and also prevents "good" LDL cholesterol from getting oxidized, thus decreasing the inflammation that occurs in atherosclerosis. Coenzyme Q_{10} levels drop when statin drugs are used, so it seems that all people who use statin drugs should also take Coenzyme Q_{10} This supplement also seems to decrease the inflammation of periodontal disease,

which has been associated with an increased risk of heart disease. Coenzyme Q_{10} seems to lower the inflammation in the brain and may ultimately delay or minimize your chances of getting Alzheimer's disease.

You have to be careful of drug supplement interactions with Coenzyme Q_{10}, because it may interfere with Warfarin and some blood thinners, and may increase the toxicity of some antidiabetic meds since CoQ_{10} actually itself lowers and controls blood sugar.

9. *Acetyl-L-Carnitine* (500–2000 mg/day). Acetyl-L-carnitine has, similar to coenzyme Q_{10}, neuroprotective, cardioprotective, antioxidant effects and prevents cell death. It is especially useful for attentional problems and memory loss due to stroke or Alzheimer's disease. In patients with mild to moderate Alzheimer's disease, there was significant improvement in cognitive abilities, and a slower rate of deterioration in memory and attention over the course of one year.

Acetyl-L-carnitine may preserve cognitive abilities, attention, and memory in normal older persons as well. Its neuroprotective effects are most helpful when used with other antioxidant supplements, including coenzyme Q_{10}. Acetyl-L-carnitine may improve levels of a key memory neurotransmitter acetylcholine.

Supplements, Medicines, and Sleep Correct Neurotransmitter Levels Critical for Memory

Most supplements and medicine treatments for memory problems focus on replacing or pumping up falling acetylcholine levels. But getting a really good night's *sleep* can also increase memory consolidation and also is a wonderful source of intuition. Every time your brain goes into the REM/dream state, acetylcholine levels go up in the hippocampus. In fact, learning is correlated with REM sleep. If you get less than six hours of sleep, you must dream less because most REM sleep occurs in the later part of the evening, that is, after seven or eight hours of sleep. In the brain, this is also when a tremendous amount of plasticity, or brain growth and repair, occurs, which is why babies sleep so much. Dreaming may be when we replay various experiences we have during the day, process their significance, and make associations with what we've learned in the past; then we file them away in memory networks all over our brain. So if you want to improve your memory if you are studying for a test, don't pull an all-nighter the night before the exam. You'll have depleted your brain's critical levels of acetylcholine by not getting your needed eight hours of sleep. There is, of course, some variation among individuals, since some people are able to get all their REM cycles in six hours of sleep, as if the brain's efficiency for acetylcholine production is greater.

On the other hand, if you can't figure out a problem after you've been puzzling over it for hours, sleep on it. During the night, plasticity, learning, associations, and connections are laid down in your brain, and chances are in the next twenty-four to forty-eight hours you'll get a rational or intuitive solution.

Some treatments for memory dysfunction and Alzheimer's disease have targeted replacing *choline* levels in the brain, since acetylcholine has two molecular parts, the acetyl part and the choline part. Unfortunately, there has been little success with this treatment route. But it is safe to try *lecithin* (or *phosphatidylcholine*) (1.8–3.0 gram per day, which is found in soybean, sunflower, and rapeseed—canola). Phosphatidylcholine is the major source of choline for the body and the brain, for production of the neurotransmitter acetylcholine but also for nerve cell membrane integrity and repair (see below). Only a few reports have indicated cognitive benefits in people with age-related memory loss and Alzheimer's disease, but no major side effects have been associated with lecithin supplementation.

CDP-choline (500–2000 mg/day) is another supplement that has been used to build up choline levels. This substance, a building block in the synthesis of phosphatidylcholine (lecithin), has two functions: It helps build up memory neurotransmitter levels of acetylcholine, and it helps build nerve cell membranes. CDP-choline has been used as a "cognitive enhancer" because it may help repair neuronal cell membranes that have been damaged by trauma, stroke, toxins, and aging.

Although CDP-choline has not been fully studied, in some studies it has been shown to help patients with brain injury and stroke recover some cognitive function, including memory. In a few studies with Alzheimer's disease, CDP slightly improved cognitive performance, especially in patients with the earlier stages of this illness. Levels of CDP-choline up to 2,000 milligrams a day have been successfully used in people with "age-related cognitive decline" to improve inefficient verbal memory. Side effects of high doses include dizziness, stomach upset, and headache. CDP-choline is usually part of a nutritional supplement blend that contains several other substances to support cognition and memory.

Acetyl-L-carnitine (see above; 500–2000 mg/day), in addition to having a neuroprotective effect and antioxidant qualities, may donate the acetyl component for formation of acetylcholine. Combining lecithin/phosphatidylcholine with tacrine or other anticholinesterases (see below) has been shown to have some success with improving memory in Alzheimer's disease.

Acetylcholinesterase Inhibitors

Once acetylcholine has been released into the space between nerve cells, the synapse, the enzyme acetylcholinesterase is available to break this neurotransmitter down into acetyl-coenzyme A and choline, thus inactivating it. One way to increase the levels of acetylcholine available for memory function is to inhibit this enzyme's activity. Current drug treatment for dementia, especially Alzheimer's disease, is limited, with the majority of medicines working by this mechanism.

Tacrine (Cognex, 10–40 mg 4x/day), *Donepezil* (Aricept, 10 mg/day), *rivastigmine* (Exelon, 1.5–12 mg/day), and *Galantamine* (Reminyl, 4–24 mg/day). None of these drugs cures the illness, but they may give some patients symptom improvement in the mild to moderate stages of Alzheimer's disease. Vitamin E, which is supposed to delay institutionalization, is often prescribed with these medicines. The downside of Tacrine (Cognex) is that it has to be given four times a day. It irritates the liver (elevates its enzymes ALT/SGPT) and can cause heart arrythmias, ulcers, nausea, and other digestive side effects. Rivastigmine (Exelon), Donepezil (Aricept), and Reminyl (Galantamine) need to be taken only once or twice a day, but they all can cause cardiac and digestive side effects.

Response to all of these drugs varies widely. Only 20 to 30 percent of patients have a positive response to tacrine, while a placebo alone gives an improvement in 10 percent of patients. These drugs may have other effects in addition to just allowing acetylcholine to sit around longer in the brain. Tacrine increases metabolism of other neurotransmitters including serotonin, norepinephrine, and dopamine; that may be important in memory function. Tacrine also seems to decrease levels of beta-amyloid protein, the neurotoxic protein associated with Alzheimer's disease.

Interestingly, there are acetylcholinesterase inhibitors in certain *vegetables* (the nightshade family). Normal dietary levels of tomato (*Lycopersicon esculentum*), potato (*Solanum tuberosum*), and eggplant (*Solanum melangena esculentum*) can theoretically increase acetylcholine in your brain since all these vegetables inhibit the enzyme that inactivates acetylcholine. Normal dietary levels (20–60 grams) cause few side effects. There are a few very rare individuals, however, who have toxic reactions of apathy, drowsiness, and visual and auditory hallucination.

Siberian Ginseng

Actually, there are seven different types of ginseng, but *Panax ginseng* (Asian ginseng) and *Eleutherococcus senticoccus* (Siberian ginseng) are used for memory. Siberian ginseng (625 mg 2/day) precipitates acetylcholine release from the brain, and increases choline uptake by the hippocampus, the key brain area for memory. Siberian ginseng has neuroprotective and antioxidant effects. It has been shown to prevent hippocampal cell loss after stroke and also scavenges free radicals, dampening the inflammation cascades that lead to nerve cell loss and degeneration. This effect has been shown in diabetic patients with small vessel disease who also have cognitive challenges.

Ginseng is also an "adaptogen," that is, it helps the body adapt to stress. It may help maintain learning and plasticity in the brain throughout its lifespan. Ginseng maintains and supports many of the nerve cellular molecular mechanisms necessary for protein production, which support nerve ending sprouting, plasticity, and laying down new nerve connections (synapses) that are critical for learning, memory, and brain repair.

Gingko Biloba

Gingko biloba (120–240 mg/day) has been very widely studied for the treatment of dementia. Gingko improves mild memory complaints in middle-aged people, ameliorating age-related verbal and nonverbal memory complaints. It also improves attention, memory function, and other cognitive abilities in patients with dementia. Its effect was substantial when compared with Aricept, and more benefit is seen the longer it is taken.

Gingko biloba was shown to delay mental deterioration in early stages of Alzheimer's disease and to protect the brain's memory area against stress. It may facilitate behavioral adaptation to stress in adverse environmental situations, and may decrease stress associated with changes in the brain.

Gingko biloba increases acetylcholine levels and improves memory and other cognitive functions by functioning as an antioxidant, similar to zinc, selenium, and alpha-tocopherol, scavenging free radicals that can set the scene for the inflammatory brain changes that precede the nerve cell death of Alzheimer's disease. Gingko biloba also affects blood vessels and ultimately increases circulation of oxygen and nutrients to the brain. This effect increases cerebral blood for the nerve cells in the memory network and improves blood flow to other areas of the body, including the coronary arteries. This is called an "anti-ischemic" effect. Ischemia, or decreased oxygenation of heart muscle, occurs prior to a heart attack. In addition to increasing blood flow in cerebrovascular (brain) and cardiovascular (heart) blood vessels, gingko biloba also increases blood flow to the ears, brain stem, and other peripheral blood vessels in the body.

If you are on an anticoagulation therapy (Coumadin) or any antiplatelet "blood thinner" (like aspirin), you should not take gingko because it can cause bleeding. Any vitamin E/alpha-tocopherol/alpha-tocotrienol supplement used with gingko can also cause bleeding, including St. John's wort, borage oil, and evening primrose oil. Other than rare bleeding complications, if combined with other "blood thinning" supplements or medicines, gingko biloba can cause mild gastrointestinal side effects, mild skin reactions and rashes, headache, dizziness, and palpitations. However, most people tolerate it very well.

Huperzine A

Chien Tseng Ta, or Huperzine A (60–200 mcg/day), an herbal supplement from the Chinese moss *Huperzia serrata,* raises acetylcholine activity in the brain, and has been shown to improve memory in Alzheimer's disease, normal aging, and multi-infarct dementia. Similar to tacrine and donepezil, this supplement may increase the memory neural network transmission in the brain. However, huperzine A is supposed to be eighty times more potent than tacrine and have fewer side effects. It has been used as a prescription drug in China since the early 1990s. Interestingly, it has also been used to treat fever and inflammation. One study showed that it prevented oxidative nerve cell death, which indicates it may reduce nerve cell degeneration. Natural forms of huperzine A (L-huperzine A) are said to be three to four times more potent than synthetic forms. Huperzine A hasn't been fully studied, but preliminary research showed significant improvement quantitatively measured on the Wechsler Memory Scale.

People with seizure disorders, heart arrhythmias, asthma, and bowel disease may have adverse effects. Nausea, diarrhea, shortness of breath, and heart arrhythmias have been seen. It is unknown whether taking huperzine A with Tacrine, Donepezil, or other drugs that increase acetylcholine can cause adverse side effects.

Nicotine

Nicotine hits the acetylcholine receptor, thus acting like acetylcholine itself in the brain, and people who smoke have been reported to have a reduced risk of Alzheimer's disease. Because of the obvious drawbacks of using this cancer-causing drug, a number of drugs are under development to mimic nicotine's action. Other drug delivery systems for nicotine treatment are also being developed, including gum, transdermal patches, and "nicotinic drug," since both smoking and chewing tobacco cause cancer.

Serotonin Drugs

Since cyclic changes in serotonin levels occur during different phases of the menstrual cycle, it makes sense that hormonal changes in a woman's body may be associated with simultaneous problems with memory and mood. In fact, low levels of the natural antidepressant *SAMe* (S-adenosyl-L-methionine) have been found in people with Alzheimer's disease. SAMe has been used for years in Europe for the treatment of depression and chronic fatigue/fibromyalgia as well as a host of other disorders. SAMe helps the function of nerve cell membranes and neurotransmitters critical for mood and sleep, and helps slow one of the inflammatory cascades behind the genesis of Alzheimer's disease.

Although studies are inconclusive, SAMe may improve memory status in patients with memory complaints. SAMe at 800 milligrams a day (with a shot of intramuscular SAMe) improved performance on a specific cognitive exam—the mini-mental-state exam—showing a capacity to "reverse or delay age-associated memory impairment."

Vitamins

Improving your general nutritional status is the easiest, most direct way of improving neurotransmitter levels for memory functions. In one study of 260 women and men over sixty years of age, people with low levels of vitamins C, B_{12}, riboflavin, and folic acid had lower memory and nonverbal abstract and frontal lobe cognitive function scores. Everyone who has memory complaints should have a work-up and blood tests to rule out B_6, B_{12}, and folate deficiency. SAMe, B_6, B_{12}, folic acid, and L-carnitine have been shown to have roles in the regulation of both memory and mood.

Interestingly, high blood homocysteine levels, which may cause oxidative injury to blood vessel walls, increase the chance of getting coronary artery disease and dementia. B_6, B_{12}, and, folic acid will decrease homocysteine levels, and hypothetically decrease your chances of getting either illness.

Supplements and Drugs for Brain Plasticity, Growth, and Repair

Low levels of DHA (docosahexaenoic acid) in your blood is a significant risk factor for Alzheimer's disease. DHA is a type of omega-3 fatty acid that is critical for nerve membrane function. In one eight-year study of 1,200 "elderly" patients, low levels of DHA increased one's chance of getting Alzheimer's by 67 percent.

Stress and irritation can imbalance the lipid composition in your nerve cell membranes (or any cell membrane in your body for that matter). DHA and omega-3 fatty acid levels are needed for lifelong plasticity, learning, memory, and other brain functions.

PHOSPHATIDYL SERINE

In seventeen double-blind studies, *phosphatidyl serine* (100–300 mg/day) has been shown to increase memory in early Alzheimer's. Phosphatidyl serine may make the membrane more fluid, and ultimately enable neurotransmitter receptors to function more efficiently in emotion, thought, and behavior.

After the "mad cow" scare, with infectious agents being transmitted in beef brain, a soy source is now used. However, phosphatidyl serine from soy is low in DHA, so authorities don't agree about whether or not soy phosphatidyl serine can significantly help memory.

ESTROGEN AND OTHER HORMONE REPLACEMENT THERAPY

A woman's risk for getting Alzheimer's is reduced by taking estrogen postmenopausally. Yet I am mentioning estrogen replacement last, at the end of a long list of other supplements and medicinal solutions for memory problems. Since menopause is a normal developmental milestone in a woman's brain and body (similar to puberty and pregnancy), it seems reasonable that its hormonal perturbations would normally encourage growth and maturity, not dementia, disease, and death.

A growing body of evidence suggests that long-term use of Provera (a combination of *synthetic* conjugated estrogens and progesterone in the form of medroxyprogesterone acetate) increases a woman's risk of stroke and breast and uterine cancer. No one knows if *bioidentical* estrogen and progesterone have the same risks. Estrogen is functionally a growth hormone that encourages, among other things, breast, uterine, and brain cell growth and development. Cancer is unbridled, out-of-control cell division. In a woman's body, the cyclic rising and falling of estrogen, progesterone, and other hormones influences a cyclic waxing and waning of the size, volume, and cellular complexity of the breast glandular tissue, uterine lining, and brain hippocampal memory areas. When a woman loses this normal cyclic nature and is given elevated levels of more potent synthetic hormones, it makes sense that the body would be subjected to unbridled growth without the wisdom of appropriately timed pruning. All cells have a genetic apparatus that controls growth and death. Giving a woman high levels of synthetic estrogen across her lifespan may bypass normal cellular controls that put the brakes on cell division and growth. HRT may encourage hippocampal cellular growth and sprouting, bypassing or overtaking the Alzheimer's pathological process/development in the brain. However, synthetic high-dose estrogen replacement may also encourage growth and "sprouting" of cells in other hormonally responsive body areas, including the breast and uterus, and lead to cancer.

You now know the risks associated with estrogen replacement, but there can also be benefits to the feminine brain. Hormones that are critical for brain function are derived from cholesterol, which is transformed to *pregnenolone,* which is then converted to *progesterone.* Both pregnenolone and progesterone have important effects on memory, mood, anxiety, and cognition. At low levels, pregnenolone calms brain excitability and prunes memory circuits. At higher levels, it increases neuronal firing, thus increasing learning and memory. Several authorities ultimately have suggested pregnenolone supplementation for people who suffer from memory complaints, but if you don't know the appropriate dose, too low a dose can actually worsen your symptoms. A higher dose may improve learning and memory and sharpen your mind, but if you are prone to anxiety and irritability, it could also overactivate your brain. And it is very possible that the dosage of the neurosteroid that you need will keep changing, since at different times and different places in the brain, neurosteroid concentrations vary according to environmental and behavioral demands.

Progesterone limits free radical damage that kills neurons, so it prevents brain cell degeneration. It has been used to promote brain cell survival and ultimately learning and memory after traumatic brain injury.

Progesterone can be converted to *DHEA.* DHEA (taken at 90–450 mg/day), similar to high-dose pregnenolone, increases brain firing, learning, and memory.

DHEA is made by both the adrenal glands and the ovaries. Levels begin to rise at puberty, reach an all-time high in adulthood at about age forty, then usually steadily decline. Some women with menopausal memory complaints have been helped with DHEA supplementation. However, if you're prone to anxiety, edginess, or irritability, or you have a history of trauma, it aggravates your brain's tendency for excitability. Excessive DHEA supplementation, some believe, causes excess production of testosterone or estrogen and some studies have noted it is addictive.

DHEA is transferred to *androstenedione,* which is then shuttled forward to and up at one of two hormonal destinations: *testosterone* and *estradiol.*

Testosterone may affect learning and memory in men, but no one really understands its impact on cognition in women. It can also be converted to *estradiol,* which may preserve attention, learning, and memory. If a woman is given estradiol after a total abdominal hysterectomy and oophorectomy (removal of the uterus and ovaries), she experiences improved cognition as well.

Estrogen replacement may either prevent the onset of dementia or delay its onset. Estrogens may have a neuroprotective effect in stroke, heart, and blood vessel disease, as well as other health conditions that result in nerve cell death. Hormonal treatment improves reaction time, memory, and learning, correcting the slowing of thoughts and movement in some women with dementia or cognitive changes.

Numerous antioxidants and neuroprotective agents, including alpha-tocotrienols, zinc, selenium, acetyl-L-carnitine, and aspirin and other NSAIDs, have many of the advantages of estrogens but not the downsides. Estrogen increases important neurotransmitter levels in the brain for attention, learning, memory, and cognition, including acetylcholine, norepinephrine, dopamine, and serotonin, but other supplements including ginseng and others may be used to increase these same substances and help memory complaints. Red wine has both a protective neuroeffect and probably increases neurotransmitter levels, since it has a substance that acts like estrogen in cognitive areas.

Soy foods, though controversial, may also be a source for estrogen-like activity without some of the detrimental effects. Rich in isoflavone phytoestrogens, soy foods have *weak* activity at estrogen receptors in the brain. High-dose soy (100 mg isoflavones/day for 10 weeks) improved "short-term" verbal memory and "long-term" memory and mental flexibility in postmenopausal women.

If you are worried about estrogen stimulation of breast, ovary, uterus, and other organs in your body, you have other options for supplements without estrogen-like activity. Although the jury is still out about how much of a growth factor effect soy has on breast, uterus, bone, and other organs, some women who were postmenopausal claim they got their periods back once they started high-dose soy. If you're worried about any estrogen-like stimulatory effect of any product—for example, if you have a first-degree relative who had breast, ovarian, or uterine cancer—don't take soy if you feel it is unsafe. The stress and its associated cortisol from taking something you're uncomfortable with won't be good for your brain and it may in fact cancel out any benefits.

Improve Your Concept of What It Is to Be an Older Adult

All the risk factors for Alzheimer's disease interfere in one way or another with plasticity, growth, and repair and there are many ways to improve these brain functions that don't involve supplements or drugs. Promoting lifelong learning, experience, and an increase in "idea density" will lower your risk of Alzheimer's disease and improve your capacity for learning, memory, and flexibility.

If your mind-set is that older is slower, weaker, and frailer, your brain will be more likely to have anatomical physiological changes that cause you to have bradyphrenia (slow thoughts), bradykinesia (slow movements), and cognitive rigidity. If your intention is always to keep things the same, and not try new experiences, the frontal lobe network for shifting perception, attention, and behavior will anatomically get "stuck in a rut." Your cognition and memory will have a parallel loss of function. Look at some Elder Role Models:

Watch movies of people who ditch a life-style in midstream and begin a new relationship, vocation, or skill. If the movies listed here seem corny and trite, substitute your own list of aging mentors:

Yoda in *Star Wars: Attack of the Clones*
Divine Secrets of the Ya Ya Sisterhood
Shirley Valentine
Guarding Tess

Read about Michelangelo, Grandma Moses, or other great geniuses and how they aged. Or work with someone who does hypnotherapy or vocalizations about your "stuck in a rut" thoughts and improve your expectations.

GET THE LEAD OUT (EXERCISE)!

Women who increase their level of baseline activity (to one hour a day or more) are less likely to develop cognitive decline.

a. *Take tai chi or qi gong classes,* which help maintain a varied repertoire of novel, smooth, balanced movement routines.
b. *Take yoga or Pilates* to increase flexibility and build muscle tone.
c. *Exercise aerobically* every morning for at least thirty minutes. *Walk* briskly outside with a friend after dinner.
d. *Take a dance class* and risk making an idiot of yourself. Make sure your class has students of many ages in it.

If you can't participate in the activities listed above, get a physical therapist, personal coach, or buddy to inspire you to build up over time your skill set in this network of your brain. Ultimately, it's not the level of your skill or physical prowess. It's the ability to grow, change, and build a continuously changing repertoire of physical goals, challenges, and skills.

SHIFT YOUR MIND-SET

Put yourself in novel situations that make you feel excited but a little on the edge, a little nervous (not too much), and that challenge and stress you. Try things you had previously deemed ridiculous, foolish, juvenile, or "out of the question."

a. Watch the top ten videos on VH1 and see what young people like in music and art.
b. Visit a new restaurant that's just opened. Try a different food.
c. Change the programmed presets on your car radio to a variety of types of music stations.
d. Have a trusted friend help you go through your closet and throw out or donate to a local charity articles of clothing that are a "rut" for you. Then have that friend help you try a new look.
e. Have a professional help you learn some new makeup routine and investigate some new beauty products. Then have a friend monitor that you really incorporate and maintain these changes into your daily repertoire.
f. Have someone do a feng shui evaluation of your house to remove clutter and areas of stagnant *qi* (stuck-in-a-rut energy).

INCREASE YOUR IDEA DENSITY. PUMP UP YOUR HIPPOCAMPAL NEURONAL TONE

Studies indicate that learning new things in the written and visual worlds lowers your risk of Alzheimer's disease.

a. Join a book club. It will force you to read a current book and discuss it with others whose views may be distinct from your own.

b. Take an art or photography class, even if you are artistically challenged. Learning about color, form, dimension, and shading will enlarge your neural perceptual sphere.

c. Teach a class in something that you are talented in. Explaining or teaching a skill or subject area and trying to activate someone else's learning of it will deepen your own knowledge. The more a brain network is used, the more associations and neural pathways are built within it. Combat disuse atrophy!

FIND SOME NEW INTERESTS

a. ***Learn the foreign language of the newest minority moving into your community.*** Not only will this increase plasticity and pump up the neurons in your language areas, but it will introduce you to a new social circle or culture. Then, as you are learning the language, volunteer in your local hospital emergency room or homeless shelter where you can use it.

b. ***Rent a video of the newest, hottest comedian.*** Keeping a healthy sense of humor is key to the health of the cardiovascular system and the brain. And current comedians will explore new ideas that are "edgy"; to understand their jokes you'll need to adapt your own mind-set.

c. ***Visit a new city and navigate with a map.*** If your vision is normal, keep driving and going out at night. Vary the routes that you use to go to familiar places.

d. ***Care for something living.*** Have a garden or a pet. Become a foster parent, grandparent, or big sister. Volunteer at your local animal shelter.

Stop Reliving Old Trauma: Listen to Your Intuition

If you keep talking over and over again (over the course of months or years) about an old abusive job, relationship, or family member, you need to see a therapist who does cognitive behavioral therapy (Chapter 8). By constantly talking about an experience, you relive it in your brain. Your body releases stress chemicals that poison your hippocampus over time, ultimately damaging your brain's memory networks. Learn to tune in to your intuition to see if you are repeating an outmoded and unhealthy pattern of behavior in your life (see Chapter 10).

Find a Life Purpose

Don't ever really "retire." If you don't want to become "reemployed," find a calling or avocation instead. Occasionally volunteering or being a professional "dabbler" won't do; you need a life purpose that makes a valuable contribution to society, permeates your thoughts upon awakening in the morning, and is still on your mind before you go to sleep. Use your unique skill and talent to make a difference in the world. The intense reward of having a life's purpose increases opiate levels in the body and helps support the key immunological elements that maintain a healthy brain.

Even though the seventy- to ninety-year-old members of the Buena Vista Social Club had all the risk factors for Alzheimer's disease and other forms of dementia, they not only survived aging, they flourished. I doubt they took gingko biloba, ginseng, selenium, DHA, or estrogen replacement to preserve their memory and brain function. Staying in touch with a passion immunized them to the societally programmed disease of aging. Remaining immersed in this lifelong love of their muse kept them moving physically, involved with people from many generations and socioeconomic backgrounds, and using a wide repertoire of social skills, and a good sense of humor. What made the members of the Buena Vista Social Club escape the ravages of aging and beat the odds of getting dementia? I don't think it was the cigars.

ELEVEN

Getting in Touch with Your Intuition: A Ten-Step Program

When I was a resident, I had a supervisor who went over my patients' cases with me in a weekly meeting. These meetings always made me nervous. Even though I was learning to become a psychiatrist, it always felt uncomfortable to sit in the room with one. One day, all of my preconceived notions about psychiatry were blown away. I was going over the issues of a particularly difficult patient, wading through the complexity of her medical problems when Dr. Brown looked over to the side and blurted out, "You know . . . do you think I should get rid of this cactus? It's all dried and spiky and lifeless-looking. When people come into the room, I think it communicates, 'You're not going to get a whole lot of nurturance here.'" I laughed. Years later, I was in London with a friend and decided to visit the Freud Museum, located in one of his former homes. We walked through the typical English fog and drizzle for hours until we finally got to the end of Freud's tree-lined street. In front of every house, except for Freud's, was a huge, leafy tree. His tree was dead and the house was empty. Obviously, we weren't going to get much out of that visit.

Intuition comes to each of us through signals in our outer and inner environment, whether it's from a cactus or a peculiar tree. It could be an inner feeling of sadness or panic, a sick feeling in our stomach, or a specific image or symbol in a dream. We get this intuitive information whether or not we are aware of it. The challenge, of course, is to become aware of it and use it. For instance, my right brain is bigger than my left brain, so my intelligence and intuition come to me primarily through visual and body senses, through clairvoyance and clairsentience. When I look at someone or hear his name, I get a visual image and a physical sense of what's going on with his emotional life and physical health. Yet hunches or flashes can also come from the body's and brain's *memories*. One you've gotten the "raw" intuitive data, it's up to you to weave the information together into a coherent message, edit out distortion, and translate elements that are encoded in symbolism.

Intuition from Left-Brain Memories

We women use both sides of our brain to speak and understand language, and so we need to use both hemispheres to be intuitive as well. Most people think you have to be a "right-brain" spacey, artsy person to be intuitive, but this is simply not true. Quite a bit of intuition comes from our left brain, but unfortunately, much of this information is lost because we don't translate it from its symbolic form and make it conscious. Here's how one woman was able to work with her intuitive symbols and interpret their meaning.

Mary-Alice, age fifty-six, was a student in an intuition class that I taught. She had been your "typical" left-brained English major in college. Always optimistic about even the most desperate situation, Mary-Alice hid her emotions behind a pleasant, brave face even when things weren't going well. It took an awful lot to upset Mary-Alice. She was strongly right-handed, couldn't read a map, and had been terrible in geometry and other visuospatial abilities. An administrative assistant to the CEO of a Fortune 500 company, she excelled at her job because she was very organized and attentive to detail. There wasn't a problem Mary-Alice couldn't solve . . . at work, that is.

But Mary-Alice had a hard time getting in touch with her intuition and said that she never got any intuitive information. She also had insomnia, and when she did get to sleep, she had terrible nightmares. In one series of dreams, Mary-Alice was trying to steer a ship that repeatedly ran aground. When she woke up, she would have a version of the Simon and Garfunkel lyric going around and around in her head, "A rock can feel no pain." Although Mary-Alice and her ex-husband had owned a sailboat that frequently went aground years ago, she hadn't been sailing in years, so she assumed the nightmares, the insomnia, and the weight she had begun to gain were due to menopause.

Mary-Alice had a twenty-four-year-old son, Sam, whom she absolutely loved. Her ex-husband, Sam's father, was an alcoholic, and had abandoned them both, so Mary-Alice had devoted herself to getting her son launched in life. More than anything Mary-Alice loved to spend time with Sam, cook his meals, and have long conversations. She thought Sam was her life's one true success story: He was charming, creative, talented, and intelligent—everything a woman could ever want. Unfortunately, Sam had not had much success himself so far. His grades had been marginal, he'd dropped out of college after two semesters, he couldn't keep a job, and he had moved back home to live with his mother. For about the same time that Sam was struggling, Mary-Alice had been having nightmares and gaining weight, yet she told me that her life would be perfect if it weren't for her sleep problems and ever-increasing waistline.

I asked Mary-Alice what her intuition was telling her was the driving force behind her mind-body problems. She couldn't think of anything except perhaps she was "disappointed" with her ex-husband for "messing up" her son's life. If her ex had been a more responsible male role model, perhaps Sam would have better self-esteem. But Mary-Alice couldn't think ill of anyone for very long, and quickly countered her criticism by saying her ex had "a good heart" and had had a "very traumatic childhood." When I pushed Mary-Alice to explain what she thought about her repeated nightmares of a boat being stranded, she immediately bristled and asked, "You're not blaming my son for my insomnia or weight problem, are you?"

Mary-Alice lived in her left brain most of the time. She rarely allowed herself to consciously feel right-brain negative emotions like sadness, anger, and fear. Any intuition that came to her through her moods and anxiety was immediately censored by her left-brain beliefs that she wouldn't be a good person, wouldn't be loved or accepted, if she got angry at someone she loved or expressed disappointment.

That old saying "Out of sight, out of mind" should really be rephrased to read, "Out of sight, out of mind, into sleep, into body." What Mary-Alice couldn't rationally see or think came out intuitively through her insomnia, her nightmares, and her weight problem. I persuaded Mary-Alice that her dreams were bringing her attention to things too uncomfortable to acknowledge when she was awake. Mary-Alice eventually realized that she was avoiding disappointment about her son's failures, because she felt she would be abandoning him like his father had. Her dreams utilized the filed-away memories of "running aground" while sailing with her ex-husband to represent symbolically her son's having run aground in his own life. The song lyrics were clearly telling her that she was stuffing her emotions so she would feel no pain. Unfortunately, once she was awake, her left brain insisted on positive emotions and censored this intuition, holding it beneath her consciousness.

Fortunately for Mary-Alice, intuition is a deeply preserved protective mechanism in our brains and bodies and will be expressed through body symptoms. Chronic insomnia and escalating weight gain were all ways that her brain and body intuitively screamed at her that something in her life was off balance. Weight gain is a health problem of the "third emotional center," indicating an issue involving responsibility and career. Mary-Alice felt overly responsible for her adult son, whose career was stalled, but learned that she could love her son but still see his faults and allow herself to feel the pain of concern about his life. She didn't have to be the "rock" in his life. After working with her dreams, getting some education on codependence, Mary-Alice worked with a counselor to create a plan to get her son out of the house. She normalized her weight and her insomnia all but vanished. A whole new world opened up for her when she also realized that her dreams were acknowledging her yearning for a new mate and adventure, which she had for so long put out of her mind.

The Left-Brain Censor: "Love Is Blind"

The rational analytical left hemisphere can frequently stand between you and your intuition, just as Mary-Alice's love for her son blinded her to his faults, and set her up to get physically sick. Nonetheless, you don't have to wait until you are asleep and dreaming to get in touch with your intuition, which can come to you through highly symbolic "flashes" of inspiration and through symptoms in your body.

A student in one of my intuition classes was quite frustrated by one of the exercises I'd given everyone. I asked them to use their intuition to figure out something about a picture of a person in a sealed envelope. I knew who it was but they didn't. Bonny couldn't get a clairvoyant picture, or a clairsentient feeling in her body for any characteristics or health problems. Everyone else in the class picked up on a physical or emotional characteristic of Mama Cass, whose picture was in the envelope, but Bonny got an image of two snakes. During the class, she wracked her brain to try to figure out the symbolic meaning of "snake," an important image in Jungian dream interpretation. Yet as Bonny was recounting to me her description of the two snakes, using her right hand to trace out their shape, she suddenly screamed, "I got it! The shape of the two snakes are the two letter S's in Mama Cass's last name! The snakes were spelling out her name for me!"

Many left-brain intuitives get partial spellings or other linguistic clues in their hunches. You may have seen some TV psychics ask questions such as, "I'm getting the name of someone, it begins with an 'S.' Is it Samuel? Stephen? Shawn? That's right, Shawn." Clearly, if you have great left-hemisphere capability for remembering names and strong linguistic skills, it makes sense that these well-developed brain pathways will be the paths that communicate to you with names or other verbal cues you can decipher. On the other hand, if you have trouble learning languages, are not good at left-brain tasks, can't remember peoples' names for the life of you, then chances are your intuition will not come to you through left-brain memories, language, and symbols, but through your other senses.

PRIMING THE INTUITIVE PUMP

An interesting feature about Bonny's story is that she realized the meaning of her intuitive image by using her right hand to trace out the pattern. To move the right hand, you must activate the left brain. This motion also stimulates the adjacent areas for language, speech, and naming. The action of tracing out the two S's with her right hand and saying them aloud primed Bonny's brain, allowing her to recognize the meaning of her hunch.

You can sometimes increase the function, or "prime" an area of the brain, by utilizing adjacent brain regions. For example, when children are practicing writing in grade school, as they carefully move their hands in their efforts to create perfect shapes, they automatically stick out their tongue. When we first learn to read, we prime our left-brain language areas by moving our lips. Once we've mastered reading and writing, we no longer need to perform these "motor overflow" movements . . . unless of course we have a unique brain organization and unusual talents and skills.

When Elton John sings and plays the piano, for instance, this modern day Mozart requires more left-hemisphere tone than his right-brained genius was probably born with. So as he sings, using his left-hemisphere language skill, and as he plays, he moves his right eyebrow upward with every two or three words. By moving the right side of his face, Elton primes his left brain, enabling him to sing and play the music simultaneously.

As we will see below, you can prompt and enhance your intuitive gifts by utilizing other functions on the same side of the brain. For example, when you write down a dream or talk about it out loud with a friend, you can find meanings that had eluded you when you simply turned it over and over in your mind. These processes help prime left-brain language areas to respond to symbolism.

Intuition from Right-Brain Memories

Everyone has had that experience of some random song playing over and over in her head for no reason whatsoever. All of a sudden, a song will pop into your head. You haven't just heard it on the radio. No one has hummed it. There may be reasons you are hearing it.

Recently, for instance, I met a friend for dinner at a local restaurant. As I approached the table, the Doors' tune for the song "Come on Baby, Light My Fire" started playing in my head. I hadn't heard the song in years, but it had been engraved in my memory after I had had to learn it as a second violin in the sixth grade in the Rhode Island All State Orchestra. I had to practice the piece several hundred times to get the notes right. Thirty years later, I was hearing the notes—though not the lyrics—in my head again, for no particular reason. It worried me.

My friend Micky looked pale. When I asked her what was wrong, Micky told me she had just gotten some terrible news: her aunt had died in an apartment fire, and the authorities suspected arson. After our lunch, I found my Doors' CD and also realized the song contained the words "funeral pyre." My right brain had signaled me about my friend's tragic loss through the song's notes, even though the full import of the left-brain lyrics didn't hit me until later.

Essentially, our brains are like intuitive jukeboxes. When we or others important to us are in danger or in distress, our minds will pull out a record of some memory to get our attention. For some of us, a musical melody will get the message across. Others, like me, won't be able to understand the full intuitive message behind the song until our left brain provides the lyrics. Right-brain intuition gives you a gestalt-like, global sense that something in your life is going poorly or well. In broad brush strokes, right-brain intuition uses past clips of something that terrified you, irritated you, or made you feel wonderful—like in the cartoons when someone gets a bright idea and a picture of a light bulb appears above the person's head or the Hallelujah Chorus plays in the background. We all have our equivalent of the Hallelujah Chorus or a light bulb when intuition gives us a spectacular idea that our intellect could not have churned up in twice the time. Intuition is speeded-up intelligence. You may get a fantastic feeling in your body as a signal that you are on the right track, or an instantaneous image in your mind, or you may hear your own special euphoric song.

I usually get intuition when I exercise. Last fall, I was thinking about what keeps us from hearing our intuition when we need it most. I put on my headphones, put disco on the CD, and started to paddle away on my elliptical trainer. About five minutes into my routine, out of the corner of my eye, through the window I saw a big white feather float down from the sky into my back yard. Seeing this feather float slowly down, side to side, evoked a memory. Somewhere I had seen that feather on the cover of a book. What was the name of that book? A mixture of excitement and curiosity washed over me. What was the name of the book? Ten minutes later, it hit me. Corny as it is, the title that came to mind was *Illusions* by Richard Bach. I got off the elliptical trainer and started to turn my house upside down to find the book and read it to see if there was something in it that could help me. I couldn't find it. Irritated, I finished my exercise routine, took a shower, and walked out the front door to see a swarm of dragonflies, flying in circles in my front yard. Actually, they appeared to be flying in figure eights. Thinking I might be hallucinating, I drove around the neighborhood to survey dragonfly behavior in other peoples' yards. I didn't see any. Feeling foolish, I asked a friend to come over to my house and tell me what she saw in my back yard. Kate drove up, and said, "Wow. Why are all those dragonflies flying in circles in your front yard?" then drove away.

Jung believes that the images in our environment, including our front yard, are frequently a symbolic communication from our unconscious. In Native American culture, too, the appearance of an animal has great value, even healing value, because it symbolizes a major characteristic or energy we need to learn to be whole. For example, the snake is a symbol of transformation; an owl, wisdom; a coyote, the trickster, the need to use your wits. So I ran downstairs to look up the meaning of dragonfly, which is to let go of old ideas: "On the psychological level, it may be time to break down the *illusions* you have held that restrict actions or ideas." When I didn't "get" the intuitive message behind the feather falling in my backyard, and the image on the cover of the book *Illusions,* I got another opportunity to hear it from the dragonflies in the front yard.

So that was the answer to the problem I had been turning over in my mind: Illusions prevent us from hearing our intuition. Illusions are thought patterns that increase our chances of having depression and anxiety as they censor our intuition. By learning what illusions we have about our life— such as "I'm not smart enough to get a better job;" "I'm not lovable enough to be in a better relationship"—we can cut through them or let go of them so we can begin to hear our intuition telling us the truth.

If an animal keeps popping up in your dreams or psyche, or keeps crossing your path in your waking life, get one of the many books or look below to examine the dream and animal symbolism so you can find what your intuition is trying to tell you.

THE SPEECHLESS RIGHT BRAIN: I'M STUCK ON A FEELING

If you're not able to translate right-brain feelings into words, you'll have a harder time comprehending your intuition's messages. When I saw the feather and the dragonflies, I got a funny feeling that they provided clues to the problem I was turning around and around in my mind, but until I was able to engage my left brain to get rational confirmation that what I was seeing was really present, and then did some reading to decipher their symbolism, my hunches were stuck at the "feeling" stage. You need both sides of your brain to gather and interpret all the information your intuition is sending you.

Attention: Roaming Intuitive Intelligence

Becoming distracted can actually be a "silent" sign from your intuition that you need to pay attention to something in your life that may not be right in front of you. Inattentiveness can signal that you're on the wrong track, that something else is more important for you to attend to, as can hyperactivity and distractibility.

HUNTING FOR CARTOONS

About two years ago, I became fixated on cartoon characters. Around the time that Charles M. Schulz died, I decided I needed to buy a print of his work, so I got on eBay and began to bid on several items, including a framed original animation illustration from *A Charlie Brown Christmas*. As I went through the hundreds of eBay listings, however, my attention kept getting distracted from Peanuts animation art and toward Bullwinkle and Tennessee Tuxedo. I had no idea why, but I was seriously distracted and I was neglecting my usual work. I found hunting for Bullwinkle and Tennessee Tuxedo so stimulating that almost everything else paled by comparison. At the same time, some friends of mine were getting involved in studying investment opportunities, but every time they tried to get me to learn about stocks and bonds to improve my financial situation, my mind would drift to an auction on eBay that would be closing in a few minutes . . . would I win the animation print of Bullwinkle flying off the high dive at 11:52 p.m. EST? I chalked up my distractibility to ADHD and possibly a form of Web addiction specific to eBay. As my friends were reading books and acquiring blue chip stocks and government bonds, I was covering my walls with framed animation art. Then one day, I flipped on the news and heard that the artist who drew Bullwinkle and Tennessee Tuxedo had died in a car accident. There was a mad dash by fans to invest in his art work, the value of which shot up in price. I realized then that my months of distractibility had been driven by my intuition.

Your attention is part of your intuitive guidance system. If you are a little spacey with ADD, or are hyperactive and motor-driven with ADHD, attention is key to your intuition. On the other hand, if you are usually able to focus when you need to but find yourself distracted and neglectful at crossroads in your life, this inattention itself may be a signal. For instance, psychotherapists are taught that if they start to get bored and distracted when a patient is talking, they need to ask if that patient is going off on a tangent and not focusing on the real crisis. You may find yourself obsessed by a "crush" at work, a sign there's a problem in your principal relationship or marriage. Or you may suddenly not be able to get your daughter out of your mind, whether you're at work, or in the supermarket, at the movies, or exercising, and get home to find a message from your daughter that she's had a car accident. A woman's right-brain emotions, attention, and intuition are so intertwined that becoming distracted is frequently a sign that something needs her attention.

Getting in Touch with Your Bodily Intuition When Your Mind Goes Blank

What do you do when you have a problem, and no matter how hard you wrack your brain, you can't see your way to the solution? You check out what's going on in your body, because, when you can't decipher your left-brain or right-brain intuition, the information gets transferred into physical symptoms.

WHEN YOUR FINGERS DO THE WALKING

Between the ages of fourteen and nineteen, I participated in yearly piano recitals. Each year, I would learn and memorize ten pieces of classical music from Mozart to Debussy. The process of learning the music was difficult enough, but the most painful aspect of auditioning was performing all of the ten pieces from memory in front of a judge. As I write this, my stomach still remembers this difficult ordeal.

Every year, the same thing would happen to me: I would start the piece, get to the third bar, and my mind would go blank. My fingers came to a screeching halt. I would look down at my hands, and tears would fall from my eyes onto the keyboard, making a "plink, plink, plink" sound. The judge would say something like, "Oh, my," come over with the music, and tell me to start again. I'd start playing with the music in front of me, but invariably after the first few bars I wouldn't need the music and would slip back into my memory, playing by heart as my fingers effortlessly flew over the keys. When I got beyond my blinding right-brain anxiety and left-brain beliefs that I was destined to screw up, I could just play the music that I memorized.

I had *brain memory* and *body memory* of all the pieces, but my brain blocked the body memory at first. Usually when your mind goes blank, body intuition will tell you what your next move is. If you stay sad, angry, or anxious and can't respond effectively, the emotions transfer from brain to body through the two-way depression-disease domino effect or anxiety-disease domino effect. If you don't pay attention to what you need to in your life, your body will speak to you in its own language, and use depression, nervousness, confusion, and memory loss to wake you up.

Ten Steps for Getting in Touch with Your Intuition

Answering the following questions will help you pinpoint how your intuition works and when it's speaking to you.

STEP 1: WHAT MAKES YOU STAND OUT FROM THE CROWD? WHAT MAKES YOU A BLACK SHEEP?

- *Do you easily get blue?* Do you tend to be moody, depressed, have PMS or perimenopausal irritability? Do you tend to be stoic? When you are around people you love, is it hard for you to know what you want and need? If so, your intuition may talk to you through your moods.
- *Are you easily shaken up?* Do you easily get nervous, anxious, and worried? Have you ever had a panic attack? Do you have to have things in your life categorized, neatly arranged, lined up, and organized? Your intuition may talk to you through anxiety.
- *Is your mind miles and miles away when you should be paying attention?* Do you have problems staying focused? Do you get stuck in a dream world? Is it hard for you not to get drawn into your loved ones' pain and suffering? Is it hard for you not to act, drive, or shop impulsively? Believe it or not, your impulsivity and distractibility may actually be the way to find and respond to your intuition.

• *Have you begun to have trouble remembering names? Addresses?* Does your mind go blank? Do you walk around like you are in a fog? You may need to give your rational mind a rest and allow intuitive wisdom to come through your right brain's daydreams or night dreams.

STEP 2: DO YOU HAVE RIGHT-BRAIN OR LEFT-BRAIN INTUITION: HOW DO YOU USE THE TWO SIDES OF YOUR BRAIN?

The Declaration of Independence says that all men are created equal, but it wasn't talking about brain organization. As you've seen, the traditional feminine brain has more connectivity between the right and left hemispheres than a man's. Genes, hormonal events in utero, and a variety of later social and environmental influences all shape a woman's brain into a traditional or not-so-traditional format. As your hormones change, the ways you use your right brain and left brain may change from puberty, to postpartum, to menopause.

Some key questions to ask:

Handedness: Are you left-handed, right-handed, or ambidextrous? Being ambidextrous or left-handed is associated with a nontraditional brain, which may increase your chances for attention deficit disorder, learning disorders, and autoimmune diseases. However, it may also increase your ability use your right-brain intuition to learn and solve problems.

Language: Do you have an easy time learning a language? Is your idea of a good time sitting down with a good, thick book? Is your speech blunt or filled with complex grammatical phrases?

If you use a varied vocabulary, complex grammatical construction, love to write in a journal, and read long books with small print, chances are you have a more compartmentalized brain. You are more likely to gain access to your intuition through symbols embedded in your day-to-day life or in dreaming. Studying the work of Jung or Native American animal totems may help you interpret the intuitions you get.

If you speak in short, simple phrases, have a difficult time learning vocabulary, and find reading a chore, you have less access to left-brain language, so you're less likely to get intuition via symbolism. When you dream of water, you'll take its message concretely. Instead of thinking that the water symbolizes emotion, you may think it's about to rain, or that you'll take a trip by boat. A more compartmentalized brain would try to examine the symbolism of the water.

Emotion: If you can hide your emotions and rarely cry in public, chances are you have a more compartmentalized brain. Your intuition is more likely to be accessible during the hormonally changeable times of PMS, pregnancy, postpartum, fertility treatments, and menopause. However, if you have always had trouble with moodiness, irritability, worry, anxiety, and panic, during these hormonal events your emotional circuits may become so loud, noisy, and active that you can't decipher the message behind the mood. If you are hyperconnected and emotionally porous, your empathy can lead to lifelong health problems. You need to keep yourself grounded more than you need to get in touch with your intuition.

Are You a Prisoner of Your Left Brain?

Do you tend to:

- Focus overly on details; talk in overly detailed, overly inclusive language
- Have difficulty saying *just* yes or no
- Have difficulty seeing the gestalt, the overarching theme, and focusing on individual "trees" and not being able to see the "forest"
- Negate or minimize painful or difficult emotions
- Censor feelings and behavior that society would condemn: "I should believe_____," or "You should feel_____"
- Focus exclusively on a personal goal and disconnect from others' feelings and thoughts

---

Are You a Prisoner of Your Right Brain?

Do you tend to:

- Talk in vague, broad terms without lots of detail
- Think in black or white, all or nothing
- Feel excessive negative emotions
- Get easily overwhelmed; unable to break down goals or problems into smaller steps
- React too much to others' feelings and thoughts
- Act immediately on a hunch without looking for supportive data or proof that it's accurate

---

Step 3: Translate the Symbols of Your Left-Brain Intuition

When you dream, your brain fires in the same electrical pattern as when you're awake. In fact, many native peoples have believed that we are more conscious when dreaming than when we are awake. Even though these ancient people didn't have electrical medical technology, their observations match what we see during an electroencephalogram (EEG) test.

This indicates to me that dream symbols are no different from those that appear when we are awake. If most of your intuition comes from left-brain symbolism, then you don't have to wait until you are asleep to get in touch with it. If you look around you during the day, you will see that the imagery and symbols that occur in your dreams appear repeatedly. The symbols that occur while you're dreaming will also pop into your mind when you are "daydreaming" or they'll materialize near you in your environment (like my feather and dragonflies). They catch our attention and communicate information, like a compass, helping us decide where to go next or what to do in our lives. The left brain can bring life and beneficial meanings to these symbols. These waking and dreaming images are part of our intuitive guidance system.

Below are some symbols that may appear in your dreams, thoughts, and environment. Your consciousness extends beyond your anatomic borders and, Jung believed, into a "universal consciousness," which contains all the spiritual and psychological information we need. But the information is in a symbolic language. When you need to learn the significance of an image or sign, look for it in the tables below or in another book, or do a Web search on your computer, but also pay attention to your dreams. The universal consciousness will insinuate the information you need in a dream or daydream, in nature, or in some aspect of your waking experience. The more desperate you are for information, the more obvious, and sometimes dramatic, the sign.

For instance, one evening last spring, I had worked all day but had not accomplished very much, and I was feeling pretty upset, because I kept falling asleep. As a result, I felt sad and depressed, as if I didn't have much to offer. So I left my office for home late at night, feeling pretty hopeless. When I turned the corner of the road, two things happened simultaneously. On my car radio, Carly Simon and James Taylor were singing "Night Owl," which mirrored what I had in fact been struggling with. And I saw by the side of the road a baby white owl standing, looking like he was waiting for a bus. I stopped for a closer look, because I thought I was hallucinating. Yes, it was indeed a baby snowy white owl standing on the edge of the road, looking like he was waiting for a bus. I'd never seen a white owl before and I haven't seen one since. I drove home and looked up the Native American meaning for white owl: It is a symbol of clairvoyance. Seeing the owl made me feel that I wasn't useless, that in fact I shouldn't focus only on my narcolepsy and what I couldn't do, but instead on what I could do with my gift of intuition.

Learning your own intuitive vocabulary can, like a street sign, steer you in the right direction when you don't know where to go next. It can help you see your way out of a blue mood or an anxious time, pull you above your individual perspective, and give you a broader view.

Intuitive Vocabulary List: Human Characters

The significance of the people who appear in our dreams may vary in meaning. The husband in your dream may actually represent your husband in your waking life or he can represent a characteristic that you're meant to use, develop, or admit to having. A dentist drilling your teeth in a nightmare may represent the professional who will be doing a root canal on you later in the week, or it may represent someone who's causing you a problem you need to get to the root of. The pregnant woman in your dream may be your sister or girlfriend or daughter who wants to have a baby, or it may be you, pregnant with an idea to which you need to give birth.

If you dream of a baby, you may be trying to figure out how to handle your naïveté and innocence in new situations—or you might really want a child. A dream about a fire may indicate that you need to examine how you control your own volatility, your potentially destructive anger, since fire symbolizes passion, love, or anger, or it could mean you should get that home fire extinguisher you keep forgetting to pick up. A nightmare in which a plumber can't seem to fix the numerous dripping faucets in your home may mean that you need help managing sadness and depression, since water can symbolize deep sadness, love, and longing, or you may have a real, physical leak in your house that needs attention. All of these symbols can have multiple meanings.

Person	Meaning
Actor	Desire for recognition
Angels	Protection
Architect	Designing a new identity
Attorney	End of a conflict
Baby	Hope, innocence, new opportunity
Bag lady, homeless person	Failure, loss of occupation or personal identity
Child	Immaturity, innocence
Enemy	A rejected or denied aspect of self
Ex-husband	Rejected masculine aspect of self

Person	Meaning
Ex-wife	Rejected feminine aspect of self
Father	Authority, guidance
Female	Receptivity (aspect of self)
Fool/clown	Unlimited possibilities, without pretentiousness
Ghosts	A part of yourself that's not developed
Giants	Someone who may dominate you
Grandparent	Gentle authority
Judge	Decision
Male	Assertiveness (aspect of self)
Masked, faceless person	Past abuse
Monster	Perpetrator, abuser
Mother	Nurturance, support
Pirate	Rejection of rules, irresponsibility
Plumber	Working on emotional health
Police	Working on self-control, guilt (if you've had a past negative experience with police), needing protection (if your past experience is positive with police)
Postman	Exciting new possibilities
Pregnant woman	Giving birth to something new
Stranger	Undiscovered, unacceptable part of self
Surgeon	Someone who is helping you heal
Unattractive/ugly person	Learning to love a rejected part of yourself
Visitor	New good news

Animal Characters

Like people, animals can also signify different meanings in our dreams. Dreams help our brain's memory system make sense and file away events of the day. So a horse, for instance, is more likely to appear in the dreams of a horse trainer because this animal is part of his daily life. Animals also have a symbolic meaning and can relate to a unique emotional feature or typical behavior. For example, since female bears are known for fiercely maternal behavior, having a bear pop up during your hike in the woods or during a dream may signify a need to get in touch with your feelings about your own mother or being a mother. Similarly, as in my story above, having an owl appear out of the blue in your life may signify an intuitive message or a need to look into areas of darkness in your life.

Animal	Meaning/Potential Ability
Bear	Maternal
Birds	Higher self, freedom
Bug, small insect	Minor problem
Butterfly	Transformation
Camel	Endurance
Chicken	Disorganization
Cow	Productive
Coyote	Trickster
Dog	Loyalty, protectiveness
Dragonfly	Illusion
Elephant	Wisdom
Fierce animals (lions, tigers)	Trying to be civilized at the expense of dignity/power
Fly	Nuisance
Frog	Transformation
Giraffe	Overview, perspective
Horse	Power, vitality, wild force of nature
Lamb	Innocence
Lion	Power, pride
Monkey/ape	Mischievous, active
Owl	Clairvoyance, seeing the mysteries of life, seeing in the dark
Ox	Burden, strength
Pets	Working on loving self
Rabbit	Fertility
Rat	Street smarts
Sheep	Conformity
Snake	Sexuality, fear about unknown power
Squirrel	Hoarding

Animal	Meaning/Potential Ability
Turtle	Protection
Whale	Deep unconscious

Inanimate Objects

Frequently, inanimate objects become "animated" in a dream, that is, they take on a quality of someone who is alive. For example, if you use a box to store or protect valuables, a box may appear in a dream signifying your need to pay attention to an area of vulnerability in your life. In many instances, objects combine with the five natural elements to convey an emotion that helps us gain insight into what we are feeling and thinking.

Over the last three years, I have been in the hormonal instability of perimenopause, with periods every eight days (yes, every eight days). I've done a lot of work to stabilize my moods, but Jung says that our external environment is a reflection of our internal emotions and never in my life have I had so many problems with the plumbing in my home. Both my downstairs and upstairs toilets constantly are running and the faucet in the downstairs shower leaks. As soon as a plumber comes and fixes one thing, something else snaps and leaks. I'm also having constant electrical malfunctions in my home, in particular with the phone lines, which seem to confound even the most seasoned electricians. Electricity and fire represent strong passion, love, and irritability, and water symbolizes moods and deep emotions, all of which tend to be volatile during the perimenopausal period. I have concluded that I won't have perfect plumbing and electrical health until I get through "the change."

Thing	Meaning
Ambulance	Rescue
Anchor	Security, stability, being tied down
Balloons	Fantasy, dreams
Blanket	Security
Book	Intellect, information
Box	Protect, store
Brakes	Proceed with caution
Bus	A shared enterprise
Candle	Looking for insight
Catalogues	Looking for options
Chair	Position

Circle	Whole
Cloak	Secrecy
Coat	Protection
Cross	Sacrifice
Crystal vase, cup, urn	Flawed or lost love
Elevator	Success with someone's help
Feathers	A lift
Garbage can	Aspect of yourself you want to transfer
Gifts that look better on the outside than the inside	A relationship that looks good superficially but has deeper problems
Gun	Violence, aggression
Hat	Options
Ladder	Climbing a ladder suggests progress toward fulfilling an ambition
Laundry	Putting in order, purification
Letter, mail	A communication between two people, expect news from someone
Lock	Negotiation in a conflict
Lost purse/empty pocket	Loss of loved one
Luggage	Plan now for a major change in the path of your life
Map	Guidance, direction
Mask	Facade, how you present yourself to the world
Mirror	Self-image
Mirror, broken	Impending potential poor health
Moon	The feminine
Mud/dirt	Messy emotions
Passport	Identity, ease of movement
Planes	Rapid progress, travel, liberation
Puppets	Lack of free choice
Ring	Promise
Skirt, trousers	Sexuality, passion
Storefront window	Unattainable things in life
Sunglasses	Mask, disguise

Thing	Meaning
Table	New relationship
Umbrella	Protecting self from emotional outburst
Underwear	Private self
Whips	Power, domination, obedience

Bodies and Buildings

Houses and your health seem to be inextricably related. How a person cares for her apartment or home is very much a reflection of how she attends to her health. Are you attentive and nurturing with your body? Do you take nutritional supplements, exercise regularly, get massages or acupuncture? If so, you're more likely to attend regularly to the upkeep and maintenance of your house and home. On the other hand, if you are more likely to ignore that broken board on the porch, turn a deaf ear to that dripping faucet, and work your way around the broken garbage disposal, then you're more likely to ignore the subtlest signs, the earliest symptoms that something is going on in your physical and emotional health.

The symbolic connection between health, houses, and emotions has long been known. One of the basic diagnostic tests in pediatric psychiatry is to have the child draw his house. The relative size, shape, texture, color, and integrity of the roof, walls, rooms, windows, and other parts of the house indicate the level of mental and emotional health of the child and his family. The "House Test" is also used to comprehend a patient's unconscious feelings about her body in many hospital center cancer treatment programs. Some individuals will dream about a house, a building, or a significant location that represents the state of their health. Buildings or places in a dream may also symbolize an event that dominates your waking life, a feeling with which you're trying to come to peace.

When a specific area in your life is out of balance, specific organs in your body may develop symptoms of illness (see Step 7, below). For example, pelvic and lower abdominal pain may be more likely to occur in a woman who is struggling with boundary and power issues in intimate relationships, or has had a past history of rape or incest. Women and men who are struggling with relationship, financial, and job-related conflicts are more likely to develop lower back pain.

Your dreams may signal a change in your physical and emotional health when body areas appear altered, animated, or with exaggerated features that further communicate a message. Losing teeth in a dream may, of course, be an intuitive warning to go to the dentist, but it may also signal a concern that your public image is distorted or spoiled somehow. Appearing naked may signal anxiety about feeling emotionally exposed. Tight clothes in a dream may signal that you feel bored or restricted in a relationship or job. Underwear in a dream may symbolize hidden feelings, and having a scarred, mutilated, slashed body may signal the presence of past trauma and abuse.

House	Meaning
House	Self
Closet	Hidden aspect of self
Room	Aspect of self
Cellar	Unconscious
Attic/roof	Spirituality
Ruins	Need to take definite action
Basement	Unconscious
Corner	No escape
Bathroom faucets	Controlling or containing emotion
Fireplace	The heart, the center
Bathroom	Areas of purification, of cleaning impurities out of self
Bedroom	Private aspect of self
Ceiling	Highest potential
Dining room	Formality
Kitchen	Nurturance
Porch	Contact with the outer world
Stairs	Goals, aspirations
Windows	Others' view of you
House without lights	Loss, especially of a loved one
Unfinished house	Work needs to be done on psyche or body
Haunted house	Fears from childhood
House on a hill	Ambition that you want to achieve
House on the water	Desire to transform life, and move forward
Locked room/dark, evil place	Fear of public exposure Public anxiety or shame

House	Meaning
Castle with a moat around it	Security Keeping others out

Building or Location	Meaning
Airport	Rapid change
Arctic	Frozen feelings
Bank	Need of preservation of resources
Boat in "huge" waves	Stormy emotional period lies ahead
Boat in dry dock	Getting stuck, not being able to move forward in life
Bridge	Overcoming problems
Buffet/banquet	Abundance in your life
Bus	Shared journey
Cliff	Challenge
Court	Place where problems are resolved
Crossroads/intersections	Making a decision
Dead end	You're on the wrong track
Desert	Isolation Determination
Fence	Boundary, separation
Fork in the road	Need to make a decision
Heaven	Spirituality, transcendence from usual reality
Hell	Spiritual suffering
Hill	Easily achieved goal
Mountain	Giant goal
On stage	Performance
Other countries	Other perspective and realities
Prison	Confinement
Road	Possible path to take in life
Road	Journey
School	Acquiring knowledge, training, discipline
Sea travel/boat	Journey into deep emotions
Shadow	Unknown, unaccepted part of self
Sky	Infinite freedom

Subway	Moving into your unconscious
Traffic	Obstacles in the path to success
Train station	Going somewhere with someone's help
Traveling in boat with others	Calm period in personal life
Zoo	Wilderness under control

Cecile, aged fifty-four, called me because she began to have some very disturbing dreams and health problems. Cecile had been the one "solid" stable person in her family to whom everyone turned to when they had a problem. Much of her self-esteem was based on being able to handle almost any problem someone handed her. However, at midlife, Cecile was feeling old, tired, and alone. Her husband had died after a long illness and she was getting tired of all the family dramas. Cecile's sister, Dora, had bipolar II and alcoholism but had been stable for about nine months. A brother had finally gotten married and was doing well in a new job.

In Cecile's dreams, her pancreas was "rotting." Moderately obese, she had struggled to lose thirty pounds but couldn't seem to do it no matter what diet plan she used. Cecile was concerned that her dream was signaling that she was developing diabetes, but doctors' tests yielded normal blood sugar levels and pancreas enzyme levels. Yet Cecile's dream symbolizes that she is having active issues in the third emotional center, since the pancreas is in the digestive tract. Cecile could always feel in her gut when her sister was beginning to drink. When she felt the first "twinges," she would call her sister and try to get her back into more regular psychotherapy sessions. Her sister had also suffered multiple episodes of pancreatitis from her alcoholism.

From her dream, Cecile realized she was beginning to carry her sister's suffering in her own body. She had long realized that her weight problem was connected to codependently carrying emotional burdens for her family. Cecile took the intuitive information from her dream and made some dramatic changes in her life. She gave up playing the martyr, and called the nearest mental health center for herself, where she signed up for her own addiction treatment for overeaters anonymous and codependency treatment.

Symbolic Actions

Everything you do in your dreams and while awake has two meanings: one symbolic and one concrete. For example, people who love flying usually take a plane ride (1) to travel to a distant location, and (2) to achieve the emotional feeling of escaping or rising above it all. If they are honest, runners will tell you that they run for two different reasons: health and a sense of escape. Actions and events also have dual meanings. Many people who've had a car accident will tell you that trauma was the catalyst they needed to reevaluate their life. Patients have frequently told me that illness and surgery helped them heal emotionally as well as physically.

In movies, directors usually incorporate a lot of symbolic events to clue in the viewer to what's going to happen next. The first time I see a movie, I am usually too dim to catch this "environmental symbolism," but by the eighth or ninth time I see it, I'll catch it. For example, it took me a long time to figure out why Cher's romantic comedy, *Moonstruck,* had that title. About the sixth time I saw the movie, I realized the importance of the cemetery scene. The old grandfather says, "Bella luna! The moon, she brings the man to the woman!"

Our feminine brain will use similar cinematography in our dreams and in real life to communicate emotions, thoughts, and intuitive advice. It is the action in scenes listed below that calls attention to what we need to think about and helps direct us to where we need to go next.

Action	Meaning
Accident	Unexpected change
Affair	Hidden, unlawful partnership
Being chased	Running away from something you fear
Being on vacation with too many things going wrong	Excess, inescapable responsibility
Being punished	You need to confront some guilt
Being rescued	Consider how you've been abandoned in your life
Cleaning	Purifying, restoring a sense of order
Climbing	Success
Climbing/hiking	Ambitions, advancement
Crash/collision	Warning to take steps to reconsider your current path in life
Dam bursting	Fury, uncontrollable anger
Death/dying	Soon being forced to end a conflict or problem

Decorating/painting	Transforming an aspect of your life
Drowning, struggling in water, flood	Being overwhelmed emotionally
Eating	Satisfaction, pleasure
Eating dessert	Indulgence
Escaping	Avoiding
Falling	Feeling out of control, out of one's league, failure
Falling but hitting something soft	Failure without long-term ill effects
Fast	Impatience, efficiency
Finding money or valuables	Hint of financial gain
Flying	Rising above circumstances Avoiding restriction Elation
Forced sex/rape	Forced intrusions in one's life
Graduation	Completion
Healing meal with someone	Shared intimacy, sexuality
Kissing	Affection, intimacy
Looking for luggage and not being able to find it	Frustration, anger
Looking in mirror	Depending on who is in reflection. Who you see is whose identity you're assuming
Losing money or valuables	Warning of future loss or theft
Missing a train, and appointment	Frustration/anger
Not being able to get a hold of someone on the phone	Assertiveness issues, not being heard, loss of intimacy
Paralysis, inability to move	Being at an impasse, not able to actively make a change
Playing	Careless, carefree activity
Pruning	Removing useless parts of life
Punishing someone	You need to learn to be more compassionate
Racing	Consider your level of competitiveness
Rape	Force in a relationship
Season change	Inner emotional transformation
Sex dreams	Attraction, love, intimacy, union

Action	Meaning
Shopping	Looking for what you want
Shrinking	Inadequacy
Stabbing	Betrayal
Storm	Forces you cannot control
Surgery	Undergoing a healing process
Taking a test or exam and not being prepared	Anticipating failure in your professional life
Trapped, struggling to find a way; lost while traveling	Trying to find direction and purpose in one's life
Vomiting	Getting rid of unacceptable thoughts or emotions
Wars, battles	Unresolved conflicts

Paint by Number

Symbols with messages can also include *colors, numbers,* and *the natural elements.* In every philosophy and theology, the basic natural elements communicate emotion. Happiness in movies is usually symbolized by sunny weather (fire), sorrow by pouring rain (water). We expect doctors, nurses, and other healing personnel to be grounded (earth), and soldiers, pilots, and other courageous individuals to have minds of "steel" (metal). These elements and the colors found in nature all appear in our dreams and communicate the same emotional tone and imagery.

Theories about the meanings of numbers are also found in most world traditions. Three—a love triangle—causes emotional conflict. There are seven virtues and seven deadly sins. Thirteen is unlucky for some, lucky for others. Numbers are imbedded in our outer and inner environment and can communicate a stage in our life's development, among other things.

Five Elements	Meaning
Fire	Strong passion
	Destruction with cleansing purification
	Strong emotion
	Spirit
Water	Love/emotion
Sea	Unconscious
Snow/ice	Obstacles in your path
Melting snow	Dissolving obstacles

Iceberg	Lack of emotional warmth
Tidal wave, drowning	Overabundance of emotions, thoughts
Avalanche	Dangerous release of emotion
Puddle	Small inconvenient emotion
Rain	Release of emotion
River	Flux, change in your life, loss of something, gain of another
Shallow water	Snap decisions
Air	Intelligence, intellect
Earth	Groundedness, nurturance
Metal	Strength, endurance

Colors	Meaning
Light illumination	Revelation, the divine
Rainbow	Reconciliation, hope
Blue	Melancholia Emotions Unconscious dreams
White	Purity
Red	Anger Passion Drive
Gray	Dull
Brown	Earth, groundedness
Orange	Fertility
Pink	Love
Yellow	Mind, intellect, wisdom
Purple	Spirituality
Green	Growth, healing, nature
Drab, colorless dreams	Depression, misery
Bright, colorful dreams	Optimism
Beige	Neutrality, absence of communication
Black	Isolation, introspection

Number	Meaning
1	New beginning, unity
2	Partnership, opposites

Number	Meaning
3	Flow; triangulation in a relationship
4	Protection, balance
5	Conflict, change
6	Peak experience
7	Karmic readjustment
8	Evolution, infinite
9	End of road
10	Major life development step
0	Unlimited potential

You don't want to interpret these symbols so strictly that you become a "Numbers Nazi" or colorphobe. Let intuition balanced with intellect guide you to make the best decision. However, to be honest, I once returned a license plate to the Registry of Motor Vehicles because I didn't like the number.

STEP 4: CHECK THE ACCURACY OF YOUR INTUITIVE VISIONS

It's almost always easier to be more intuitive about others' lives at a distance than to have insight about your own life; in other words, we tend to be intuitively "far-sighted." Changes in the vision in your eyes tend to your shifting intuitive abilities as you age. Before the age of forty, people are far more likely to develop a problem with nearsightedness than farsightedness. However, once they hit midlife, the incidence of farsightedness begins to climb. Before and during puberty, we tend to act impulsively and blurt out our intuition—since brain circuits for inhibiting impulses aren't fully wired and up and running. Once you're about age ten, these frontal lobes start to come on board. You're less likely to say automatically what's on your mind and more likely to think before you voice an opinion. At puberty, you also become more able to think in metaphors and use symbolic thought to communicate to others. Brain pathways develop that help you contain your emotions and mold your thoughts and behavior at a more mature level. Developing self-control is a necessary part of socialization, but frontal lobe censorings make it harder to hear our intuition as it comes through our emotions or thoughts. Learning and practicing Step 5 in Chapter 8 may help you to identify the thought patterns that mute your intuition. These patterns are usually based on past failures or painful experiences.

"I can't change a relationship."

"I can't change my job."

"God has it in for me."

We are likely to develop a warped perception of our own lives as we accumulate a lifetime of emotional bruises, disappointments, and mental scars. However, when it comes to someone else's life, we are less likely to be so pessimistic. Unless we're true narcissists, it's almost always easier to say to someone else, "I have a hunch you should quit that job. You have so much to offer, but you just don't see it."

What You See Is What You Get: Concrete Intuition

What does the following phrase mean to you: "People who live in glass houses shouldn't throw stones."

1. Don't break the glass
2. If something is fragile, you shouldn't throw stones at it
3. If you're vulnerable, you shouldn't attack or criticize others

If you picked (1) or (2), then your thinking and possibly your intuition are concrete. If you picked (3), your brain is capable of more symbolism. For example, in a symbolic dream, a glass house might communicate your hidden feelings of vulnerability. However, if your mind is more concrete, a dream about glass may mean that you need to wash your windows.

Since I easily get bored at cocktail parties because I don't drink, I ask people how they brush their teeth. Usually they will accurately pantomime their usual routine of holding a toothbrush, applying toothpaste, and vigorously cleaning their teeth. The capacity to pantomime, to use space symbolically, creating the illusion of a toothbrush and toothpaste, for example, demonstrates more advanced frontal lobe brain development. On one hand, this means you can see the world in a more abstract way, but unfortunately it also means that you are more likely to censor your intuition.

However, if the person uses his finger (body part as object) instead of pantomiming a toothbrush in space, he has just demonstrated that his thoughts and intuition are more concrete, less likely to be censored, and his actions more impulsive. The constant stream of intuitive information would make it harder for him to be "socially appropriate."

If You Have Intuitive Farsightedness

If you keep your intuition at arm's length from your consciousness, this blocking of perception may help you fit into a high-powered job and be diplomatic during a complicated social situation, but it may lead to problems in your personal life. This sort of "psychic blindness" can make your relationships stagnate, give you difficulty with your children, and make it hard for you to see the subtle first signs of problems in your closest relationships. What's the solution? Get a friend or counselor with good common sense who's going to be honest with you and deliver his perspective gently but directly. When you begin to get dreams or symptoms in your body that something is "off," schedule an appointment with a friend who can give you her intuitive perception and objective point of view. Some friends or loved ones may be too close to you to provide accurate insight, which is why people have always sought out shamans, spiritual counselors, and advisers to get untarnished, level-headed, "objective" perspectives on their lives. The best psychics can give you intuitive information at a distance knowing only your name and age. Other intuitives need more information to prime their psychic machinery; some need to see you or hold something that has a concrete connection to your life. Yet if the psychic knows anything about your life, the information can bias him or her. Anyone close to you might have intuitive farsightedness.

A modern, licensed psychotherapist can give you a neutral, unbiased opinion and teach you how to make appropriate changes in your life. (See Chapter 8.)

STEP 5: CHECK YOUR PLUMBING: KEEPING THE INTUITIVE PIPELINE OPEN AND OPERATING

Intuition comes through a combination of feelings, thoughts, and body sensations.

> *Feelings:* The five basic emotions of fear, anger, sadness, love, and joy, and their derivatives, including depression, worry, panic, irritability, euphoria, and bliss.
> *Thoughts:* The ideas that enter and exit your stream of consciousness when you are awake or dreaming, images (clairvoyance), and sounds (clairaudience).
> *Body sensations:* Symptoms of health, disease, and clairsentience.

The way to keep your intuition circuits firing to their maximum capabilities is to keep your brain and body functioning smoothly. For example, if you have severe depression, panic, or irritability, you would have trouble hearing subtler intuitive signals underlying the louder, pervasive, disordered mood. ADHD, forgetfulness, dyslexia, and other learning disorders can disrupt your life. If you are in chronic pain or suffer from a disabling, life-threatening illness, the financial frustrations, the numerous doctors' visits, and the relationship fallout all make intuition difficult to hear amid the constant health crises.

Medical and Nutritional Support for Maintaining Stable Mind-Body Pathways for Intuition

- *Treat depression, moodiness, and irritability* with appropriate nutritional or medical supplements. (See Chapter 5.)
- *Minimize anxiety and panic* with appropriate nutritional and medical supplements. (See Chapter 7.)
- *Manage attention deficit disorder* and other attention and memory disorders with appropriate nutritional and medical supplements. (See Chapters 9 and 10.)
- *Obtain treatment and appropriate medical management* for physical illnesses, especially pain disorders.
- *Take a minimal number* of medicines and nutritional supplements to treat above syndromes. Multiple medicines, herbs, and vitamins lead to side effects that can be confused with body intuition. In addition, overmedication *numbs* you so you don't experience symptoms of emotional and physical distress or intuition. Medical and nutritional treatment should not totally eradicate symptoms, but get them down to a manageable level so that you can hear the intuition signals embedded in your distress.
- *Long-term maintenance program for healthy intuition:* Nutritional supplements can help keep your mind-body path healthy. Take the supplements for your unique brain problems, whether depression and moodiness (Chapter 4), fear and anxiety (Chapter 6), or attention and memory. (Chapters 9 and 10.)

Vitamins for a Healthy Mind and Clear Intuition

Vitamin B_1 (thiamine)	27 mg
Vitamin B_2 (riboflavin)	27 mg
Vitamin B_3 (niacin)	40 mg
Vitamin B_6 (pyridoxine)	27–40 mg
Vitamin B_{12}	60 mcg
Biotin	300 mcg
Pantothenic acid	90 mg
Folic acid	1000 mcg

Found in any "megavitamin," these individual vitamins help your body and brain make more serotonin.

DHA (docosahexaenoic acid, 300–3000 mg/day), an omega-3 fatty acid, is a mood stabilizer and prevents inflammation in both brain and body.

Phosphatidylcholine, derived from lecithin (15–30 mg/day), provides appropriate insulation of nerve pathways in the brain and body.

Magnesium (citrate 900–2500 mg/day) and *calcium* (citrate or carbonate 900–4100 mg/day). Both mineral supplements help stabilize mood and are important for the electrical stability of cell membranes.

Acupuncture will balance your immune system and buffer stress levels. Acupressure or shiatsu massage are also helpful for milder physical and emotional imbalances.

Exercise. Regular exercise (at least thirty minutes a day, five or six days a week) improves mental and physical health and helps you gain access to your right brain-body network that's so important for intuition.

STEP 6: CUT BACK IF YOU ARE OVEREXTENDED INTUITIVELY

Medical people have a term for someone who comes into the hospital emergency room with a plethora of psychiatric, physical, and social problems: "train wreck."

Bettina, for instance, was one of the most intuitive women I have ever met, but her brain and body were extremely fragile. Bettina was so emotionally thin-skinned that she could almost always feel what a loved one was thinking or feeling. She was intuitively overextended. Modern psychiatry had diagnosed her as having major depression, panic disorder, attention deficit disorder, chronic fatigue/fibromyalgia, and irritable bowel syndrome, but Bettina really suffered from psychic overload. She was so keyed in to others' emotions and thoughts, she had none of her own. Other people's fear, anger, and sadness invaded her psyche and made it toxic. Utterly dependent on everyone else's happiness and approval, Bettina's health had become completely depleted.

I'll explain how you can keep your brain and body healthy while you are intuitively connected to others' distress, but first see if the following statements apply to you. If so, you may be at risk for emotional overload and having blurred personal boundaries between you and other people.

- ❏ If I lose someone, I will feel weak and vulnerable.
- ❏ I usually get rejected and abandoned by friends and family.
- ❏ People usually find me unattractive and uninteresting.
- ❏ I don't have the ability to support myself in the world.
- ❏ I am uncomfortable accepting help . . . it's easier to give than to take.
- ❏ I easily get scapegoated in my family and other organizations.
- ❏ People try to control me and make demands.
- ❏ I feel empty and alone unless I am with someone.
- ❏ No matter what I do, I always manage to have disasters.
- ❏ If I try my best and succeed, I lose the love of those closest to me.
- ❏ I have trouble making decisions.
- ❏ I blame myself for things that go wrong around me. Other people's happiness and well-being are my responsibility.
- ❏ Whatever I do, I will never be good enough.
- ❏ I am not valuable unless I'm taking care of other people's needs.
- ❏ I can't tolerate pain and unpleasant emotions.

Now, to see if your intuition is apt to get derailed, please check what your automatic response would be to the following situations?

1. You have just picked up your best friend, Cathy, to go to lunch. Even though you're on time, she looks angry. What do you do first?
   - ❏ Take a personal "tick check," figure out if there was something you did that could have aggravated her.
   - ❏ You wait for your friend to get around to telling you why she's angry. However, on the way to the restaurant, you notice you're starting to get tense and your stomach is starting to feel queasy.
   - ❏ You ask your friend why she seems upset.

2. You can't help yourself. You finally ask Cathy why she's upset. She says she appreciates your asking, but she doesn't want to talk about it. What do you do next?

❏ Try to make small talk during lunch, but can't help but obsess about what could possibly be bothering Cathy. Through the appetizer, main course, and dessert, you try to perform an emotional "search and rescue" for what's bothering your friend.

❏ Change the subject and talk about other things, but realize that you are not really remembering what you're eating and your stomach is getting even more upset.

❏ You know your friend's upset but are able to go on with the lunch because you know that eventually she's going to snap out of it.

If you checked the first response to both questions, chances are you are so intuitively keyed in to others' emotions, it's almost impossible for you to hear your own emotions. If you chose the second response, you may be able to redirect your feelings and thoughts after you have noticed a loved one is upset, but your body intuition will still be keyed into your friend's distress and likely to get overloaded.

However, if you checked the third response, you are one of those unusual women who can readily separate someone else's pain from your own thoughts and feelings. Congratulations, you're rare! You have either had a lot of psychotherapy and codependence treatment or your brain is non-traditional, more compartmentalized.

Most women with the hyperconnected feminine brain will have a hard time being able to simultaneously (1) have healthy emotions, clear thinking, good physical health, and ready access to intuition; and (2) be emotionally and intuitively keyed in to another's pain. Nonetheless, you can learn to unclog your intuitive pipeline and keep it open. The following section will help.

Minimize Identity Diffusion: Identify and Shore up Your Personal Boundaries

A kind of bi-location occurs when you are intuitively picking up someone's pain at a distance. You're in two places at once: Part of your energy is with your loved one and the rest is within your own mind and body. If you are good at dividing your attention among several different goals, keeping several balls in the air, then being intuitively plugged in to many people's lives simultaneously will not affect your emotional or physical health or prevent you from having access to your own intuition. However, if like Bettina you have ADD (attention deficit disorder), are prone to depression and anxiety, and have a history of severe trauma, being intuitively plugged in to so many people's lives may cause identity confusion and diffusion. This can blur your emotions, too, and you begin to lose the ability to know where your life ends and someone else's begins. Their anger becomes your anger. When they're depressed, you're depressed. You have intuitively "spread yourself too thin."

The two best treatments for being too intuitively keyed in to others' lives are *codependence treatment* and dialectic behavioral therapy (DBT). DBT teaches how to identify those thoughts, feelings, and sensations that are coming from the left brain's "reasonable" mind and those coming from the right brain's "emotional" mind and to balance them. When you identify which events have precipitated your own mood, anxiety, or symptoms, you develop a firmer awareness of your own self-concept and boundaries. (This process is shown in Chapter 8.) You also learn how not to respond compulsively to intuitive information about loved ones. DBT is invaluable in helping you maintain healthy emotional, physical, and mental boundaries. It is the treatment of choice to prevent you from reacting and overreacting to your intuition.

STEP 7: SCAN YOUR BODY

If you don't pay attention to the intuition behind your mood, anxiety, or distractibility, you will get physical symptoms. You can often figure out what part of your life is out of balance by scanning your body. The health of seven body regions, or "emotional centers," is influenced by a corresponding life problem.

To do an intuitive body scan on yourself, check out each of these centers and their related issues. Where do you tend to get health problems? If you tend to have problems in your lower back, then you're more likely to struggle with second emotional center issues, that is, in your intimate relationships or with money and finances. If you have developed high blood pressure or hypercholesterolemia, these classic fourth emotional center symptoms may indicate unexpressed, unresolved problems with frustration, anger, and other emotions that you need to get "off your chest." On the other hand, if you have a problem at work, your first intuitive signals may have been emotional—frustration, fear, and anxiety—but perhaps you ig-

Body Area	Meaning
First Emotional Center	
Blood	Family
Bones	A sense of support
Joints	Organizations that make us feel safe and
The immune system	secure and give us a sense of belonging
Second Emotional Center	
Lower back, pelvis	Intimate and financial relationships
Reproductive organs: uterus, ovaries,	Money
cervix, vagina, prostate, testes	Finances
Lower urinary tract	Creativity
Third Emotional Center	
Digestive tract	Intuition, gut sense
Kidneys	Self-esteem
Weight, eating	Responsibility
	Work, competition
	Addiction
Fourth Emotional Center	
Heart, blood vessels	Emotional expression
Lungs	Partnership
Breasts	Nurturance
	Passion
Fifth Emotional Center	
Mouth, jaw, teeth	Communication
Thyroid	Will
Neck	Timing
Sixth Emotional Center	
Eyes, ears, nose	Perception
Brain	Thought
	Morality
Seventh Emotional Center	
Life-threatening health problems	Purpose in life
	Connection with spirit/the divine

nored them and now you have the much more uncomfortable symptom in the third emotional center: an ulcer. Most of us ignore or censor the earliest forms of intuition because they could cause us to examine an area in our life that we don't want to make the effort to change. But the more you ignore, the more problems you create: Your body will continue to throw one health problem after another at you until you *have* to stop and examine what is wrong with your life.

STEP 8: THE ABCs OF TAKING CARE OF BUSINESS

Once you've heard what your intuition is telling you, you next need to do the groundwork to make the changes it's asking you to make. The seven basic areas that your intuition may ask you to address parallel the seven emotional centers. You may be asked to:

1. Change your relationship to a family or other organization that's supposed to make you feel safe, secure, and give you a sense of belonging . . . but isn't.
2. Change the dynamics between you and a partner; change how you go after money or property. Investigate how you are tapping into your creativity.
3. Improve the setting in which you work, or how you handle responsibility.
4. Change how you express your emotions in a partnership; investigate how you nurture yourself or others.
5. Change how you communicate and assert your point of view in relationships and at work.
6. Evaluate the flexibility and power of your intellect, your opinions, and your reasoning abilities.
7. Improve your relationship with spirituality and a higher power.

How do you implement the changes your intuition is asking for?

A. *Check Your Facts*

Intuition helps you figure out problems and make decisions even when you don't have enough concrete, rational information. But after you've had a hunch, dream, or flash of what to do, you want to check it out and confirm its accuracy. For example, if you have a dream that warns you of a problem with your pancreas, go to the doctor and get a thorough checkup and appropriate lab work. If your pancreas is fine, then check out other interpretations of the dream. Alternatively, if you have a sense that a friend is in danger, call her up and find out subtly how she is feeling. *Don't* say, for example, "Hey, I had a dream you died of a heart attack. Have you been having any chest pains or shortness of breath?" This approach could scare and offend her, although I'm sure you've run across the well-meaning soul who does this—the "Psychic from Hell."

B. *Do Your Homework*

Write down the problem and bring it to a second pair of eyes—an objective psychotherapist, counselor, friend, or spiritual authority—someone who has no vested interest in how you conduct your life. Get the appropriate training to initiate the change in the family, relationship, or job. Lasting change cannot occur overnight. Like orthodontic work that straightens and corrects your teeth, it takes a series of subtle, persistent, unrelenting adjustments to your thoughts and behavior. A coach or trained psychotherapist should follow you weekly to orient your stepwise journey and evaluate your progress.

C. Clean House

It's no wonder we frequently don't listen to our intuition. The number one reason we get a hunch or an intuitive warning is that we need to look at some aspect of our life that demands growth and development. Change almost always involves losing something you thought you needed, whether it is a job, a dead-end relationship, or a way of thinking. Change also almost always brings a mixture of fear, terror, uncertainty, but ultimately relief and exhilaration. Pregnancy, labor, and childbirth are the ultimate symbols of growth and development in life and show that, to get anything of value, you must invest time, energy, patience; you must learn to tolerate emotional discomfort and pain when necessary.

A Dress Rehearsal for Change: Emotional Feng Shui for Your Life

Making changes in your living space is a dress rehearsal for changing the energy of your life. What do pregnant women do right before they are ready to deliver their baby? Besides getting a nursery ready, most women feel compelled to clean out a room, closet, or drawer—a symbolic preparation for making room for a new member of the family. Before final exams, many students I've known have found security and confidence by clearing off a desk or cleaning out drawers. In the art of feng shui, you superimpose a three-by-three grid on the architectural layout of your house and locate nine different subsections, each of which has a symbolic function or meaning:

- Wealth and prosperity
- Fame and reputation
- Love and marriage
- Health and family
- Earth and groundedness
- Children and creativity

- Knowledge and self-development
- Career
- Helpful people and places

Changing your living environment will create an energy blueprint for changes you want to make in other life areas. For example, the act of throwing out clutter or useless articles in the "love and marriage" area of your house will create intention and attention to those areas in your relationship that are stagnant. Looking for leaky faucets and other metaphors for waste in your wealth and property area can help reorganize and reorient you to examining patterns of economic inefficiency in your life. By gaining mastery on a small scale—over your immediate physical environment—you create a template for successful changes on a grander scale.

How Much Change Do You Need? Minor Repairs or Total Renovation

Some people are comfortable with throwing things out and metaphorically burning bridges. Others crave the stability and security of holding on to the familiar. Stable, gradual changes, whether to a relationship, family, or career, are the least disruptive and more likely to last. For instance, work with a vocational counselor or career coach before you quit a job outright. If you've just found out your husband is having an affair, see a marriage therapist before you call a divorce lawyer. (On the other hand, if you've been in marriage therapy for seven years, and your husband is on his third affair, a more radical approach is needed—perhaps "a radical husbandectomy.")

If you are already an impulsive bridge burner, you want to try to change your way now and make slower, more subtle changes in your life. Ask stabilizing individuals in your life to help you draw up a more gradual timeline to accomplish your goal. If you are compulsive or indecisive, you may need to import a very energetic, pushy, inspiring support person to get you to act.

STEP 9: ASSERTIVENESS: HAVING A SAY, TAKING A STAND

One of the biggest blocks to using your intuition is the reluctance to open your mouth and talk about it out loud. You should be able to talk about the feelings and thoughts that are the basis of your intuition, so they don't go to waste, and so they don't fester and ultimately increase your chance of becoming ill.

I was on *The Oprah Winfrey Show* in 1993 to talk about listening to your intuition. After my segment, a woman who had been in a plane crash said that, before she got on the plane with her husband and her baby, she had gotten a bad feeling about the flight. Although she had flown many times before without feeling nervous, this time she got a feeling that something bad was going to happen. The plane crashed; luckily everyone survived. Oprah asked me what I thought of the woman's story. I replied, "Why didn't she say something? Why did she get on the plane?" And Oprah said, "That's what I was thinking." Everyone gets intuitions, but if you don't say them out loud and respond to them, they remain just that, a feeling and a thought.

Women don't voice their intuition for a variety of reasons. Saying something might:

1. Disrupt your family
2. Disrupt a relationship with a partner; threaten your financial security
3. Threaten job security
4. Make you look angry, unpleasant, or difficult to get along with
5. Not be appreciated by others, inconvenience others
6. Make you look stupid or foolish
7. Be considered antisocial, rude, immoral, disrespectful, or judgmental

Assertiveness is the ability to skillfully give voice to feelings, thoughts, and, of course, your intuition. I have yet to meet someone who has problems voicing his or her intuition who doesn't also suffer from problems with assertiveness. To be assertive, you must keep in mind the four rights to a healthy intuitive voice. You must say:

1. The *right* statement
2. To the *right* person
3. At the *right* time
4. At the *right* intensity

The Right Statement

For healthy intuition, one must confidently, briefly, and in a nonjudgmental way state what you are feeling or thinking.

"I've got a feeling this plane might crash."
"It just occurred to me that you might be in pain."

Not

"If I were you, I'd get off this plane because it's going to crash."
"Why are you in pain again? Don't you know how to take care of yourself?"

The Right Person

Frequently, it's hard to talk directly to someone who can judge and control us. In the old television show *Leave It to Beaver,* when the Beaver was afraid to tell his father something, he would run crying to his mother, who, acting as go-between, would talk to her husband. In Catholicism, we call this the "To Jesus through Mary" maneuver, the classic triangular communication style of someone who lacks assertiveness. Having historically had low social status, women have become socialized to communicate through intermediaries. For example, when we're mad at our boss, we bitch and moan to a co-worker. If we're mad at a partner, instead of saying something to him or her directly, we may sound off with a close friend on the phone.

If you have all your left-brain facts in line to support your intuition, if the issue is important enough to your self-respect, and if you have the appropriate social relationship to deal directly with the individual, you must learn to speak directly—without anger or blaming—to him or her. That is skillful, healthy assertiveness.

The Right Time

To be effective when you are assertive, you must speak at the appropriate moment. If your boss seems to be in a bad mood when she comes in to work, maybe waiting a little to talk to her would be more effective.

Many people have "communication diarrhea" and impulsively blurt out whatever comes into their minds. They don't generally find a receptive audience. Most women, however, suffer from communication blockages. If something bothers them, they're likely to say nothing and let their emotions and feelings simmer until all of a sudden they boil over and blurt out what's on their mind. Poorly timed assertiveness will also have a negative reception.

The Right Intensity

People who have problems with assertiveness tend to have one of two different modes of communication. They may state their position firmly and
emphatically, with no hint of negotiation or flexibility. Or they may give a
lot of nonverbal hints or cues without ever directly saying what they're
thinking or feeling. For example, a woman who has a bad feeling about
going on a plane is likely to procrastinate about packing, lose the plane
tickets, make everyone late, and use other passive maneuvers to somehow
prevent everyone from going.

The simple truth is that most of us don't assertively express our feelings, thoughts, and intuition because we are afraid of making people angry
at us. However, using an indirect, triangular communication style is irritating to everyone. Speaking your mind too abruptly or too late, yelling, or
dropping vague hints is also unlikely to make people happy. Simple, effective, timely communication of your intuition may be difficult, but in the
long run it preserves relations, it doesn't destroy them.

Women who have been raised in a physically or emotionally abusive
environment are more likely to have unhealthy communication styles. As
a result, they are more likely to have difficulty hearing and expressing their
intuition. *Dialectic behavioral therapy* (DBT) can help them find their emotional and intuitive voice (see Resource Guide).

STEP 10: STEP OUT IN FAITH

After you have (a) identified what your intuition is trying to tell you, (b)
checked the facts to be sure your intuition is accurate, and (c) identified
what you need to change in your life . . . what do you do next?

Once you have all the information you need, you simply move, step
out in faith. Close your eyes, say a prayer, take a chance, and move.

Every once in a while, I get someone in a reading who really has all the
information she needs. She's learned the language of her intuition, found
rational data to support her hunch, gotten people to help guide her to
make the change in her life. But she can't take the next step. Her progress
has come to a screeching halt because she is afraid to move to the next
level—to get that new job, to go back to college, to begin a new relationship or end a dead-end one. Here's what I learned about how to get yourself to take the plunge.

When I was in middle school, my sister and I took Red Cross swimming lessons at the navy base pool, a place that seemed harsh and forbid-

ding, although my memories may be slightly distorted by my immense terror and discomfort. Three hundred noisy kids stood waiting and shivering by the side of the pool until the doors to the dressing room would swing open and the instructor, a "seasoned" veteran with a bathing cap with the ears flipped up, would walk out, turn on her heel, and in a stiff pose, suddenly blow a loud whistle and yell, "Everyone in the pool!" I'd stand frozen while everyone around me jumped in. Eventually, the instructor would guide me to the side of the pool and I would painfully, slowly slide my feet, then my knees, then thighs, then trunk into the water. But to pass the ten-week class in which I was enrolled, Advanced Beginner, I would have to learn how to dive into the pool.

Twenty-nine weeks later, I was still entering the pool in the same phobic fashion. I repeated the class three times because I could not bring myself to dive. Session after session, I would freeze. My parents were getting sick and tired of paying for swimming lessons, and the week before my third and final chance to take the final exam and pass Advanced Beginner, they took action.

Motivational Factor #1 for Change: Time and money have run out.

"Time's up," they told me. "We have no more money to invest in these lessons." On a Saturday, they took me to a local Howard Johnson's pool, paid the five-dollar fee, and walked me to the diving board. "Jump," they said.

I stood on the end of the diving board for what seemed like hours, but was probably only forty minutes. While I stared down at the water in the dark, scary recesses of the deep end of the pool, people were beginning to go up to my family, asking questions. Soon everyone was watching.

Motivational Factor #2: Tell as many people as possible what you need to do.

Although this may feel like it's putting pressure on you to perform, the presence of others can cheer you on and make it too embarrassing to back out of your goal.

I stood on that board with my arms outstretched. A bunch of alternate scenarios flashed through my mind.

Motivational Factor #3: Do you want to be left behind? A competitive spirit and fears of abandonment can be very motivating.

I realized that if I stopped going to swimming lessons, the world of swimming would not come to a screeching halt without me. All my friends were enrolled in the classes, and I would have to watch them move forward as I remained hopelessly behind. It wasn't the swimming I hated, so was I really going to let this diving phobia prevent me from progressing?

Motivational Factor #4: You can't stay where you are.

After twenty-nine weeks, I had become the oldest student in Advanced Beginner. During the class, I would watch my friends at the far end of the pool learn new swimming strokes that I couldn't learn. I began to feel like a plant that was "potbound," too overgrown to stay in the same small container.

As I stood on the diving board at the Howard Johnson's, I contemplated what my life would be like in five years: a high school student swimming with prepubertal middle-schoolers. The image wasn't pretty.

Motivational Factor #5: You don't have to be perfect. In life, we are all graded on a PASS–FAIL basis.

I began to realize that I didn't have to do the best dive, I just had to do "a" dive off the board.

Motivational Factor #6: Failure is not as frightening as regret.

I realized if I didn't take the plunge, I would have no respect for myself. Everyone around the pool was cheering me on. I didn't want to be left behind and I couldn't stay on that diving board for the rest of my life.

I closed my eyes.

Said a little prayer.

Stepped forward in faith.

And I jumped.

Of course, after I came back up to the surface of the water and looked at all the people around the edge of the pool who were soaking wet, I realized I had done the biggest belly flop imaginable. However, even though it wasn't pretty, it was, in fact, a dive. I had succeeded. I did the same belly flop the next Wednesday at the final exam, and I passed. I didn't go on to an Olympic career in swimming or diving, but I did become a lifeguard and swimming instructor.

In facing subsequent struggles with fear, failing, and getting stuck, I've worked through these same steps. Fear—especially fear of failing—prevents most of us from acting on our intuition. Most people tell me that if they could get over their fear and were *guaranteed* success, they would readily move forward and realize their potential in jobs, relationships, and life in general. You can do it. Use the steps. Take the plunge.

Heavy Traffic at Intersections in Your Life

When I was doing my doctoral studies in Boston, I didn't have my driver's license so I rode my bike everywhere. Through winter, spring, summer, or fall, I pedaled a racing bike through the heavily trafficked streets of the inner city and surrounding suburbs. Even though I was on a bicycle, I followed the traffic rules . . . mostly. One cold day, during rush hour, black ice on Huntington Avenue coated the road and trolley tracks in the middle of the street. I came to an intersection and had to take a left-hand turn. I saw a break in the traffic so, instead of stopping, I gunned it, only to hit the icy rail of the trolley tracks and fall smack in the middle of the intersection. Heavy traffic was bearing down on me from five directions, and a trolley was heading right toward my head. The wind had been knocked out of me and I was disoriented so I couldn't figure out what direction I needed to go, but I had no time to think, anyway. Something deep inside me shoved me up and onto my feet and I got on the bike and bolted to safety just as the train whooshed past.

I'm sure you have your own equivalent to this story. Somewhere in your life, you got to a fork in the road, and under crisis conditions were forced to make a decision. Maybe you'd run out of money and time. Maybe you were at risk for losing someone close to you. You were at a busy intersection and traffic was bearing down upon you. Indecisiveness was not an option. It was do-or-die time. After my fall on the trolley tracks, I took stock of myself and my bike and, unbelievably, both of us had gotten away without a scrape and were still headed in the right direction. Somehow in these forced-choice situations, we almost always make the right decision. Since there's no time for fear, you step out in faith.

After you've done the appropriate planning and preparation for changing your life, faith will override fear every time, allowing you to use your intuition to make the best decision. Yet in most situations, we are not forced by external pressures to make a decision. How then do we call on our intuition to help us? Because anxiety and fear often underlie indecision, you can work on reducing them with the supplements, medicines, and therapies that can restore your sense of passion and potential. And you can spark the faith you need to propel you forward.

Getting in Touch with Faith

Although you can get in touch with faith in physical places like churches and memorials, true faith is an inside job. To remind yourself of your own innate faith or restart your faith if it has stalled, here are some suggestions that have worked for me, my friends, and my patients.

- Recall times when you have been up the creek without a paddle and have gotten through safely. Recall how you were feeling, who appeared out of nowhere, and how it all "came together" for survival and even success.
- Do a little of something you are good at, that you feel competent about, that gives you a sense of competency and fulfillment.
- It sounds slightly sappy, but it works. Watch inspiring movies of people who have experienced tragedy and transcended it:
  > *Rudy*
  > *Resurrection*
  > *The Sound of Music*
  > *Seabiscuit*
  > *The Miracle*
  > *Erin Brockovich*
  > *Heaven Can Wait*
  > *Steel Magnolias*

Suppose you do all your homework, you get loving, expert instruction and support, you take the plunge, and you fail? Sometimes you're meant to fail and you learn something important for your next goal. Failing is just redirection, a road sign indicating another route. It's *not* the end of the road. One of my favorite comediennes is Ellen DeGeneres, whose career has had both glowing successes and glaring public failures. In a recent monologue, she noted how all of us are a product of both our successes and failures. She said that if it weren't for her first television show, which was canceled, she wouldn't have gotten her second television show, which was canceled, but which led to her daytime talk show, which is an incredible, award-winning success. It's very easy to enjoy success, but it's painful to be in the intermediary disappointments before a success.

In the year after graduating from college, I had to leave a research job because of a medical problem. At the time, I felt like a complete failure. I wanted to get into medical school and do research, and the one job that could help me achieve my goal had just gone up in smoke. I had a lot of student loans to pay, so I went to a temp agency and chose a job "at random" as a switchboard operator at an investment company. So, in an uncomfortable office uniform, I answered phones and simultaneously studied for both the MCAT (medical school entrance exam) and GRE (graduate school entrance exam). For nearly two weeks, with a mixture of humiliation, embarrassment, and despair, I studied, prayed, and answered the phones over and over, "Quality Properties. May I help you?"

There was nothing else for me to do but move forward in faith and play the hand I had been dealt. Then one day, a man who had been watching me answer the phones and study for exams came up to my desk and said, "You're a very interesting person. What do you eventually want to do?" I rather self-consciously told him I wanted to be a physician and a scientist, and he told me he knew the dean of a medical school. I brushed him off. But the next day, I found a note on my telephone switchboard. The man had made an appointment for me with the chairman of the M.D./Ph.D. program and the dean of admissions at Boston University's School of Medicine, where I eventually applied and from which I successfully graduated. My failure had led to a success.

Since that time, my life has had many failures, interspersed with successes. All of them are part of a perfect path on which I'm guided by intellect, intuition, and faith. I hope I have helped you see how your life can be helped by intuition as well as by using the amazing strengths of your New Feminine Brain. Learn how to cultivate the unique genius behind the flaws in your feminine brain. Your combination of intellect and intuition is as perfect as the smile on the *Mona Lisa*.

"Nothing in life is to be feared. It is only to be understood."
—Marie Curie, who had one of the first New Feminine Brains way back when

Resource Guide

Light

Most artificial light, including both regular incandescent and standard fluorescent lighting, lacks the full and balanced wave light spectrum found in sunlight—which in the proper amounts is considered a nutrient. Using natural lighting in your home optimizes your health in many ways, most notably enhancing mood and fertility. Sources of products for natural lighting include:

Day-Light Technologies, Inc.
Halifax, N.S., Canada

Light for Health
P.O. Box 1760
Lyons, CO 80540
Phone: 800-468-1104
www.lightforhealth.com

Natural Lighting
1939 Richvale
Houston, TX 77062
Phone: 888-900-6830
www.naturallighting.com

Ott-Lite Technology
P.O. Box 172425
Tampa, FL 33672-0425
Phone: 800-842-8848
www.ottlite.com/wtb.asp

Varilux Company
9 Viaduct Road
Stamford, CT 06907
Phone: 800-786-6850
www.verilux.net

Supplements

DAILY SUPPLEMENTAL VITAMINS AND MINERALS:

Daily vitamin and mineral supplements are vital at any time in your life. Make sure your supplements are guaranteed potency and manufactured according to GMP (good manufacturing processes) standards, a term that denotes high quality. I recommend USANA, which has "pharmaceutical-grade" vitamins, made from the highest-quality ingredients.

USANA's Essentials: Actually two different high-potency supplements, USANA's Mega Antioxidant Vitamin supplements and USANA's Chelated Mineral supplements, taken together as a daily regimen. These products provide optimal, balanced amounts of the essential vitamins and minerals, along with fifteen potent antioxidants (including olivol, or olive fruit extract, a recent addition). For information, contact:

> USANA
> 3838 West Parkway Boulevard
> Salt Lake City, UT 84120
> Phone: 888-950-9595
> www.usana.com

Verified Quality's Super Multi-Complex: This daily supplement has twenty-eight vitamins and minerals, but contains no coatings, binders, or fillers. It's also free of dairy, wheat, eggs, soy, yeast, commercial sugars, starch, preservatives, and hydrogenated oil.

Council for Responsible Nutrition (CRN): a Washington-based trade association representing ingredient suppliers and manufacturers in the dietary supplement industry. CRN's website contains detailed information on supplements, including basic information on and links to studies about a wide array of herbs and botanicals. One page (www.crnusa.org) gives clear and detailed information on how to read a supplement label. The council's downloadable publication, *The Benefits of Nutritional Supplements,* is a particularly enlightening document that shares much research that supports taking nutritional supplements at higher levels than the RDA to prevent chronic disease. For more information, contact:

> Council for Responsible Nutrition (CRN)
> 1828 L Street NW, Suite 900
> Washington, DC 20036-5114
> Phone: 202-776-7936
> www.crnusa.org

Omega-3 Fatty Acids/DHA

The main sources of omega-3 essential fatty acids (EFAs) in our diets are fatty fish and green leafy vegetables such as spinach, broccoli, cabbage, and lettuce. Unprocessed vegetable oils—especially flaxseed oil—are also rich sources of EFAs, although the refining process used for many commercial oils (including soybean and canola oils) removes nearly all the essential omega-3 fatty acids.

Docosahexaenoic acid (DHA) is an omega-3 fatty acid essential to human brain and eye development and function. Most of us don't get nearly enough of this vital nutrient (the National Institutes of Health recommends consuming 300 milligrams a day). The best sources of DHA include eggs from chickens raised on DHA-rich food, wild (not farm-raised) cold-water fish such as salmon and sardines, and supplements made from algae.

Healthwell, a website operated by New Hope Natural Media (the leading publisher of natural products magazines and producer of natural products trade shows and conferences in the United States), offers an excellent and detailed article about DHA at the following link:

www.healthwell.com

Martek Biosciences Corporation (888-OK-BRAIN; www.dhadepot), a manufacturer of microalgae products, operates a site called DHA Depot with lots of detailed information about this nutrient—including its importance for pregnant and lactating women and infants. The site also features a calculator that allows you to figure out how much DHA you get in a typical day's meals and snacks.

Some sources of these essential fats that I particularly recommend include:

Wild Alaskan salmon is a rich source of omega-3 fatty acids. The Vital Choice Company now offers a variety of its salmon product combinations designed specifically for new mothers. All Vital Choice salmon is naturally organic and free of antibiotics, growth hormones, and artificial coloring. It comes vacuum-packed and frozen. Vital Choice also sells salmon fillets and salmon burgers separately. For more information, contact:

Vital Choice Seafood
605 30th Street
Anacortes, WA 98221
Phone: 800-608-4825
www.vitalchoice.com

Neuromins from Nature's Way: These gelcaps contain a vegetable source of DHA that closely matches the DHA in human breast milk and is specially formulated for maternal nutrition.

USANA's OptOmega essential fatty acid oil: Contains an ideal ratio of the two essential fatty acids known as alpha-linolenic acid (an omega-3 fatty acid) and linoleic acid (an omega-6 fatty acid) that are important to cardiovascular health. In addition, these fatty acids also promote healthy immunity, mental sharpness, and healthy skin. This all-natural, vegetarian product is produced from certified organic, unrefined cold-pressed flaxseed, sunflower seed, pumpkin seed, and extra-virgin olive oils and contains no trans fatty acids.

USANA's BiOmega-3: These capsules contain 1000 milligrams of cold-water fish oil, including the important omega-3 fatty acids EPA and DHA, in a natural form that is easily absorbed by the body. For more information, contact USANA. Whole Flax Seed from Cathy's Country Store is organically grown in North Dakota and has an especially nutty and delicious flavor. For more information, contact Emerson Ecologics.

FiProFLAX (ground flax) is cold milled by Health from the Sun from premium quality flax with a high oil content. Alternatively, you can take certified organic flaxseed oil from a bottle (although the shelf life is short, so keep it in your refrigerator for maximum longevity) or in gel capsules. For more information, contact Emerson Ecologics.

Omega Smart Bars: This totally organic vegan product not only delivers a healthy dose of omega-3s, but it's also high in fiber and has a low glycemic index. The ingredients (which are all organic) include ground flaxseed, figs, agave nectar, a number of dried fruits, soy flour, toasted soy nuts and either almonds or walnuts, plus a little cinnamon and other organic spices. This product contains no artificial flavorings, dairy or whey, hydrogenated oils, processed sugar, wheat, synthetic vitamins, eggs, predigested hydrolyzed or soy protein isolates or caseinates. For more information, contact Emerson Ecologics.

Mind-Body Makeover

In the *Mind-Body Makeover Oracle Cards* (Mona Lisa Schulz, M.D., Ph.D., Hay House, 2005) I teach you how to rewire seventy different thought patterns that tend to create emotional and physical distress. Whether you are having problems with depression, anxiety, low self-esteem, difficulties with work, or your physical health, you can learn to recognize the unhealthy thought pattern, on one side of the round card, and then turn the thought around to the healthier mind-set on the reverse side of the card.

Psychotherapy and Support Groups
Cognitive Behavioral Therapy

The National Association of Cognitive-Behavioral Therapists is an organization dedicated solely to the teaching and practice of cognitive-behavioral psychotherapy—which holds that our own thoughts cause our feelings and behaviors (as opposed to external things like other people or situations). CBT therapists teach patients that even if they can't change a situation, they can change the way they think about it, helping them to become calmer and at peace with life's challenges. The organization's website not only has an extensive description of this type of therapy, it also has a search page that provides names of certified CBT therapists in your area. For more information, contact:

> The National Association of Cognitive-Behavioral Therapists
> P.O. Box 2195
> Weirton, WV 26062
> Phone: 800-853-1135
> www.nacbt.org

DIALECTIC BEHAVIORAL THERAPY (DBT):

Described as "an eclectic mix of cognitive-behavioral techniques, skills training, Zen, and existentialism," DBT can be extremely helpful for anyone dealing with extreme emotional reactions (which, when left unaddressed, can lead to a number of serious mental and physical health problems). I believe that everyone with somatic illness of any kind, particularly a chronic illness, can benefit from the skills discussed in the Linehan approach, even though they were designed for those suffering from a specific mental health problem. Most major mental health centers now offer DBT groups.

RECOMMENDED READING ON DBT:

Marsha M. Linehan, Ph.D., *Skills Training Manual for Treating Borderline Personality Disorder* (Guilford Press, 1993); www.behavioraltech.com and http://faculty.washington.edu/line han

Dr. Linehan is a professor of psychology and an adjunct professor of psychiatry and behavioral sciences at the University of Washington, Seattle. She is also director of the Behavioral Research and Therapy Clinics.

Scott E. Spradlin, *Don't Let Your Emotions Run Your Life: How Dialectical Behavior Therapy Can Put You in Control* (New Harbinger Publications, 2003)

POSTPARTUM DEPRESSION (PPD) INFORMATION:

Depression After Delivery, Inc., is a national, nonprofit organization that provides support for women suffering from depression during or after delivery. Its focus includes education, information, support groups, telephone support, and professional referral for women and their families (including names of local support groups for PPD). For more information, contact:

> Depression After Delivery (D.A.D.)
> Box 1282
> Morrisville, PA 19067
> Phone: 800-944-4773
> www.depressionafterdelivery.com

Postpartum Support International is an educational, referral, and advocacy group devoted to increasing awareness about and discussion of postpartum depression. Its website has lots of background information, as well as a bookstore, Internet forums and chat rooms, links to local support groups across the country, and a self-assessment test. For more information, contact:

> Postpartum Support International
> 927 North Kellogg Ave.
> Santa Barbara, CA 93111
> Phone: 805-967-7636
> www.postpartum.net

Assertiveness Training

Paul Schenk, Psy.D., *Great Ways to Sabotage a Good Conversation* (Standard Press, 2002); www.drpaulschenk.com

In this helpful book, written with a sharp sense of humor, Dr. Schenk (a clinical psychologist in private practice in Atlanta) outlines how we often fall into language traps while talking with children, mates, friends, co-workers, and others that sabotage what we mean to say. By shifting our choice of words, he explains, we will not only boost our communication skills but greatly improve our relationships.

Imagery and Visualization

Louise Hay's *Overcoming Fears* audio program: This popular visualization program (available on audiocassette and CD) from Louise Hay will help you transform your deeply held beliefs that the world is an inescapably stressful place. This audio program directs you in changing your perception and biochemistry over time so that you begin to attract experiences of safety, security, and peace. As you feel safer and more peaceful more often, your stress hormone levels will level off, and so will your tendency to store fat as "protection." You will experience noticeable results in how you feel and think about yourself and your life after just one month of listening to this program consistently each day. Louise Hay is also the author of twenty-seven books, including *You Can Heal Your Life* (Hay House, 1987) and *Empowering Women* (Hay House, 1997). For more information, contact:

> Hay House, Inc.
> P.O. Box 5100
> Carlsbad, CA 92018-5100
> Phone: 800-654-5126
> www.Hayhouse.com

Belleruth Naparstek's audio program: I am uplifted and inspired every time I listen to it. If you listen consistently at least once per day, you will experience noticeable results in how you feel and think about yourself and your life in one month. This product doubled weight loss in a placebo-controlled pilot study at Canyon Ranch. For more information, contact:

> Health Journeys
> 891 Moe Dr., Suite C
> Akron, OH 44310
> Phone: 800-800-8661
> www.healthjourneys.com

Creating Happiness

Maria Rodale and Maya Rodale, *It's My Pleasure* (Free Press, 2005)
     Rodale and Rodale give you several different routes to import happiness into your life ultimately, which helps you utilize all of your brain potential.

Acupuncture and Traditional Chinese Medicine

Gary F. Fleischman, O.M.D., and Charles Stein, *Acupuncture: Everything You Ever Wanted to Know* (Barrytown, 1998); www.AcupunctureNewHaven.com
     This easy-to-read guide is useful for patients and medical professionals alike; it discusses the fundamentals of traditional Chinese medicine as well as sharing information on how TCM is used to treat various conditions. Dr. Fleischman is a board-certified acupuncturist practicing in New Haven, CT, who earned his degree from the China Institute of Acupuncture and the Guangdong Provincial Hospital of Traditional Chinese Medicine in Guangzhou, China.

Ruth Kidson, M.Sc., M.B., B.S., *Acupuncture for Everyone: What It Is, Why It Works, and How It Can Help You* (Healing Arts Press, 2000)

If you have ever wondered how and why acupuncture works, this book by a British doctor is an excellent place to begin your reading. Dr. Kidson demonstrates how an acupuncturist makes his or her diagnosis and how the patient is then treated. For the person drawn to this modality yet wary of the experience, this text makes going to an acupuncturist much less intimidating.

To find a practitioner of Traditional Chinese Medicine (Acupuncture):

Traditional Chinese Medicine (TCM), a 3000-year-old health and wellness system, is based on the idea that all illness stems from imbalances of ch'i, or life energy, in the body. Its primary focus is prevention, although its therapies (including acupuncture as well as the use of Chinese herbs and bodywork) also treat pain, illness, and disease. It's ideal to get a referral to an acupuncturist or TCM practitioner from your health care practitioner, but if you can't find one this way, contact:

> The National Certification Commission for Acupuncture and Oriental Medicine
> 11 Canal Center Plaza, Suite 300
> Alexandria, VA 22314
> Phone: 703-548-9004
> www.nccaom.org

Naturopathic Medicine

Naturopathic doctors (NDs) are physicians who rely mostly on natural methods to help the body heal itself. They focus on the underlying cause of illness instead of relying mainly on the treatment of symptoms. They usually incorporate a variety of types of alternative or complementary medicine in their practice, although they may also use conventional medicine, depending on the individual patient. For more information on naturopathic physicians or to find one in your area who specializes in pediatrics, contact:

> The American Association of Naturopathic Physicians
> 3201 New Mexico Avenue NW, Suite 350
> Washington, DC 20016
> Phone: 866-538-2267 or 202-895-1392
> www.naturopathic.org

Exercise and Fitness

John Douillard, Ph.D., *Body, Mind, and Sport: The Mind-Body Guide to Lifelong Health, Fitness, and Your Personal Best* (Harmony Books, 1994, revised edition, Three Rivers Press, 2001); www.lifespa.com

Dr. Douillard is a former professional athlete who applies mind/body principles to fitness in this book, designed to help readers determine which sport (and so which diet and exercise program) they are best suited for, depending on their individual nature. The suggested fitness programs include both plans for the competitive athlete as well as plans for the rest of us. The revised edition includes forewords by tennis stars Billie Jean King and Martina Navratilova.

Mari Winsor, *The Pilates Powerhouse: The Perfect Method of Body Conditioning for Strength, Flexibility, and the Shape You Have Always Wanted in Less Than an Hour a Day* (Perseus Books, 1999)

Pilates is an excellent way to strengthen your core muscles and also increase flexibility because it engages your mind, muscles, breathing, and stretching all at once. Pilates has influenced and improved the way I perform every other activity, including walking!

To keep track of your Pilates workouts, I also recommend Mari Winsor's *The Pilates Workout Journal* (Perseus Books, 2001).

Brooke Siler, *The Pilates Body: The Ultimate At-Home Guide to Strengthening, Lengthening, and Toning Your Body—Without Machines* (Broadway Books, 2000).

Brooke Siler is one of the most sought-after Pilates instructors in the country, and for good reason. Extremely well-organized and easy to use, this book is great for at-home practice as well as travel, whether you are just starting out or a seasoned Pilates practitioner.

Miriam E. Nelson, Ph.D., *Strong Women Stay Young* (Bantam, revised edition, 2000); www.strongwomen.com.

This book is great for learning the basics of strength training. Dr. Nelson's program is scientifically proven to build muscle and bone mass in midlife women. The Strong Women Stay Young program consists of two forty-minute weight-training sessions per week in which you work opposite muscle groups together, which not only builds strength but also improves balance (something women start to lose in their forties). It's simple; you can do it at home or in the gym and, regardless of your current fitness level, you'll obtain results quickly. In one study, Dr. Nelson found that the elderly patients who participated in her program significantly improved their strength and decreased their falls in just a few weeks.

Peggy W. Brill, P.T., *The Core Program: 15 Minutes a Day That Can Change Your Life* (Bantam Books, 2001).

Over the years, scores of women have complained to me about their aching backs, sore necks, hip pain, shoulder pain, and so on. Though stretching and exercise usually help alleviate most common aches and pains, not all methods help all people. This book gives you a simple fitness routine developed expressly for women that works regardless of your age, shape, or starting point. Because it takes only fifteen minutes per day, just about everyone can benefit.

Diet, Weight, and Healthy Eating

H. Leighton Steward, Morrison Bethea, Sam Andrews, and Luis A. Balart, *The New Sugar Busters: Cut Sugar to Trim Fat* (Ballantine Books, 2003); www.sugarbusters.com

The basic equation in this easy-to-understand book is simply put: Too Much Sugar = Too Much Insulin. Excess sugar consumption has been linked to myriad health problems, including depression, impaired immune function, and weight gain. If you suspect your diet may contain too much sugar or that you are sugar-sensitive, this book can help you evaluate your dietary needs more clearly. It contains meal plans and recipes that have helped many people lose or maintain their weight, as well as balance hormones, insulin, and eicosanoid levels.

Geneen Roth, *When Food Is Love: Exploring the Relationship Between Eating and Intimacy* (Dutton, 1991); www.geneenroth.com

If you are facing the emotional dimensions of overeating, read this book. No one has ever written more eloquently or helpfully on the subject of eating and emotions.

Geneen Roth, *Appetites: On the Search for True Nourishment* (Dutton, 1996); www.geneen roth.com.

What do women *really* want? Using eating as a metaphor for feminine desire in contemporary American culture, Geneen Roth examines the depths of our search for true nourishment, intimacy, friendship, health, and success.

Ray Strand, M.D., a family physician in South Dakota and the author of *Releasing Fat: Developing Healthy Lifestyles that Have a Side Effect of Permanent Fat Loss* (Health Concepts Publishing, 2003); www.bionutrition.org

Dr. Strand, a specialist in nutritional medicine, presents cutting-edge medical evidence explaining why so many diets don't work. He's been applying these truths in his private medical practice for over eight years. Not only are insulin-resistant patients improving their health and lifestyles, they are beginning to release fat for the first time in their lives.

Dr. Strand's website offers information about beating insulin resistance, including instructions on eating a healthy diet, following the right exercise program, and taking dietary supplements. The site includes detailed information about the glycemic index as well as recommended foods to help you prevent insulin resistance and maximize your health.

The National Eating Disorders Association (NEDA)
NEDA, the largest not-for-profit organization in the United States, works to prevent eating disorders and to provide treatment referrals to those suffering from anorexia, bulimia, and binge eating disorder and those concerned with body image and weight issues. NEDA's website offers tons of information on eating disorders, and includes an Eating Disorders Survival Guide, links to treatment providers in your area. For more information, contact:

> The National Eating Disorders Association (NEDA)
> 603 Stewart St., Suite 803
> Seattle, WA 98101
> Phone: 206-382-3587
> www.edap.org

Medical Intuition

For more information or to make a medical intuitive appointment, call Mona Lisa Schulz at 207-846-6497 or visit her website, www.drmonalisa.com.

Addiction

Andrew Weil, M.D., and Winifred Rosen, *From Chocolate to Morphine: Everything You Need to Know About Mind-Altering Drugs* (Houghton Mifflin, 2004); www.drweil.com

This recently revised book aimed at parents and their children gives an unbiased description of the ways a wide variety of drugs affect the mind and body and discusses the difference between drug use and drug abuse. The information includes side effects, precautions, and alternatives for legal drugs like caffeine and antihistamines as well as the illegal variety.

Nancy Goodman, *It Was Food vs. Me . . . and I Won* (Viking Press, 2004)
A former binge eater shares the story of how she overcame a lifelong obsession with food. This candid book gives advice on separating food and emotion, taking the fear out of food by learning to safely feed your cravings, how to redirect your energy from what you eat and how much you weigh to who you really are—and how to learn to love that person.

QUITTING SMOKING

Gotta Quit: a website (www.gottaquit.com) from the Monroe County, NY, Department of Health. The site offers lots of information about how to quit smoking and offers powerful tools such as goal-setting opportunities that make use of emailed reminders containing information you provide and quit coaches trained by the University of Rochester Medical Center who are available for live chat.

DRUG AND ALCOHOL ADDICTION AND ABUSE

Alcoholics Anonymous: the group that's been helping alcoholics stop drinking, one day at a time, ever since the 1930s. One page on AA's website specifically addressed to teens gives a quiz designed to help them decide if drinking has become a problem for them. The site also gives contact information on local chapters across the country and has a link to the text of "The Big Book," what AA members call the text *Alcoholics Anonymous* (Alcoholics Anonymous World Services, revised edition, 2000). For more information, contact:·

Alcoholics Anonymous General Service Office
P.O. Box 459, Grand Central Station
New York, NY 10163
Phone: 212-870 3400
www.aa.org

COMPULSIVE EATING

Overeaters Anonymous (OA): This worldwide, twelve-step fellowship and recovery program from compulsive overeating is modeled after Alcoholics Anonymous. OA addresses more than just weight loss and also promotes physical, emotional, and spiritual well-being. OA doesn't promote any particular eating plan or diet, but members (not all of whom are obese) are encouraged to develop their own food plan with a health care professional and a sponsor. For more information, contact:

Overeaters Anonymous
World Service Office
P.O. Box 44020
Rio Rancho, NM 87174-4020

Phone: 505-891-2664

Website: www.overeatersanonymous.org

Margaret Bullitt-Jonas, *Holy Hunger: A Woman's Journey from Food Addiction to Spiritual Fulfillment* (Vintage, 2000); www.holyhunger.com

Episcopal minister Bullitt-Jonas's incredibly touching memoir shares the story of how her economically privileged childhood with an alcoholic father and an emotionally reclusive mother spawned a food addiction, and how she eventually recovered—through her faith in a higher power and help from the twelve-step program Overeaters Anonymous.

Herbert Benson, M.D., with Miriam Z. Klipper, *The Relaxation Response* (updated and expanded edition, Quill, 2001); www.herbertbenson.com

First published in 1975, this groundbreaking book demystified meditation and brought it from the realm of the gurus to within reach of the general public. The authors cite studies showing that the relaxation response not only reduces stress but also lowers blood pressure and helps reduce risk for heart disease. The technique Benson, a Harvard researcher, teaches is simple and requires just ten to twenty minutes a day. Although a plethora of good books about meditation exist today, this classic is still excellent for a basic understanding of the techniques and instructions for how to get started.

Fatigue

Jacob Teitelbaum, M.D., *From Fatigued to Fantastic!* (Avery Pub. Group, 2001); www.endfatigue.com

Dr. Teitelbaum is not only a leading researcher in the field of chronic fatigue and fibromyalgia, but he's suffered from both conditions himself. In this updated and revised edition of his book, he discusses the newest findings about these conditions and his treatment advice, which combines over-the-counter drugs, diet modification, vitamin and mineral supplements, acupuncture, massage, chiropractic medicine, herbal supplements, and psychotherapy.

Back Pain

Ronald D. Siegel, Psy.D., Michael H. Urdang, and Douglas R. Johnson, M.D., *Back Sense: A Revolutionary Approach to Halting the Cycle of Chronic Back Pain* (Broadway Books, 2001); www.backsense.org

I highly recommend this wonderful book, written by three men who are themselves former chronic back pain sufferers, to everyone with chronic back problems. The first of my patients who read this book got out of bed and off narcotics for the first time in months. The authors assert that truly bad backs are rare, and that many back problems may well begin with an injury, but they become chronic conditions because of stress (which causes painfully tight muscles) and inactivity (which makes you lose conditioning, leaving you more vulnerable to additional injury).

Women's Health

Dr. Christiane Northrup is probably America's number one women's doctor. In addition to *Women's Bodies, Women's Wisdom* (Bantam, 1994), *The Wisdom of Menopause* (Bantam, 2001), and *Mother-Daughter Wisdom* (Bantam, 2005), her free monthly e-letter and subscription newsletter are available through her website, www.drnorthrup.com. I consider her website and periodicals akin to a national clearinghouse for up-to-date and accurate information about women's health.

Notes

Chapter One

20 *The traditional male brain:* Wooley CS, et al (1997). Estradiol increases the sensitivity of hippocampal CA, pyramidal cell to NMDA receptor-mediated synaptic input correlates with dendritic spine density. *J Neurosci,* 17:1848–1859; Phoenix CH, et al (1959). Organizing action of prenatally administered testosterone proprimate in the tissues mediating mating behavior in the guinea pig. *Endocrinology,* 65:369

21 *They also provide insight into:* Jacobs B, et al (1977). Lifespan dendritic and spine changes in areas 10 and 18 in human cortex. *J Child Neurol,* 386:661–680; Rabinowicz T, et al (1998). Gender differences in the human cerebral cortex: More neurons in males: more processes in females. *J Child Neurol,* 14(2):98–107; deCourten-Myers G (1999). The human cerebral cortex: Gender differences in structure and function. *J Neuropath Exp Neurol,* 58:217–226; Esposito G, et al (1996). Gender differences in CBF as a function of cognitive state of PET. *J Nucl Med,* 37:559–564

21 *The traditional female brain:* Jacobs B, et al (1993). A quantitative dendritic analysis of Wernicke's area in humans. II. Gender, hemisplenic, and environmental factors. *JCN,* 327:97–111.

22 *How fast a girl matures:* Garcia-Segura LM, et al (1974). Gonadal hormone regulation of glial fibrillary acidic protein and glial ultrastructure in the rat neuroendocrine hypothalamus. *GLIAI,* 10:59–69.

22 *Hormones even govern:* Wooley CS, et al (1997). Estradiol increases the sensitivity of hippocampal CA, pyramidal cell to NMDA receptor-mediated synaptic input correlates with dendritic spine density. *J Neurosci,* 17:1848–1859; Jung-Testas I and Baylieu EE (1998). Steroid hormone receptors and steroid action in rat glial cells of the central and physical neurosystems. *J Steroid Biochem Mol Biol,* 65:243–251; Garcia-Segura LM, et al (1996). Endocrine glial cells in the brain actions of steroid and thyroid hormones and in the regulation of hormone secretion. *Front Neuroendocrinol,* 17:180–211; Garcia-Segura LM, et al (1996). Gonadal hormones as promoters of structural synaptic plasticity. *Prog Neurobiol,* 44:279–307; Naftolin F, et al (1993). Estrogen induces synaptic plasticity in adult primate neurons. *Neuroendocrinology,* 57:935–939; Goodman CS and Schatz CJ (1993). Developmental mechanisms that generate precise patterns of neuronal connectivity. *Cell 72/Neuron 10* (suppl): January 77–98; McEwen BS, et al (1991). Steroid hormones as mediators of neural plasticity. *J Steroid Biochem Mol Biol,* 39:223–232;

Matsumoto A (1992). Hormonally-induced synaptic plasticity in the adult neuroendocrine brain. *Zool Sci,* 9:679–695.

23 *You might "throw":* Phoenix CH, et al (1959). Organizing action of prenatally administered testosterone proprimate in the tissues mediating mating behavior in the guinea pig. *Endocrinology,* 65:369.

24 *The previously unused visual area:* Sadato, N et al (1996). Activation of the primary visual cortex by Braille reading in blind subjects. *Nature* 380: 526–528.

26 *Handedness is in part genetic:* Annett M (1985). *Left, Right, Hand, and Brain: The Right Shift Theory.* Hillsdale, NJ, Erlbaum.

26 *There is an association:* Orsini DL and Satz P (1986). A syndrome of pathological 1-handedness and correlates of early left hemisphere injury. *Archives of Neurology,* 43:333–337; Geschwind N and Galaburd AM (1987). *Cerebral Lateralization: Biological Mechanisms, Associations, and Pathology.* Cambridge, MA, MIT Press; Geschwind N and Behan P (1982). Left handedness immune disease, migraine, and developmental learning disorder. *Proc Nat Acad Sci,* 79:5097–5100.

26 *So, if you are left-handed:* Aboitiz FP, et al (1992). Individual differences in brain asymmetries and fiber composition in the human corpus callosum. *Brain Research,* 598:151–154; Geschwind N and Galaburda AM (1985). Cerebral lateralization: Biological mechanisms association and pathology I to II. *Archives of Neurology,* 42:428–459, 521–552, 632–654.

27 *Since the traditional man's brain is more compartmentalized:* Kimura D (1973). Manual activity during speaking. *Neuropsychologica,* 71:45–50; Laveigne F and Kimura D (1997). Hand movement asymmetry during speech. *Neuropsychologica,* 25:689–694; Denckla MB and Rudel R (1974). Rapid "automatized" naming of pictured objects, colors, letters, and numbers. *Cortex,* 10:186–202.

27 *Having language in both hemispheres:* Levy J (1972), in *The Biology of Behavior* (ed. Kiger J). Corvallis, Oregon State University; Hampson E and Kimun D (1972), in *Behavioral Endocrinology,* eds. Becker J, Breedlove S, and Crews D, pp 357–398, Cambridge, MA, MIT Press; Shaywitz BA, et al (1995). Sex differences in the functional organization of the brain for language. *Nature,* 373:607–609; Edward S, et al (1976). Language and intelligence in dysphasia: Are they related? *Brit J of Disorders of Communication,* 11:83–94; McGlone J and Kertesz A (1973). Sex differences in cerebral processing of visuospatial tasks. *Cortex,* 9:313–320.

27 *Yet, when women speak:* Aboitiz FP, et al (1992). Individual differences in brain asymmetries and fiber composition in the human corpus callosum. *Brain Research,* 598:151–154, Shall SA and Kim KL (1990). Androgen receptors are differentially distributed between right and left cerebral hemispheres of the fetal male rhesus monkey. *Brain Research,* 516:122–126; Marcoby E and Jacklin C (1974). *The Psychology of Sex Differences.* Stanford University Press; Galaburda AL, Rosen GD, and Sherman GF (1990). Individual variability in cortical organization: Its relationship to brain laterality and implications to function. *Neuropsychologia,* 28:529–546; Witelson SF (1989). Handedness and sex differences in the isthmus and splenum of the corpus callosum in humans. *Brain,* 112:799–835; Aboitiz FP, et al (1992). Fiber composition of the human corpus callosum. *Brain Research,* 598:143–153

27 *Therefore, women may be anatomically encouraged to talk:* Denckla MB and Rudel R (1974). Rapid "automatized" naming of pictured objects, colors, letters, and numbers. *Cortex,* 10:186–202; Kimura D (1999). Chapter 8, Verbal Abilities. In:

Sex and Cognition, Cambridge, MIT Press, p 93; Harshman R, Hampson E, and Berenbaum S (1983). Individual differences in cognitive abilities and brain organization. Part I: Sex and handedness differences in ability. *Can J Psychology,* 37:144–192; Kimura D (1994). Body asymmetry and intellectual pattern. *Personality and Individual Differences,* 17:53–60.

28 *Connections for language, perception, and attention:* Ward SL, Newcombe N, and Overton WP (1986). Turn left at the church or three miles north: A study of direction-giving and sex differences. *Environment and Behavior,* 18:192–213.

28 *Women's brains generally have a better capacity:* Duggan L (1950). An experiment in immediate recall in secondary school children. *Brit J Psychol,* 40:149–154; Blecker ML, Bolla-Wilson K, and Meyers BA (1988). Age-related sex differences in verbal memory. *J Clin Psychol,* 44:403–411.

29 *Dyslexia can take a different form in women:* Baynes K, Tram MJ, and Gazziniga MS (1992). Reading with a limited lexicon in the right hemisphere of a cellosotomy patient. *Neuropsychologia,* 30:187–200; Hellige JB (1993), Ch. 2, Behavioral Asymmetrics in Humans, in JB Hellige *Hemispheric Asymmetry: What's Right and What's Left.* Cambridge, Harvard University Press.

29 *Most dyslexic adults have more difficulty with writing:* Geschwind N and Galaburda A (1987). Chapter 7, Pathology of Asymmetry in Developmental Learning Disorders. In Geschwind N and Galaburda A, Cambridge, MA, MIT Press, p 66; Galaburda AM and Kemper TL (1979). Cytoarchitecture abnormalities in developmental dyslexia: A case study. *Ann Neurol,* 6:94–100; Gordon HW (1983). Cognitive asymmetry in dyslexic families. *Neuropsychologica,* 18:645–656; Sano F (1918). James Henry Pullen: The Genius of Earlswood. *J Mental Sci,* 64:251–267; Rimland B (1978). The autistic savant. *Psychology Today,* August 69–80; Geschwind N and Galaburda A (1987), Chapters 7–9, in: *Cerebral Lateralization: Biological Mechanisms, Associations, and Pathology,* Cambridge, MIT Press.

31 *Left-brain language in isolation:* Moscavitch M and Olds J (1982). Asymmetrics in spontaneous facial expression and their possible relation to hemispheric specialization. *Neuropsychologie,* 20:71–82; Kaplan JA, et al (1990). The effects of right hemisphere damage on the pragmatic interpretation of conversational remarks. *Brain and Language,* 38:315–333; Ley RG and Bryden MP (1982). A dissociation of right and left hemispheric effects of recognition of emotional tone and verbal content. *Brain and Cognition,* 2:3–9.

31 *After ovulation, the right brain dominates:* Altemus M, et al (1989). Neuropsychological correlates of menstrual mood changes. *Psychosom Med,* 51:329–336; Sackeim HA, et al (1982). Hemispheric asymmetry in the expression of positive and negative emotions: Neurologic evidence. *Arch Neurol,* 39:210; Davidson R and Fox M (1983). Asymmetrical brain activity discriminates between positive and negative affective stimuli in human infants. *Science,* 218:1235–1237; Sackheim HA and Gur RC (1978). Lateral asymmetry in intensity of emotional expression. *Neuropsychologia,* 16:473.

33 *Women tend to have a keener sense than men:* Argyle M, Salter V, Nicholson H, Williams M, and Burgess P (1970). The communication of inferior and superior attitudes by verbal and non-verbal signals. *Br J Soc Clin Psychol,* 9:222–231; Hall J (1984). *Nonverbal Sex Differences,* Baltimore, Johns Hopkins; Kimura D (1999), *Sex and Cognition,* Cambridge, MA, MIT Press, p 89, Chapter 7, Perception.

34   *Testosterone and progesterone lower the immune system's ability:* Kimura D (1999). *Sex and Cognition,* Cambridge, MA, MIT Press, p 89, Chapter 7, *Perception;* Kimura D (1987). Are men's and women's brains really different? *Can Psychol,* 28(2):133–147.

34   *Women with excessively high estrogen and lower testosterone:* Delgado AR and Prieto G (1996). Sex differences in visuospatial ability. *Memory and Cognition,* 24(4):504–510.

34   *When androgen (testosterone) concentrations were higher:* Watson NV and Kimura D (1991). Non-trivial sex differences in throwing intercepting: Relation to psychometrically defined spatial functions. *Personality and Individual Differences,* 12:375–385; Galea LAM and Kimura D (1973). Sex differences and route learning. *Personality and Individual Differences,* 14:53–56; Beatty WW and Troster AI (1987). Gender differences in geographical knowledge. *Sex Roles,* 16:565–590.

37   *This skill can be seen today in women's:* Kimura D (1987). Are men's and women's brains really different? *Can Psychol,* 28(2):133–147; Delgado AR and Prieto G (1996). Sex differences in visuospatial ability. *Memory and Cognition,* 24(4):504–510; Watson NV and Kimura D (1991). Non-trivial sex differences in throwing intercepting: Relation to psychometrically defined spatial functions. *Personality and Individual Differences,* 12:375–385.

37   *Some have argued that women's advantage:* Hall JAY and Kimura D (1995). Sexual orientation and performance on sexually dimorphic motor tasks. *Archives of Sexual Behavior,* 24:395–407; Nicholson KG and Kimura D (1996). Sex differences for speech and manual skill. *Perceptual and Motor Skills,* 82:3–13.

37   *Scientists have found that men and women:* Delgado AR and Prieto G (1996). Sex differences in visuospatial ability. *Memory and Cognition,* 24(4):504–510.

38   *Perhaps traditional women's way of compensating:* Watson NV and Kimura D (1991). Non-trivial sex differences in throwing intercepting: Relation to psychometrically defined spatial functions. *Personality and Individual Differences,* 12:375–385; Galea LAM and Kimura D (1973). Sex differences and route learning. *Personality and Individual Differences,* 14:53–56; Beatty WW and Troster AI (1987). Sex differences in geographical knowledge. *Sex Roles,* 16:565–590.

38   *Today, for instance, if you can't find the ketchup:* Eals M and Silverman I (1994). The hunter-gatherer theory of spatial sex differences: Proximate factors mediating female advantage in recall of object arrays. *Ethology and Sociobiology,* 15:95–105; McBurney DH, Gawlin SJC, Devinin IT, and Adams C (1997). Spatial memory of women: Strong evidence for the gathering hypothesis. *Evolution and Human Behavior,* 18:165–174.

38   *Again, not all women and men are the same:* Ghent-Braine L (1961). Developmental changes in tactual thresholds on dominant and non-dominant sides. *J Comp Physiol Psych,* 54:670–673; Weinstein S and Sersen EA (1961). Tactual sensitivity as a function of handedness and laterality. *J Comp Physiol Psych,* 54:665–669.

38   *In contrast, premenstrually:* Vandenberg SG and Kuse AR (1978). Mental rotations, a group test of 3 dimensional spatial visualization. *Perception and Motor Skills,* 47:599–601.

40   *For some ADHD women at menopause:* Hampson E and Kimura D (1988). Reciprocal effects of hormonal fluctuations on human motor and perceptual-spatial skills. *Behavioral Neuroscience,* 102:456–459; Voeller KK (2001). ADHD as a Frontal Subcortical Disorder. In: Lichter D and Cummings DL, eds, *Frontal Subcortical Circuits in Psychiatric and Neural Disorders,* New York, Guilford Press.

41   *Women also have a more sensitive:* Ghent-Braine L (1961). Developmental changes in

tactual thresholds on dominant and non-dominant sides. *J Comp Physiol Psych*, 54:670–673; Weinstein S and Sersen EA (1961). Tactual sensitivity as a function of handedness and laterality. *J Comp Physiol Psych*, 54:665–669.

41 *so we have a lower threshold:* Rose RM, et al (1975). Consequences of social conflict on plasma testosterone levels in Rhesus monkeys. *Psychosom Med*, 37(1):50–61.

41 *Pain and any other uncomfortable body feeling:* Schulz ML (1998). *Awakening Intuition: Using Your Mind-Body Network for Insight and Healing.* New York, Crown.

Chapter Two

51 *When a woman's social status rises:* Mason JW (1968). Organization of psychoendocrine mechanisms. *Psychosom Med*, 30:565–580; Sade DS (1964). Seasonal cycle in size of testes of free ranging *Macaca malatta. Folia Primat*, 2:171–180; Gordon JP, et al (1973). Seasonal changes in sexual behavior and plasma testosterone levels of group living monkeys. *Am Zool*, 13:1267; Wild RA, et al (1985). Lipoprotein lipid concentrations and cardiovascular risk in women with polycystic ovary syndrome. *J Clin Endocrinol Metab*, 61:946; Coulan CB and Anneger JF (1982). Breast cancer and chronic anovulated syndrome. *Surgical Forum*, 33:474; Coulan CB, et al (1983). Chronic anovulation syndrome and associated neoplasia. *Obstet Gynecol*, 61:403; Krieg JC (1991). Eating disorders as assessed by cranial computerized tomography (CT). *J Adv Experi Med Biol*, 291:223–229.

51 *androgens that masculinize:* Naftolin F (1981). Understanding the basis of sex differences. *Science*, 211:1263–1264; Hazeltine FP and Ohno S (1981). Mechanism of gender differentiation. *Science*, 211:1272–1278

52 *women's degree of masculinization increased:* Twenge, JM (1997). Changes in masculine and feminine traits over time: A Meta-analysis. *Sex Roles*, 36(5–6):305–325.

52 *Some people erroneously generalize this finding:* Weisz J, et al (1982). Maternal stress decreases steroid armatase activity in brains of male and female rat fetuses. *Neuroendocrinology*, 35:374; Ward IL and Weisz J (1980). Maternal stress alters plasma testosterone in fetal males. *Science*, 207:328; Ward IL and Weisz J (1984). Differential effects of maternal stress on circulating levels of corticosterone, progesterone, and testosterone in male and female rat fetuses and their mothers. *Endocrinology*, 114:1635; Dorner G, et al (1980). Prenatal stress as possible etiologic factor of homosexuality in human males. *Endokrinologie*, 75:365; Ellis L, et al (1988). Sexual orientation of human offspring may be altered by severe maternal stress during pregnancy. *J Sex Res*, 25:152.

52 *Some but not all women whose brains were masculinized:* Baron-Cohen S, et al (2004). *Prenatal Testosterone in Mind: Amniotic Fluid Studies.* Cambridge, MIT Press, pp. 34–35.

52 *Scientists have shown that our femininity:* Hines M (2000). Gonadal hormones and sexual differentiation of human behavior: Effects on psychosexual and cognitive development. Chapter 14, in: *Sexual Differentiation in the Brain,* New York, CRC Press, pp. 266–267

52 *But hormones do shape our brains:* Stumf WE, et al (1976). The anatomical substrate of neuroendocrine regulation as defined by autoradiography with H-estradiol, [3H]testosterone, and [3H]progesterone. In: *Neuroendocrine Regulation of Fertility International Symposium,* Basel, Karger; Raisman G and Field PM (1971). Sexual dimorphism in the preoptic area of the rat. *Science*, 173:731–733.

53 *DES daughters have an increased frequency:* Hines M (1982). Prenatal gonadal

hormones and sex differences. *Psycho Bull,* 92:56–60; Nichols PL and Chen TC (1981). *Minimal brain dysfunction: A prospective study.* Hillsdale, NJ, Lawrence Erlbaum.

54 *Just as sex hormones administered to a pregnant woman:* Berenbaum SA and Hines M (1992). Early androgens are related to sex-typical toy preference. *Psychol Science,* 3:203–206; Leverani CH and Berenbaum SA (1998). Early androgen effects on interests in infants. *Developments in Neuropsychology,* 14:321–340.

55 *Environmental xenoestrogens may increase the incidence:* Gellert RG, et al (1978). Kepone, Mirex, Dieldrin, and Aldrin: Estrogenic activity and the induction of persistent vaginal estrus and anovulation in rats following neonatal treatment. *Environ Res,* 16:31; Kelce WR, et al (1995). Persistent DDT metabolite P_1P_1DDE is a potent androgen receptor antagonist. *Nature,* 375:581; Wong CI, et al (1995). Androgen receptor versus agonist activity of the fungicide Vinclozolin relative to hydroxyflutamine. *J Biol Chem,* 270:19998–20003; Fry D and Mandtoone CK (1991). DDT-induced feminization of gull embryos. *Science,* 213:922; Crews D, et al (1995). The role of estrogen in turtle sex determination and the effect of PCB's. *Environ Health Perspect,* 103(suppl 7):73; Korach KS, et al (1998). Estrogen receptor-binding activity of polychlorinated hydroxybiphenils. *Mol Pharmacol,* 33:120.

55 *Alcohol, cocaine, and monosodium glutamate (MSG):* Ohe E (1994). Effects of aromatase inhibitor on sexual differentiation for SON-POA in rats. *Acta Obstet Gynecol Japan,* 46:227; Dohler KP, et al (1984). Differentiation of the sexually dimorphic nucleus in the preoptic area of the rat brain is inhibited by postnatal treatment with an estrogen antagonist. *Neuroendocrinology,* 38:297; Ahmad II, et al (1991). Prenatal ethanol and the prepubital sexually dimorphic nuclei of the preoptical area. *Physiol Behav,* 79:427; Hsieh YL, et al (1997). The neonatal neurotoxicity of MSG in the sexually dimorphic nuclei of the preoptic area in rats. *Dev Neurosci,* 19:342.

57 *Hyperinsulinism and obesity increase the chances:* Wild RA, et al (1985). Lipoprotein lipid concentrations and cardiovascular risk in women with polycystic ovary syndrome. *J Clin Endocrinol Metab,* 61:946; Coulan CB and Anneger JF (1982). Breast cancer and chronic anovulated syndrome. *Surgical Forum,* 33:474; Coulan CB, et al (1983). Chronic anovulation syndrome and associated neoplasia. *Obstet Gynecol,* 61:403; Krieg JC (1991). Eating disorders as assessed by cranial computerized tomography (CT). *J Adv Experi Med Biol,* 291:223–229.

58 *Now, many scientists believe that:* Speroff L, et al. *Clinical Gynecologic Endocrinology and Infertility.* 4th Edition, Baltimore, Williams and Wilkins, pp. 220–225; Northrup C (1998). *Women's Bodies, Women's Wisdom.* New York, Bantam, pp. 220–224.

59 *So it's not surprising that CT brain scans:* Krieg JC (1991). Eating disorders as assessed by cranial computerized tomography (CT). *J Adv Experi Med Biol,* 291:223–229; Kornreich L, et al (1991). CT and MR evaluation of the brain in patients with anorexia nervosa. *Am J Neuroradiology,* 12(6):1213–1216; Hoffman GW, et al (1989). Cerebral atrophy in anorexia nervosa: A pilot study. *Biol Psychiatry,* 23(3)321–324; Wu JC, et al (1990). Greater left cerebral hemispheric metabolism in bulimia assessed by positron emission tomography. *Am J Psychiatry,* 147(3):309–312.

60 *To find out what style of brain you have for perception:* Vandenberg SG and Kuse AR (1978). Mental rotations, a group test of 3 dimensional spatial visualization. *Perception and Motor Skills,* 47:599–601; Silverman I and Eals M (1992). Sex differences in spatial abilities, evolutionary theory, and data. In JH Burkan, L

Cosmides, and J Tooby (eds), *The Adapted Mind.* New York, Oxford Press, pp. 533–549.

60   *Traditional women have been shown:* Baenninger M and Newcomb N (1989). The role of experience in spatial performance. *Sex Roles,* 20:327–344.

60   *Some have suggested that differences:* Feingold A (1988). Cognitive gender differences are disappearing. *American Psychologist,* 43:95–103; Masters MS and Sanders B (1993). Is the gender difference in mental rotation disappearing? *Behavior Genetics,* 23:337–341.

62   *Now look at Figure 3:* Osterrieth PA (1944). Le Test de copie d'une figure complexe. *Archives de Psychologie,* 30:206–356, translated by J Corwin and FW Bylsma (1993), *The Clinical Psychologist,* 7:9–15; Rey, A (1941). L'examen psychologique dans les d'encephalopathie traumatique. *Arch Psychol,* 28:112; Rey, A. (1970). *L'examen clinique en psychologie.* Presses Universitaires de France, Paris.

62   *This mirrors the order in which the brain:* Best CT, et al (1988). The emergence of cerebral asymmetries in early human development. In: *Brain Lateralization in Children.* DL Molfese, ed., New York, Guilford Press.

63   *This exercise gives you a good idea:* Kaplan E (1989). A process approach to neuropsychological assessment. In: *Clinical Neuropsychology and Brain Function* (pp. 125–168), Washington DC, American Psychological Association.

63   *Generally speaking, someone majoring:* Dabbs J (1980). Left-right differences in cerebral blood flow and cognition. *Psychophysiology,* 17:548–551.

Chapter Three

67   *Almost Famous;* TM & © 2001 Dreamworks LLC and Columbia Pictures Industry, Inc. All rights reserved. 100 Universal City Plaza, Universal City, CA 91608.

67   *Emotions have always been an issue for women:* Brody LR (1993). Understanding gender differences and expression of emotion. In: S Ablou et al, eds. *Human Feelings: Exploration and Affect, Development and Meaning,* pp. 89–122, Hillsdale, NJ, Analytic Press; Lennon R and Eisenberg N (1987). Gender and age differences in empathy and sympathy. In: N. Eisenberg and J. Strayers, eds. *Empathy and Its Development,* pp. 195–217, Cambridge, England, Cambridge University; Brody LR (1999). *Gender, Emotion and the Family,* Cambridge, MA, Cambridge University Press; Allen J and Halloun D (1976). Sex differences in emotionality: A multidimensional approach. *Human Relations,* 29:711–720; Scherer K, Walbott H, and Somerfield A (1986). *Experiencing Emotion: A Cross-Cultural Study.* Cambridge, England, Cambridge University Press; Fergusen TJ and Crowley S (1997). Gender differences in the organization of guilt and shame. *Sex Roles,* 37:19–44.

68   *Optimism and love enhance the immune system:* Shaver PR, et al (1996). Is love a "basic" emotion? *Personal Relationships,* 3:81–96; Panksepp J, et al (1998). The quest for long term health and happiness: To play or not to play. *Psychol Inquiry,* 9:56–66.

68   *These circuits in the brain and brain stem help:* Linehan M (1993). *Skills Training Manual for Treating Borderline Personality Disorder,* New York, Guilford Press, p. 143; Damasio AR (2000). Subcortical and cortical brain activity during the feeling of self-generated emotions. *Nature Neuroscience,* 3(10):1049–1056; Panksepp J (2000). Ch. 9, Emotions as natural kinds within the mammalian brain. In: *Handbook of Emotions,* 2nd ed., New York, Guilford Press; Scherer KR and Wallbutt HG (1994). Evidence for universality and cultural variation of differential emotional response patterning. *J Personal Soc Psych,* 26:310–328.

69 *The five basic emotions parallel:* Kaptchuk TJ (2000). *The Web that Has No Weaver,* Chicago, Contemporary Books, pp. 157–160.

69 *Emotional disharmony can induce:* Aron A and Aron E (1991). Love and sexuality. In K. McKinney and S Sprechter, eds. *Sexuality in Close Relationships,* Hillsdale, NJ, Erlbaum, pp. 25–48.

70 *Like fear, love makes your heart beat faster:* Damasio AR (2000). Subcortical and cortical brain activity during the feeling of self-generated emotions. *Nature Neuroscience,* 3(10):1049–1056.

70 *The neurochemical changes that love causes:* Shaver PR, et al (1996). Is love a "basic" emotion? *Personal Relationships,* 3:81–96; Panksepp J, et al (1998). The quest for long term health and happiness: To play or not to play. *Psychol Inquiry,* 9:56–66 Panksepp J, et al (1984). The psychology of play: Theoretical and methodological perspectives. *Neurosci and Biobehav Reviews,* 8:465–492; Aron A and Aron E (1991). Love and sexuality. In: K. McKinney and S Sprechter, eds. *Sexuality in Close Relationships,* Hillsdale, NJ, Erlbaum, pp. 25–48.

77 *Depression, irritability, anxiety, and panic:* National Institutes of Health Conference/NIH Pain Research Consortium (1998). "Gender and Pain: A Focus on How Pain Impacts Women Differently than Men." Bethesda, Maryland, April 7–8; Keogh E and Holdcroft A (2002). Sex differences in pain: Evolutionary links in facial pain expressions. *Behav Brain Sciences,* 25(4):465.

80 *The following medical intuitive reading:* All case studies in this book are "composite" histories of patients or medical intuitive clients. No case is an actual specific individual but a composite of many different individuals. If you're thinking you recognize yourself in this story, that's great, because you fit the prototype and hopefully the case study will help you understand something about your own emotions and health. However, no person described, Betty-Ann or anyone else, is an actual living individual.

85 *Neuronal pathways in the anger highway:* Traxler BG, et al (1977). The association of elevated plasma cortisol and early atherosclerosis as demonstrated by coronary angiography. *Atherosclerosis,* 26:151–162; Sklar LS and Arlsman H (1981). Stress and cancer. *Psychol Bulletin,* 89:369–406; Ironson G, et al (1992). Effects of anger on left ventricle ejection fraction in coronary artery disease. *Am J Cardiol,* 70: 281–285; Leventhal H and Patrick-Miller L (1993). Emotions and illness: The mind is in the body. In: M Lewis and JM Haviland, eds. *Handbook of Emotions,* New York, Guilford Press, pp. 365–379; Leventhal H and Patrick-Miller L (2000). Ch. 33, *Emotions and physical illness: Causes and indicators of vulnerability.* In: *Handbook of Emotions,* 2nd ed., New York, Guilford Press, pp. 523–537.

86 *Chronically elevated cortisol levels increase your risk:* Traxler BG, et al (1977). The association of elevated plasma cortisol and early atherosclerosis as demonstrated by coronary angiography. *Atherosclerosis,* 26:151–162; Sklar LS and Arlsman H (1981). Stress and cancer. *Psychol Bulletin,* 89:369–406; Ironson G, et al (1992). Effects of anger on left ventricle ejection fraction in coronary artery disease. *Am J Cardiol,* 70: 281–285; Leventhal H and Patrick-Miller L (1993). Emotions and illness: The mind is in the body. In: M Lewis and JM Haviland, eds. *Handbook of Emotions,* New York, Guilford Press, pp. 365–379; Leventhal H and Patrick-Miller L (2000). Ch. 33, *Emotions and physical illness: Causes and indicators of vulnerability.* In: *Handbook of Emotions,* 2nd ed., New York, Guilford Press, pp. 523–537.

86 *you do not get something you want:* Linehan M (1993). *Skills Training Manual for Treating Borderline Personality Disorder,* New York, Guilford Press, 143; Damasio AR

(2000). Subcortical and cortical brain activity during the feeling of self-generated emotions. *Nature Neuroscience,* 3(10):1049–1056; Panksepp J (2000). Ch. 9, Emotions as natural kinds within the mammalian brain. In: *Handbook of Emotions,* 2nd edition, New York, Guilford Press; Scherer KR and Wallbutt HG (1994). Evidence for universality and cultural variation of differential emotional response patterning. *J Personal Soc Psych,* 26:310–328.

86 *your point of view in a conflict can be right:* Linehan M (1993). *Skills Training Manual for Treating Borderline Personality Disorder,* New York, Guilford Press, p. 143; Damasio AR (2000). Subcortical and cortical brain activity during the feeling of self-generated emotions. *Nature Neuroscience,* 3(10):1049–1056; Panksepp J (2000). Ch. 9, Emotions as natural kinds within the mammalian brain. In: *Handbook of Emotions,* 2nd edition, New York, Guilford Press; Scherer KR and Wallbutt HG (1994). Evidence for universality and cultural variation of differential emotional response patterning. *J Personal Soc Psych,* 26:310–328.

88 *And if the emotions are neutralizing:* Plutnik R (1983). Emotion in early development: A psychological evolutionary approach. In: R Plutnic and H Kellerman, *Emotion: Theory, Research, and Experience,* Vol. 2, pp. 221–257, New York, Academic Press; Plutnik R (1980). *Emotion: A Psycho-evolutionary Synthesis.* New York, Harper and Row; Schulz ML (1998). *Awakening Intuition,* New York, Harmony/Crown.

91 *All emotions use the body as their theater:* Linehan M (1993). *Skills Training Manual for Treating Borderline Personality Disorder,* New York, Guilford Press, p. 143; Damasio AR (2000). Subcortical and cortical brain activity during the feeling of self-generated emotions. *Nature Neuroscience,* 3(10):1049–1056, Panksepp J (2000). Ch. 9, Emotions as natural kinds within the mammalian brain. In: *Handbook of Emotions,* 2nd edition, New York, Guilford Press; Scherer KR and Wallbutt HG (1994). Evidence for universality and cultural variation of differential emotional response patterning. *J Personal Soc Psych,* 26:310–328; Traxler BG, et al (1977). The association of elevated plasma cortisol and early atherosclerosis as demonstrated by coronary angiography. *Atherosclerosis,* 26:151–162; Sklar LS and Arlsman H (1981). Stress and cancer. *Psychol Bulletin,* 89:369–406; Ironson G, et al (1992). Effects of anger on left ventricle ejection fraction in coronary artery disease. *Am J Cardiol,* 70: 281–285; Leventhal H and Patrick-Miller L (1993). Emotions and illness: The mind is in the body. In: M Lewis and JM Haviland, eds. *Handbook of Emotions,* New York, Guilford Press, pp. 365–379; Leventhal H and Patrick-Miller L (2000). Ch. 33, *Emotions and physical illness: Causes and indicators of vulnerability.* In: *Handbook of Emotions,* 2nd ed., New York, Guilford Press, pp. 523–537.

Chapter Four

97 *depression occurs twice as often in women:* Kessler RC (2000). Gender differences in major depression. In Frank E, ed. *Gender and Its Effects in Psychopathology,* pp. 61–84, Washington, DC, APA Press, Garvey MJ and Tollefson OD (1984). Post-partum depression. *J Reprod Med,* 29:113–116; Rausch JL and Parry BL (1993). Treatment of premenstrual mood symptoms. *Psych Clin NA,* 16:829–839; Cullbery J (1972). Mood changes and menstrual symptoms with different gestagen/estrogen combinations. *Acta Psychiatr Scand,* 236:1–86; Janowsky DS, et al (1996). Association among ovarian hormones, other hormones, emotional disorders, and neurotransmitters. In: Jensvold MF, et al, *Psychopharmacology and Women: Sex, Gender, and Hormones,* Washington, DC, APA Press, pp. 85–106.

97   *That's right, 25 percent of all women:* Blazer DG, et al (1994). The prevalence and distribution of major depression in a national community sample: The National Co-morbidity Survey. *Am J Psychiatry,* 151:979–986.

100   *The sadness and anger brain circuit connections:* Ironson G, et al (1992). Effects of anger on left ventrical ejection fraction in coronary artery disease. *Am J Cardiol,* 70:281–285; Koskenhuo M, et al (1988). Hostility as a risk factor for mortality and ischemic heart disease in men. *Psychosom Med,* 50:163–164; Denollet J, et al (1996). Personality as independent predictor of long-term mortality in patients with coronary artery disease. *Lancet,* 347:417–421; Domar A, et al (1992). The prevalence and predictability of depression in infertile women. *Fertil and Sterility,* 58:1158–1163; Goodkin K, et al (1986). Stress and hopelessness in the promotion of cervical intraepithelial neoplasms in invasive squamous cell carcinoma of the cervix. *J Psychosom Res,* 30:67–76; Pinter EJ, et al (1967). The influence of emotional stress on fat mobilization: The role of endogenous catecholamine and ß-adrenergic receptors. *Am J Med Sci,* 254:634; Werkman SL and Greenberg SS (1967). Personality and interest patterns in obese adolescent girls. *Psychosom Med,* 29(1):72–78; Nerem RM, et al (1980). Social environment as a factor in diet-induced atherosclerosis. *Science,* 208(4451):1475–1476; Parkes CM, et al (1969). "Broken Heart." *Brit Med J,* 1:740; Mittleman MA, et al (1995). Triggering of acute MI onset by episodes of anger. *Circulation,* 92:1720–1725.

102   *Anger is usually easier for you to express and resolve:* Brady LR (1993). On understanding gender differences in the expression of emotions. In: S Ablou et al, eds. *Human Feelings,* Hillsdale, NJ, Analytic Press, pp. 89–121; Frost W and Averill J (1982). Differences between men and women in everyday experience of anger. In: J Averill, *Anger and Aggression,* New York, Springer Verlag, pp. 281–316; Coats EJ and Feldman RS (1996). Gender differences in non-verbal correlations of social status. *Personal Social Psychol Bull,* 22:1014–1022; Knudsen B (1996). Facial expression of emotion influence interpersonal trait inferences. *J of Non-Verbal Behav,* 20:165–182.

102   *In an extreme stuck case, the combined emotions:* Knudsen B (1996). Facial expression of emotion influence interpersonal trait inferences. *J of Non-Verbal Behav,* 20:165–182; MacAndrew FT (1986). A cross-cultural study of recognition thresholds for facial expression of emotion. *J of Cross-Cultural Psychol,* 17:211–224; Averill JR (1997). The emotions: An integrative approach. In: R Hogan, et al, *Handbook of Personal Psychology,* San Diego, CA, Academic Press, pp. 513–541.

105   *Yet in spite of the range of severity:* American Psychiatric Association (2000). *Diagnostic Criteria from DSM-IV-TR,* APA Press, Washington, DC.

107   *Without the maximal use of frontal lobe pathways:* Berman KF, et al (1997). Modulation of cognition-specific cortical specific activity by gonadal steroids: A positron-emission tomography study in women. *Proc Natl Acad Sci,* 94:8836–8841; Arpels JC (1996). The female brain hypoestrogenic continuum from premenstrual syndrome to menopause. *J Reprod Med,* 41:633–639; Schmidt PJ, et al (1998). Different behavioral effects of gonadal steroids in women with and in those without premenstrual syndrome. *N Eng J Med,* 338:209–216.

107   *PMS may exaggerate normal:* Sackheim H, et al (1982). Hemispheric asymmetry in the expression of positive and negative emotions, *Archiv Neurol,* 39:210–218; Bogousslausky J, et al (1988). The syndrome of unilateral tuberothalamic artery territory infarction. *Stroke,* 17:434–441; Cummings JL and Mendez MF (1984). Secondary mania with focal cerebrovascular lesions. *Am J Psychiatry,*

141:1084–1087; Mendez MF, et al (1989). Neurobehavioral changes associated with caudate lesions. *Neurology,* 39:349–354; Starkstein SE, et al (1987). Comparison of cortical and subcortical lesions in the production of post-stroke mood disorders. *Brain,* 110:1045–4059.

108 *So, the right-brain emotion of fear:* Anderson PA and Guerrero LK, eds. (1998). Ch. 1, Communication and emotion: Basic concepts and approaches, In: *Handbook of Communication and Emotion,* pp. 5–24. Boston, Academic Press.

109 *Its untreated mini-depressive episodes:* Herzog A (1997). Ch. 27, Neuroendocrinology of epilepsy. In: SC Schacter and O Devinsky, eds., *Behavioral Neurology: The Legacy of Norman Geschwind,* pp. 223–242, New York, Lippincott-Raven; Himmelhoch JM and Garfinkel ME (1986). Sources of L.CO₂ resistance in mixed mania. *Psychopharmacol Bull,* 22:613–620; Raleigh MJ, et al (1984). Social and environmental influences in blood serotonin concentrations in monkeys. *Archiv Gen Psychiatry,* 41:505–510; Depue RA and Spoont MR (1986). Conceptualizing a serotonin trait: A behavioral dimension of constraint. *Annals of NY Acad Sciences,* 487:47–62; Abplanalp J, et al (1979). Psychoendocrinology of the menstrual cycle. *Psychosom Med,* 41:605–615.

111 *The right temporal lobe, hypothesized to be critical:* Parkinson B, et al (1996). *Changing Moods: The Psychology of Mood and Mood Regulation.* New York, Longman.

112 *When your brain holds an emotion long enough:* Parkinson B, et al (1996). *Changing Moods: The Psychology of Mood and Mood Regulation.* New York, Longman; Davidson RJ, et al (2000). Human EEG. In: JT Cacioppo, et al, eds. *Principles of Psychophysiology,* 2nd edition, Cambridge, MA, Cambridge University Press; Channon S and Green PSS (1999). Executive function in depression, *J Neurol Neurosurg Psychiatry,* 66:162–171; Carter CS, et al (1998). Anterior cingulate cortex error detection and on-line monitoring of performance. *Science,* 280:747–749.

116 *She began to head bake sales and bazaars:* American Psychiatric Association (2000). *Diagnostic and Statistical Manual of Mental Disorders,* 4th edition, text revisions. Washington, DC, APA Press.

117 *Transient changes in levels of norepinephrine:* Devinsky O, et al (1995). The contribution of anterior cingulate to behavior. *Brain,* 118:297–306.

117 *Depressive brain changes are the opposite:* Damasio AR, et al (2000). Subcortical and cortical brain activity during the feeling of self-generated emotions. *Nature Neuroscience,* 3(10):1049–1056.

117 *It may also be key to:* Mayberg HS (1999). Reciprocal limbic-cortical function and negative mood: Converging PET findings in depression and normal sadness. *Am J Psychiatry,* 156(5):675–682.

117 *Interestingly, when a sad person's transient mood:* Lawrence AD and Grasby PM (2001). Ch. 10, The functional neuroanatomy of emotional disorders: Focus and depression and PTSD. In: G Gainotti, ed., *Handbook of Neuropsychology,* 2nd ed., vol. 5, *Emotional Behavior and Its Disorders,* New York, Elsevier; Raiche ME (1998). Behind the scenes of functional brain imaging. *Proc Natl Acad Sci USA,* 95:765–772; Mayberg HS (1997). Limbic-cortical dysregulation: A proposed model of depression. *J Neuropsychiatry and Clinical Neurosc,* 9:471–81.

117 *However, if the "sadness" brain circuit:* Lee JM, et al (1999). The changing landscape of ischemic brain injury. *Nature,* 399(suppl.):A7–A14

124 *Many women, like Brenda:* Siever LJ and Davis KL (1985). Overview: Toward a dysregulation hypothesis of depression. *Am J Psychiatry,* 142:1017–1031.

126 *Some people, however, can't escape:* Willner P (1997). Validity, reliability, and utility of

the chronic mild stress model of depression. *Psychopharmacology*, 134:319–329; Willner P, et al (1992). Chronic mild stress-induced anhedonia. *Neurosci Biobehav Rev*, 16:525–534; Meerlan P, DeBoer SF, et al (1996). Changes in daily rhythms of body temperature and activity after a single social defeat in rats. *Physiol Behav*, 59:735–739; Ladd CO, et al (2000). Long-term behavioral and neuroendocrine adaptation to adverse early experience. *Prog Brain Res*, 122:81–103; Shaffery I, et al (2003). The neurobiology of depression. *The Neuroscientist*, 9(1):82–98.

128   *Symptoms usually begin in the fall:* Boehnert CE and Alberts RA (2003). Seasonal affective disorder in women. *Women's Health in Primary Care*, 6(1):32–36; Rosenthal NE, et al (1984). Seasonal affective disorder: A description of the syndrome and preliminary finding with light therapy. *Arch Gen Psychiatry*, 41:72–80; American Psychiatric Association (2000). *Diagnostic and Statistical Manual of Mental Disorders*, 4th edition, text revisions. Washington, DC, APA Press, pp. 425–427.

128   *Women and men with this disorder:* Lingjaerde O, et al (1999). Characteristics of patients with otherwise typical winter depression, but with incomplete summer remission. *J Affect Disorder*, 53:91–94.

128   *The brain circuits for happiness, love, bonding, eating, and sex:* Most notably, the bed nucleus of the stria terminalis is anatomically different in women and men. The ventral medial nucleus of the hypothalamus and the preoptic areas are wired differently in men and women for eating food, craving love and sex. Becker JB, et al, eds. (1992). *Behavioral Endocrinology*, Cambridge, MA, MIT Press; Panksepp J (1998). *Affective Neuroscience: The Foundation of Human and Animal Emotion*, New York: Oxford University Press, pp. 125–320; Moss RL and Dudley CA (1984). The challenge of studying the behavioral effects of neuropeptides. In: LL Iversen, et al, eds. *Handbook of Psychopharmacology*, Vol. 18, pp. 397–454, New York, Plenum; Peterson CA, et al (1992). Oxytocin in maternal sexual and social behaviors. *Annals NY Acad Sci*, 652.

129   *The same neurotransmitters:* Panksepp J (1998). *Affective Neuroscience: The Foundation of Human and Animal Emotion*, New York: Oxford University Press, pp. 125–320.

129   *Testosterone is also critical for:* Aron A and Aron E (1991). Love and sexuality. In: K. McKinney and S Sprecher, eds. *Sexuality in Close Relationships*, Hillsdale, NJ, Erlbaum, pp. 25–48; Shaver, PR, et al (1996). Is love a basic emotion? *Personal Relationships*, 3:81–96.

133   *Authority figures in my life:* Post RM, et al (1982). Kindling and carbamazepine in affective illness. *J Nerv Mat Dis*, 170:717–731.

134   *I feel physically attractive:* Busco MR and Rush AJ (1998). *Cognitive Behavioral Therapy for Bipolar Disorder*, New York, Guilford Press.

141   *When your physical health changes:* Mesulam MM and Mufson EJ (1982). Insula of the old world monkey. III. Efferent cortical output and comments on function. *Journal of Comparative Neurology*, 212:38–52; Penfield W and Faulk ME (1955). The insula: Further observations on insula function. *Brain*, 78:445–470; Hoffman BL and Rasmussen T (1953). Stimulation studies of insular cortex of Macaca mulatta. *J Neurophysiol*, 16:343–351; Kalia M and Mesulam MM (1980). Brainstem projections of sensory and motor components of the vagus complex in the cat. *J Comp Neurol*, 193:435–466; Kalia M and Mesulam MM (1980). Brainstem projections of sensory and motor components of the vagus complex in the cat. *J Comp Neurol*, 193:467–508; Beckstead RM, et al (1980). The nucleus of the solitary tract in the monkey: Projections to the thalamus and brain stem nuclei. *J*

Comp Neurol, 190:259–282; Mufsun et al (1981). Insular interconnections with the amygdala in the rhesus monkey. *Neuroscience,* 6:1231–1248.

137 *Depending on your unique feminine brain wiring:* Oppenheimer SM, et al (1992). Cardiovascular effects of human insular cortex stimulation. *Neurology,* 42:1727–1732; Pool JL and Ransohoff J 1949. Autonomic effects on stimulating rostral portion of cingulate gyrus in man. *J Neurophysiol,* 12:385–392; Showers M and Lauer EW (1961). Somatovisceral motor patterns in the insula. *J Comp Neurol,* 117:107–116; Sugar O, et al (1948). A second motor cortex in the monkey (Macaca mulatta). *J Neuropath Exp Neurol,* 7:182–189; Henke PG (1982). The telencephalic limbic system and experimental gastric pathology. *Neurosci Biobehav Rev,* 6:381–390; Henke PG (1992). Stomach pathology and the amygdala. In: JP Aggleton, ed. *The amygdala,* New York: Wiley-Liss, pp. 324–338; Clause, RE and Custman PJ (1983). Psychiatric illness and contraction abnormalities of the esophagus. *New Eng J Med,* 309:1337–1342; Lown B, et al (1976). Basis for recurring ventricular fibrillation in the absence of coronary heart disease and its management. *New Eng J Med,* 294:623–629; Damasio AR (1995). On some functions of the human prefrontal cortex. *Ann NY Acad Sci,* 769:241–251; Ramirez-Amaya V, et al (1996). Insular cortex lesions impair the acquisition of conditional immunosuppression. *Brain Behav Immun,* 10:103–114; Rogers MP and Fozdar M (1996). Psychoneuroendocrinology of autoimmune disorders. *Adv Neuroimmunol,* 6:169–177; Mesulam MM (2000). Ch. 1, Behavioral Neuroanatomy: Large scale networks, associating cortex, frontal syndromes, the limbic system, and hemisphere specializations. In: *Principles of Behavioral and Cognitive Neurology,* 2nd ed., New York, Oxford University Press; Wall PD and Davis GD (1951). The cerebral cortex systems affecting autonomic function. *J Neurophysiol,* 14:508–517; Aziz Q, et al (1997). Identification of human brain loci processing esophageal sensation using positron emission tomography. *Gastroenterology,* 113:50–59; Willett CJ, et al (1986). Cortical projections to the nucleus of the tractus solitarius—An HRP study in the cat. *Brain Res Bul,* 16:497–505; Hull RE and Cornish K (1977). Role of the orbital cortex in cardiac dysfunction in anesthetized rhesus monkey. *Exp Neurol,* 56:289–297; Chapman WP, et al (1950). Effect upon blood pressure of electrical stimulation of tips of temporal lobes in man. *J Neurophysiol,* 13:65–71; Hoffman BL and Rasmussen J (1953). Stimulation studies of insular cortex of *Macaca mulatta. J Neurophysiol,* 16:343–351; Kaada BR, et al (1949). Respiratory and vascular responses in monkeys from temporal lobe, insula, orbital surface, and cingulate gyrus. *J Neurophysiol,* 12:348–356.

140 *Interestingly, the abnormalities weren't everywhere in her brain:* Thomas AJ, et al (2002). Ischemic basis for deep white matter intensities in major depression. *Arch Gen Psychiatry,* 59:785–792.

140 *doctors question whether depression causes:* Alexopoulos GS, et al (1997). Vascular depression hypothesis. *Arch Gen Psychiatry,* 54:915–922.

140 *On the other hand, depression causes:* Ford DE, et al (1998). Depression is a risk factor for coronary artery disease in men. *Arch Intern Med,* 158:1422–1426; Everson SA, et al (1998). Depressive symptoms and the increased risk of stroke mortality over a 29 year period. *Arch Intern Med,* 158:1133–1138; Jonas BS, et al (1997). Are symptoms of anxiety and depression risk factors for depression? *Arch Fam Med,* 6:43–49; Tracey KJ (2002). The inflammatory reflex. *Nature,* 420:853–859.

140 *Many treatments that successfully beat depression:* Coussens LM, and Werb Z (2002).

Inflammation and cancer. *Nature*, 420:860–867; Libby P (2002). Inflammation and atherosclerosis. *Nature*, 420:869–874; Hart BL (1988). Biological behavior of sick animals. *Neurosc Biobehav*, 12:123–137; Baumann H and Gaudia J (1994). The acute phase response. *Immunol Today*, 15:74–80; Kant S, et al (1992). Sickness behavior as a new target for drug development. *Trends Pharmacol Sci*, 13:24–28; Patterson P, et al, eds. (2000). *Neuroimmune Interactions and Neurologic and Psychiatric Disorders*, Berlin: Springer, pp. 79–88, 169–184; Reaver EM (1988). Lecture 1988. Role of insulin resistance in human disease. *Diabetes*, 37:1595–1607; Lustman PJ, et al (2000). Fluoxetine for depression in diabetes. *Diabetes Care*, 23:618–623; Maheux P, et al (1977). Fluoxetine improves insulin sensitivity in obese patients with NIDDM independent of weight loss. *Int J Obes Relat Metab Disord*, 21:97–102; Despres JP (1993). Abdominal obesity as an important component of insulin resistance syndrome. *Nutrition*, 9:452–459; Visser M, et al (1993). The effect of fluoxetine on body weight, body composition, and visceral fat accumulation. *Int J Obes Relat Metab Disord*, 17:247–253; Sehab J, et al (1993). Vitamin status and intake as primary determinants of homocysteinemia in an elderly population. *JAMA*, 270:2693–2698; Schub J (1999). Homocysteine metabolism. *Ann Rev Nutr*, 19:217–246; Suscovick DS, et al (1995). Dietary intake and cell membrane levels of long chain c-3 polyunsaturated fatty acids and the risk of primary cardiac arrest. *JAMA*, 274:1363–1367; Adams PB (1996). Arachidonic acid to eicosapentanoic acid ratio in blood correlates positively with clinical symptoms of depression. *Lipids*, 31(suppl):sup 157–161; Edwards R, et al (1998). Omega-3 polyunsaturated fatty acid levels in the diet and RBC membranes of depressed patients. *J Affect Disorder*, 48:149–155; Peet M, et al (1998). Depletion of omega-3 fatty acid levels in RBC membranes of depressive patients. *Biol Psychiatry*, 43:315–319; Bottiglier J, et al (2000). Homocysteine, folate, methylation, and monoamine metabolism in depression. *J Neurol Neurosurg*, Coppen A and Bailey J (2000). Enhancement of the antidepressant action of fluoxetine by folic acid. *J Affect Disorder*, 60:121–30; Fava M, et al (1977). Folate, vit. B$_{12}$, and homocysteine in major depressive disorder. *Am J Psychiatry*, 154:426–428.

Chapter Five

148   *Once your brain's mood brake is disengaged:* Soares C, et al (2001). Efficacy of estradiol for the treatment of depressive disorders in perimenopausal woman. *Arch Gen Psychiatry*, 58:529–534.

148   *So when you take an SSRI:* Klein P, et al (1999). Mood and menopause. *Brit J Ob-Gyn*, 106:1–4.

152   *In contrast, the older, less selective antidepressant:* Wagner KD (1996). Major depression and anxiety disorders associated with Norplant. *J Clin Psychiatry*, 57:152–157; Mayos AL, et al (1986). The effects of norethisterone and post-menopausal women on estrogen replacement. *Br J Obstet Gynecol*, 93:1290–1296; Sharriff S, et al (1995). Mood disorder in women with early breast cancer taking Tamoxifen, and estradiol receptor antagonist. *Ann NY Acad Sci*, 761:365–368; Love RR, et al (1991). Symptoms associated with Tamoxifen treatment in post-menopausal women. *Arch Inter Med*, 151:1842–1847; Roca CA, et al (2000). Effects of progestins on mood during hormone-replacement therapy. Abstracts of the *39th Annual Meeting of the American College of Neuropsychopharmacology*, San Juan, PR.

152   *depending upon the woman's irritability:* Writing Group for Women's Health

Investigators (2002). Risks vs. benefits of estrogen plus progestin in healthy post-menopausal women. *JAMA*, 288:321–333.

152   *Sure, 50 percent of the people:* Majewska MD, et al (1990). The neurosteroid DHEA is an allosteric antagonist of GABA, receptor. *Brain Research*, 526:143–146.

152   *Ten to 15 percent will show no improvement:* Morales AJ, et al (1994). Effects of replacement dose of DHEA in men and women of advancing age. *J Clin Endocrinol Metab*, 78:1360–1367.

152   *When a patient develops a supportive relationship:* Bloch M, et al (1999). DHEA treatment of midlife dysthymia. *Biol Psychiatry*, 45:1533–1541; Donnet KA and Brown, RP (1990). Cognitive effect of DHEA replacement therapy. In: Kalami MY, ed. *The Biological Role of DHEA,* New York, Walter de Gruyter, pp. 65–74; Wolkowitz O, et al (1999). Double blind treatment of DHEA. *Am J Psychiatry*, 156:646–649.

155   *For some women:* Roca CA, et al (2000). Effects of progestins on mood during hormone-replacement therapy. Abstracts of the *39th Annual Meeting of the American College of Neuropsychopharmacology,* San Juan, PR.

156   *Older But Very Potent Antidepressants:* Muller WE, et al (1997). Effects of hypericum extract on biochemical models of antidepressant activity. *Pharmacopsychiatry*, 30:102–107; Teufal-Mayer R, and Gleitz J (1997). Effects of long term administration of hypericum extracts in affinity and density of central $5HT_{1A}$, $5HT_{2A}$ receptors. *Pharmacopsychiatry*, 30:113–116; Graff A, et al (1997). St. John's wort, Hypericum perforatum, in: Upton R, ed. *American Herbal Pharmacopoeia and Therapeutic Compendium,* Santa Cruz, CA, American Herbal Pharmacopoeia; Kasper S (1997). The treatment of seasonal affective disorder with Hypericum extract. *J Geriatri Psychiatry Neurol*, 7(suppl 1):sup29–sup33.

158   *In 1997, there were 8,986 reported adverse side effects:* Braun RP and Gerbary PL (2000). Ch. 1, Interactive psychopharmacology, in: PR Muskin, ed. *Complementary and Alternative Medicine and Psychiatry,* Washington, DC, APA Press.

158   *Constant paranoia isn't good for your mood:* Braun RP and Gerbary PL (2000). Ch. 1: Interactive Psychopharmacology, in: PR Muskin, ed. *Complementary and Alternative Medicine and Psychiatry,* Washington, DC, APA Press.

158   *Higher doses of St. John's wort:* Vorbach EU, et al (1997). Efficacy and tolerability of St. John's wort extract LI 160 vs. Imipramine in patients with severe repressive episodes according to ICD-10. *Pharmacopsychiatry*, 10:81–85; Gaster B and Holroy IJ (2000). St. John's wort for depression. *Arch Intern Med*, 160:152–156; Linde K, et al (1996). St. John's wort for depression: An overview and metaanalysis for randomized clinical trials. *BMJ*, 313: 253–258.

158   *Sometimes, at higher dose levels:* Hyman SE et al (1995). Ch. 3, Antidepressant drugs. In: *Handbook of Psychiatric Drug Therapy*, 3rd edition, Boston, Little Brown; DeMott K (1998). St. John's wort tied to serotonin syndrome. *Clin Psychiatry News,* March 1998, p. 28; LeCrubier Y, et al (2002). Efficacy of St. John's wort extract WS 5570 in major depression: A double-blind, placebo-controlled trial. *Am J Psychiatry*, 159:1361–1366; DeSmet PAGM and Nolan WA (1996). St. John's wort as an antidepressant. *BMJ*, 313:241–242; Kendrick T (1997). Meta-analysis Hypericum extracts (St. John's wort) are effective in depression. *Evidence-Based Med,* 2:24.

159   *If you take St. John's wort with another SSRI:* Piscatelli SC, et al (2000). Indinivir concentration and St. John's wort. *Lancet,* 355:547–548.

159   *St. John's wort can alter the blood levels:* Miller, LG (1998). Herbal medicinals: Selected

clinical considerations, focusing on known or potential drug–herb interactions. *Arch Intern Med,* 158:2200–11.

159   *Serotonin is synthesized:* Hyman SE and Nestler EJ (1993). Ch. 3, "Overview of neuropsychopharmacology." In: *The Molecular Foundations of Psychiatry,* Washington DC, APA Press, pp. 80–83.

159   *Good sources of tryptophan:* Murray MD (1998). *5-HTP: The Natural Way to Overcome Depression, Obesity, and Insomnia,* New York, Bantam Books, pp. 22–33.

160   *Taking six grams of tryptophan alone:* McGrath RF, et al (1990). The effect of L-tryptophan on seasonal affective disorder. *J Clin Psychiatry,* 51:162–163.

160   *Improvements were made in the production:* Kilborne EM, et al (1996). Tryptophan produced by Shana Denko and epidemic eosinophilia-myalgia syndrome. *J Rheumatology,* 46 (suppl):81–88; Belongia EA, et al (1990). An investigation of the cause of eosinophilia–myalgia syndrome associated with tryptophan use. *New Eng J Med,* 323:357–365.

161   *Some sources say that:* Murray MD (1998). *5-HTP: The Natural Way to Overcome Depression, Obesity, and Insomnia,* New York, Bantam, pp. 31–34.

161   *5-HTP also raises levels:* Van Praag HM and Lemus C (1986). Monoamine precursors in the treatment of psychiatric disorders. In: RJ Wurtman and JJ Wurtman, eds. *Nutrition and the Brain,* Vol. 7, New York, Raven.

161   *5-HTP is rapidly taken up:* Miyakoshi N, et al (1974). Distribution and metabolism of L 5-hydroxy-tryptophan-^{14}C in cat brain after intravenous administration. *Japanese J of Pharmacol,* 24:1424.

161   *5-HTP has also been helpful:* Byerley WF (1987). 5HTP: A review of its antidepressant efficacy and adverse effects. *J of Clin Psychopharm,* 7:127–137; van Hiele JJ (1980). L-5-hydroxytryptophan in depression: The first substitution therapy in psychiatry. *Neuropsychology,* 6:230–240; Goldblum DS, et al (1996). The hormonal response to IV-5HTP in bulimia nervosa. *J of Psychosom Research,* 40(3):289–297; Zarcone VP and Hoddes E (1975). Effects of 5-HTP in fragmentation of REM sleep in alcoholics. *Am J of Psychiatry,* 132(1):74–76; Guilleminault C, et al (1973). Effects of 5-HTP on sleep of a patient with a brain stem lesion. *Electroenceph Clin Neurophysiol,* 34:177–184; deBenedittis G and Massei R (1985). Serotonin precursors in chronic primary headache. *J Neurosurg Science,* 29:239–248; Titus F, et al (1986). 5-HTP vs. methysergide in the prophylaxis of migraine. *Eur Neurol,* 25:327–329; van Prang HM (1981). Management of depression with serotonin precursors. *Biol Psychiatry,* 16:291–310; Mendlewicz J and Youdin MB (1980). Antidepressant potentiation of 5-HTP by L-deprenil in affective illness. *J of Affective Disorders,* 2:137–146; Puttini PS and Carusi I (1992). Primary fibromyalgia syndrome and 5-HTP. *J Int Med Res,* 20(2):182–189; Canglano C, et al (1992). Eating behavior and adherence to dietary prescriptions in obese adult subjects treated with 5-HTP. *Am J Clin Nutrition,* 56(5):863–867.

161   *Gingko Biloba (240 mg/day) is an herbal supplement:* Ramassamy C, et al (1992). The ginkgo biloba extract EGL.761 increase synaptosomal uptake of 5-hydroxytryptamine. *J Pharm Pharmacol,* 44(11):943–945.

161   *it may also interrupt the domino effect:* Sheline YI, et al (1996). Hippocampal atrophy in recurrent major depression. *Proc Natl Acad Sci USA,* 93(9):3908–3913; DeKloat ER, et al (1999). Stress and cognition: Are corticosteroids good or bad guys? *Trends Neurosci,* 22(10):422–426.

161   *Gingko biloba has a similar mechanism:* Cohen AJ and Bartlik B (1998). Ginkgo

biloba for antidepressant-induced sexual dysfunction. *J Sex Marital Therapy,* 24:139–143.

161 *Women who took this supplement:* Cohen AJ and Bartlik B (1998). Ginkgo biloba for antidepressant-induced sexual dysfunction. *J Sex Marital Therapy,* 24:139–143; Lavoisier P, et al (1995). Clitoral blood flow increases after vaginal pressure stimulation. *Arch Sex Behavior,* 24(1):37–45; Rajfer J, et al (1992). Nitric oxide as a mediator of relaxation of corpus cavernosum in response to non-adrenergic, non-cholinergic neurotransmitters. *New Eng J Med,* 326:90–94.

162 *Studies suggest that all blood thinners:* Voelker R (1999). Herbs and anesthesia. *JAMA,* 281:1882.

162 *Siberian ginseng (625 mg 2x/day):* Itoh T, et al (1989). Effects of Panax ginseng root in the vertical and horizontal motor activities and on brain monoamine-related substances in mice. *Planta Med,* 55(5):429–33.

162 *This type of ginseng:* Wang A, et al (1995). Effects of Chinese ginseng root, stem, leaf saponins on learning, memory, and biogenic monoamines in the brain of rats. *Chung Kyo Chung Tao Tsa Chih,* 20(8):493.

162 *Like gingko biloba, Siberian ginseng:* Kim HS, et al (1992). Antagonism of 4–50, 488H-induced antinocioception by ginseng total saponins is dependent on serotonin mechanisms. *Pharmacol Biochem Behav,* 42(4):587–593; Koi SR, et al (1996). Comparative study on the essential oil components of panax species. *Korean J Ginseng Sci,* 20:42–48.

163 *Ginseng also inhibits:* Kim DH et al (1998). Inhibition of stress-induced plasma corticosteroid levels by ginsenosides in mice. *Neuro-Report,* 9(10):2261–2264.

163 *Since it has mild stimulating qualities:* Vogler BK, et al (1999). The efficacy of ginseng: A systematic review of randomized trials. *Eur J Clin Pharmacol,* 55:567–575.

163 *If you are taking other sedative or stimulant medicines:* Brinker F (1998). *Herb Contraindications and Drug Interactions,* 2nd edition, Sandy, OR, Eclectic Medical Publications.

164 *The next week, you add a pill:* Agnoli A, et al (1976). Effect of SAMe upon depressive symptoms. *J Psychiatr Res,* 13:43–54; Fava M, et al (1990). Neuroendocrine effects of SAMe; a novel putative antidepressant. *J Psychiatr Res,* 24:177–184; Otero-Losadai MD and Rubio MC (1989). Active changes in serotonin metabolism after SAMe administration. *Gen Pharmacol,* 20:403–406; Bottiglieri T (1997). SAMe Neuropharmacology. *Expert Opinion on Investigational Drugs,* 6:417–426; Reynolds EH, et al (1987). Transmethylation and neuropsychiatry in biochemical, pharmacological clinical aspects of transmethylation. *Cell Biol Reviews,* 2:93–100; Bell KM, et al (1994). SAMe plasma levels in major depression and changes with drug treatment. *Act Neurol Scand,* 154:15–18; Salmaggi P, et al (1993). Double-blind, placebo-controlled study of SAMe in depressed post-menopausal women. *Psychother Psychosom,* 59:34–40; Bressa GM (1994). SAMe as an antidepressant: Meta-analysis of clinical studies. *Acta Neurol Scand Suppl,* 154:7–18; Cerutti R, et al (1993). Psychological stress during puerperium: A novel treatment approach using SAMe. *Current Therapeutic Res Clin and Experimental,* 53:707–716; Rosenbaum JF, et al (1990). The antidepressant potential of oral SAMe. *Acta Psychiatr Scand,* 81:432–436; Janicak PG, et al (1988). SAMe in depression: A literature review and preliminary report. *Ala J Med Sci,* 25:306–313; Bell KM, et al (1988). SAMe treatment of depression: A controlled clinical trial. *Am J Psychiatry,* 145:1110–1114; Fava M, et al (1995).

Rapidity of onset of antidepressant effect of parenteral SAMe. *Psychiatry Res,* 56:295–297.

164 *People with bipolar/manic depressive illness:* Criconia AM, et al (1994). Results of treatment with SAMe in patients with major depression and internal illnesses. *Current Therapy Research Clin Experimental,* 55:686–674; DeVanna M and Rigamonti R (1992). Oral SAMe in depression. *Curr Ther Res Clin Experimental,* 52:478–485; Berlanga C, et al (1992). Efficacy of SAMe in speeding onset of action of Imipramine. *J Psychiatr Res,* 44:257–262; Benedetto P, et al (1993). Clinical evaluation of SAMe vs. transient electrical nerve stimulation in primary fibromyalgia. *Current Therapy Research Clin Experimental,* 53:222–229; Grassetto M and Varitto E (1994). Primary fibromyalgia is responsive to SAMe. *Current Therapy Research Clin Experimental,* 55:797–806; Volkmann H, et al (1997). Double blind, placebo-controlled crossover study: IV SAMe in patients with fibromyalgia. *Scand J Rheumatol,* 26:206–211; Berger R and Nowak H (1987). New medical treatment of osteoarthritis. *Am J Med,* 83:84–88; Di Padova C (1987). SAMe in the treatment of osteoarthritis. *Am J Med,* 83:60–65; Brown RP and Gerbary PL (2000). Ch 1, Integrative psychopharmacology: A practiced approach to the herbs and nutrients in psychiatry. In: PR Muskin, ed., *Complementary and Alternative Medicine and Psychiatry,* Washington, DC, APA Press.

165 *No other medicine could prevent:* Schulz ML (1998). *Awakening Intuition: Using Your Mind-Body Network for Insight and Healing.* New York, Crown Publishing.

166 *There is evidence that medicines and supplements:* Kapur S and Mann JJ (1992). Role of dopaminergic system. *Biol Psychiatry,* 32:1–17; Beyer P and Lecrubier Y (1996). Atypical antipsychotic drugs in dysthymia. *European Psychiatry,* 11(sup 3):135sup–140sup; Klimek V, et al (2002). Dopaminergic abnormalities in amygdaloid nuclei in major depression. *Biol Psychiatry,* 52:740–748; Simonson M (1985). Letter. *J Clin Psychiatry,* 46(8):355; Beckman H, et al (1979). DL Phenylalanine vs Imipramine: A double-blind controlled trial. *Arch Psychiatr Nervenke,* 227(1):49–58.

166 *PEA and phenylalanine may also help:* Kitada T, et al (1990). Studies on the enhanced effect of acupuncture analgesia and acupuncture anesthesia by D-phenylalanine (2nd report)—schedule of administration and clinical effects in low back pain and tooth extraction. *Acupunct Electrother Res,* 15(2):121–135; Walsh NE, et al (1986). Analgesic effectiveness of D-phenylalanine in chronic pain patients. *Arch Phys Med Rehabil,* 67(7):436–439; Mitchell MJ, et al (1987). Effect of L-tryptophan and phenylalanine on burning pain threshold. *Phys Ther,* 67(2):203–205.

167 *You can get the same or similar effect:* Spatz H and Spatz N (1978). Urinary and brain phenylethylamine levels under normal and pathological conditions. In: Mosnaim and Wolf, eds. *Noncatecholic Phenylethylamines,* Part I, New York, Marcel Dekker, pp. 447–474; Beckmann H (1983). Phenylalanine in affective disorders. *Adv Biol Psychiatry,* 10:137–147.

167 *For some, chocolate use:* Weil A and Rosen W (1993). *From Chocolate to Morphine: Everything You Need to Know About Mind-Altering Drugs.* Boston, Houghton-Mifflin, pp. 43–44.

167 *Folic acid and vitamin B_{12} help convert:* Abou-Saleh MT and Coppen A (1986). The biology of folate in depression. *J Psychiatr Res,* 20(2):91–101; Shorvon SD, et al (1980). The neuropsychiatry of megaloblastic anemia. *Br Med J,* 281:1036–1042; Godfrey PSA, et al (1990). Enhancement of recovery from psychiatric illness by methylfolate. *Lancet,* 336:392–95; Bell I, et al (1990). Vit B_{12} and folate status in

acute geropsychiatric inpatients. *Biol Psychiatry,* 27(2):125–137; Coppen A (1967). The biochemistry of affective disorders. *Br J Psychiatry,* 113:1237–1264.

167 *Women on "the Pill":* Adams PW, et al (1974). Vit B$_6$, depression, and oral contraception. Letter, *Lancet,* 3:516–517; Sterner RT and Price WR (1973). Restricted riboflavin. *Am J Clin Nutr,* 26:150–160; Carney MW, et al (1982). Thiamine, riboflavin, and pyridoxine deficiency in psychiatric in-patients. *Br J Psychiatry,* 141:271–272.

167 *Low folic acid levels:* Fava M, et al (1997). Folate, vitamin B$_{12}$, and homocysteine in major depressive disorder. *Am J Psychiatry,* 154(3):426–428.

167 *Low and high blood levels of calcium and magnesium:* Lindner J, et al (1989). Calcium and magnesium concentrations in affective disorder. *Psychiatr Scand,* 80:527–537; Bowden CL, et al (1988). Calcium function in affective disorders and healthy controls. *Biol Psychiatry,* 23(4):367–376; Hall RC and Joffe JR (1973). Hypomagnesemia: Physical and psychiatric symptoms. *JAMA,* 224(13): 1749–1751; Frizel D, et al (1969). Plasma calcium and magnesium in depression. *Br J Psychiatry,* 115:1375–1377.

168 *These neuroprotective agents:* Sapolski RM (2003). Neuroprotective gene therapy against neurological insults. *Neuroscience Reviews,* 4:61; Lee JM, et al (1999). The changing landscape of ischemic brain injury mechanisms. *Nature,* 399(suppl):A7–A14.

171 *but studies suggest that people who have problems with anger:* Peet M, et al (1998). Depletion of omega-3 fatty acid levels in red blood cell membranes of depressive patients. *Biol Psychiatry,* 43:315–319; Maes M (1998). Fatty acids, cytokines, and major depression. *Biol Psychiatry,* 42:313–314.

171 *Omega-3 fatty acids and DHA:* Stoll AL (1999). Omega-3 fatty acids in bipolar disease. *Arch Gen Psychiatry,* 56:407–412.

171 *Studies report few side effects to:* Ariza-Ariza R, et al (1998). Omega-3 fatty acids in rheumatoid arthritis. *Semin Arthritis Rheum,* 27:366–370; Belluzi A, et al (1996). Effects of enteric coated fish oil preparation on relapses in Crohn's disease. *New Eng J Med,* 334:1557–1560; Curtis CL, et al (2000). Omega-3 fatty acids specifically modulate catabolic factors involved in articular cartilage degradation. *J Biol Chem,* 275:721–724; Grapinski JP, et al (1993). Preventing restenosis with fish oil following coronary angioplasty. *Arch Intern Med,* 153:1595–1601.

171 *The other available options:* Stevens LJ, et al (1995). Essential fatty acid metabolism in boys with ADHD. *Am J Clin Nutrition,* 62:761–768; Crawford MA, et al (1993). Nutrition and neurodevelopmental disorders. *Nutrition and Health,* 9:81–97; Jensen, et al (1996). Biochemical effects of dietary linoleic/alpha-linolenic acid ratio in term infants. *Lipids,* 31:107–113; Mellerup ET, and Plenga P (1988). Imipramine binding in depression and other psychiatric conditions. *Acta Psychiatric Scand,* 78(supp 345):61–68; Ellis PM and Salmoud C (1999). Is platelet imipramine binding decreased in depression? *Biol Psychiatry,* 36:292–299; Simopoulos AP (1991). Omega-3 fatty acids in health and disease and in growth and development. *Am J Clin Nutr,* 54:438–463; Hibbeln JR, et al (1989). Are disturbances in lipid-protein interactions by phospholipas-A$_2$ a predisposing factor in affective illness? *Biol Psychiatry,* 25:945–961; Hibbeln JR and Salem N (1995). Dietary polyunsaturated fatty acids and depression: When cholesterol does not satisfy. *Am J Clin Nutr,* 62:1–9; Schubert DS (1993). Depression in multiple sclerosis: A meta-analysis. *Psychosomatics,* 34(2):124–130;

Gersh B, et al (1965). Alteration in myelin fatty acids and plasmalignan in multiple sclerosis. *Ann Nat Acad Sci,* 405–407.

171 *Omega-6 fatty acids:* Miller LG (1998). Herbal medicinals: Selected clinical consideration focusing on known and potential drug-herb interactions. *Arch Intern Med,* 158:2200–2211.

172 *Since a higher ratio of omega-6 fatty acids:* Hibbeln JR (1998). Fish consumption and major depression. *Lancet,* 351:1213; Maes M, et al (1996). Fatty acid composition in major depression. *J Affect Dis,* 38:35–46; Adams PB, et al (1996). Arachidonic acid to eicosapentanoic acid ratio in blood correlates positively with clinical symptoms in depression. *Lipids,* 31(suppl): sup157–supl61; Weidner G, et al (1992). Improvements in hostility and depression in relation to dietary change and cholesterol lowering. *Ann Intern Med,* 117(10):820–825.

172 *In combination with lithium:* Stoll AL, et al (1996). Omega fatty acid in bipolar disorder: A preliminary double-blind, placebo-controlled trial. *Arch Gen Psychiatry,* 56:407–412; Stoll AL, et al (1996). Choline in the treatment of rapid-cycling bipolar disorder: Clinical and neurochemical finding in lithium-treated patients. *Biol Psychiatry,* 40:382–388.

172 *This may strengthen the membrane:* Cohen BM, et al (1982). Lecithin in the treatment of mania: Double-blind, placebo-controlled trials. *Am J Psychiatry,* 139:1162–1164.

172 *Lecithin may also be helpful:* Schreier HA (1982). Mania responsive to Lecithin in a 13 year old girl. *Am J Psychiatry,* 139:108–110; Cohen BM, et al (1980). Lecithin in mania: A preliminary report. *Am J Psychiatry,* 137:242–243.

172 *It is important to take:* Tamminga C, et al (1976). Depression associated with oral choline. Letter, *Lancet,* ii: 905.

172 *Inositol:* Benjamin J, et al (1995). Inositol treatment in psychiatry. *Psychopharmacol Bull,* 31(1):167–175.

172 *Inositol has successfully treated:* Levine J, et al (1995). Double-blind, controlled trial of Inositol treatment of depression. *Am J Psychiatry,* 152(5):792–794.

172 *It may also improve cognitive disorders:* Fux M, et al (1996). Inositol treatment of obsessive-compulsive disorder. *Am J Psychiatry,* 153(9):1219–1221; Barak Y, et al (1996). Inositol treatment of Alzheimer's disease. *Prog Neuropsychopharmacol Biol Psychiatry,* 20(4):729–735.

172 *Too little or too much progesterone:* Rubinow DR, et al (1998). Estrogen serotonin interactions: Implications for affective regulation. *Biol Psychiatry,* 44:839–850; Duman RS, et al (1997). A molecular and cellular theory of depression. *Arch Gen Psychiatry,* 54:597–606; McEwen BS, et al (1984). Towards a neurochemical basis of steroid hormone action. In: C Martin, ed. pp. 1153–1176, *Frontiers of Neuroendocrinology,* New York, Raven Press.

173 *For women whose estrogen drops suddenly:* Bloch M, et al (2000). Effects of gonadal steroids in women with a history of post-partum depression. *Am J Psychiatry,* 157:824–830; Sichel DA, et al (1995). Prophylactic estrogen in recurrent post-partum affective disorder. *Biol Psychiatry,* 38:814–818; Gregoire AJ, et al (1996). Transdermal estrogen for the treatment of severe post-natal depression. *Lancet,* 347:930–933.

173 *However, they must also take progesterone:* Bernardi M, et al (1989). Influence of ovariectomy, estradiol, and progesterone on the behavior of mice in an experimental model of depression. *Physiol Behavior,* 45:1067–1068.

173 *Some women with PMS:* Ganger K, et al (1989). Symptoms of estrogen deficiency

associated with supraphysiologic plasma estradiol concentrations in women with estradiol. *Br Med J,* 299:601–602.

173 *For women who are perimenopausal:* Soares C, et al (2001). Efficacy of estradiol for the treatment of depressive disorders in permimenopausal women. *Arch Gen Psychiatry,* 58:529–534; Klein P, et al (1999). Mood and menopause, *Brit J Ob-Gyn,* 106:1–4.

173 *Synthetic progesterone:* Wagner KD (1996). Major depression and anxiety disorders associated with Norplant. *J Clin Psychiatry,* 57:152–157; Mayos AL, et al (1986). The effects of norethisterone and post-menopausal women on estrogen replacement. *Brit J Ob-Gyn,* 93:1290–1296.

173 *Tamoxifen and other SERMs:* Sharriff S, et al (1995). Mood disorder in women with early breast cancer taking Tamoxifen, and estradiol receptor antagonist. *Ann NY Acad Sci,* 761:365–368.

174 *If you have had serious irritability and depression:* Love RR, et al (1991). Symptoms associated with Tamoxifen treatment in post-menopausal women. *Arch Inter Med,* 151:1842–1847; Roca CA, et al (2000). Effects of progestins on mood during hormone-replacement therapy. Abstracts of the *39th Annual Meeting of the American College of Neuropsychopharmacology,* San Juan, PR.

174 *The Women's Health Initiative:* Writing Group for Women's Health Investigators (2002). Risks vs. benefits of estrogen plus progestin in healthy post-menopausal women. *JAMA,* 288:321–333.

175 *After DHEA treatment some women:* Donnet KA and Brown RP (1990). Cognitive effect of DHEA replacement therapy. In MY Kalami, ed. *The Biological Role of DHEA,* pp. 65–74, New York, Walter de Gruyter.

175 *Some studies suggest:* Majewska MD, et al (1990). The neurosteroid DHEA is an allosteric antagonist of GABA$_A$ receptor. *Brain Research,* 526:143–146; Morales AJ, et al (1994). Effects of replacement dose of DHEA in men and women of advancing age. *J Clin Endocrinol Metab,* 78:1360–1367; Bloch M, et al (1999). DHEA treatment of midlife dysthymia. *Biol Psychiatry,* 45:1533–1541.

175 *If your depression occurs:* Wolkowitz O, et al (1999). Double blind treatment of DHEA. *Am J Psychiatry,* 156:646–649.

176 *Doses begin at 1–2 milligrams:* Bartlik B, et al (1999). The combined use of sex treatment and testosterone replacement for women. *Psychiatric Annals,* 29:27–33; Northrup, C (2003). *The Wisdom of Menopause.* New York, Bantam, pp. 282–283; Rako S (1999). Testosterone deficiency and supplementation for women: Matters of sexuality and health. *Psychiatric Annals,* 29:23–26; Sarrel P, et al (1998). Estrogen and estrogen-androgen replacement in post-menopausal women dissatisfied with estrogen only therapy. *J Reprod Med,* 43(10):847–856.

176 *After high levels of DHEA:* Mortola SF and Yen SSC (1990). The effect of oral DHEA on endocrine metabolic parameters in post-menopausal women. *J Clin Endocrinol Metab,* 71:696–704; Baulieu EE (1996). DHEA: A fountain of youth. *J Clin Endocrinol Metab,* 81:3147–3151; Rubinow DR and Schmidt PJ (1996). Premenstrual syndrome. *Endocrinologist,* 2:47–54.

176 *Since hypothyroidism and depression:* Massondi MS (1985). Prevalence of thyroid antibodies among healthy middle-aged women. *Ann Epidemiol,* 5(3):229–233; Arem R (1999). *The Thyroid Solution,* New York, Ballantine Books.

176 *Studies don't agree:* Arem R (1999). *The Thyroid Solution,* New York, Ballantine Books.

177 *Frequently, antidepressant therapy:* Reed K and Bland RC (1977). Myxedema madness. *Acta Psychiatr Scand,* 56:421–426; Tachman ML and Guthrie GP (1984). Hypothyroidism: Diversity of presentation. *Endocr Rev,* 5:456–465.

177 *Combinations of T₄ (Synthroid) and T₃ (Cytomel):* T₃ may have different effects on brain function than T₄. Bunevicious R, et al (1999). Effects of thyroxine (T_4) as compared with thyroxine plus triodothyronine (T_3) in patients with hypothyroidism. *New Eng J Med,* 340:424–429.

177 *The depression associated with:* Haggerty JJ, et al (1990). Subclinical hypothyroidism: A review of neuropsychiatric aspects. *Int J Psychiatry Med,* 20:193–208.

177 *Even if a woman's blood test:* Targum SD, et al (1984). Thyroid hormone and the TRH stimulation test in refractory depression. *J Clin Psychiatry,* 45:345–347; Hyman SE, et al (1995). Ch. 3: Antidepressant drugs, pp. 55–67. In: SE Heyman, et al, eds. *Handbook of Psychiatric Drug Therapy,* Boston, Little Brown.

177 T_3, 25–75 milligrams a day can "augment": Studies suggest that 50–60% of patients benefit from this approach. Esposito S, et al (1997). The thyroid axis and mood disorders. *Psychopharmacol Bull,* 33:205–217; Joffee RT, et al (1993). A placebo controlled comparison of lithium and T₃ augmentation of tricyclic antidepressants in unipolar refractory depression. *Arch Gen Psychiatry,* 50:387–393.

177 *Interestingly, adding thyroid hormone:* Gittlin MJ, et al (1987). Failure of T₃ to potentiate tricyclic antidepressant response. *J Affective Disorders,* 13:267–272.

177 *Neuroscientists believe that:* Joffe R (2002). Ch. 82: Hypothalamic pituitary thyroid axis, p. 873. In: *Hormones, Brain, and Behavior,* Vol. 4, New York, Elsevier Science.

178 *Side effects can include:* Hoberg E, et al (2000). Quantitative high performance liquid chromatographic analysis of diterpenoids in agni-casti fructus. *Planta Med,* 66(4):352–355; Loch EG, et al (2000). Treatment of PMS with a phytopharmaceutical formulation (containing Vitex agnus-castus). *J Women's Health Gend-based Med,* 9(3):315–320; Lauritzen C, et al (1997). Treatment of PMS with Vitex agnus-castus: Controlled, double-blind study vs. pyridoxine. *Phytomedicine,* 4:183–189; Muehlenstedt D, et al (1978). Short-lived phase and prolactin. *Int J Fertil,* 23(3):213–218; Klepser T and Nisley N (1999). Chaste tree berry for PMS. *Alternative Medicine Alert,* 2(6):61–72.

178 *Black cohosh has few side effects:* Genazzani E and Sorrentino L (1962). Vascular action of acteina, active constituent of Actaes racemosa. *Nature,* 194:544–545; Jarry H and Harnisdifeger G (1985). Studies on the endocrine effects of the contents of cimicifuga racemosa. *Planta Med,* 1:46–49; Jarry H, et al (1985). Studies on the endocrine effects of the contents of Cimicifuga racemosa: 2. In vitro binding of compounds to estrogen receptors. *Planta Med,* 4:316–319; Gruenfeld J (1998). Standardized black cohosh (Cimicifuga) extract clinical monograph. *Quarterly Rev Nat Med,* Summer:117–125; Stolz H, et al (1982). An alternative to treat menopausal complaints. *Gyne,* 1:14–16; Vorberg G (1984). Treatment of menopause symptoms. Successful hormone-free therapy with Remifemin®. *ZFA,* 60:626–629.

178 *If estrogen levels are low:* Newall CA, et al (1996). *Herbal Medicine: A Guide for Healthcare Professionals:* London, UK, The Pharmaceutical Press.

178 *In addition to acting as an antidepressant:* Armanini D, et al (1999). Reduction of serum testosterone in men by licorice. *New Eng J Med,* 341:1158.

178 *It may also inhibit:* Tyler VE (1994). *Herbs of Choice.* Binghamton, NY, Pharmaceutical Products Press; Eagen PK, et al (2000). Medicinal herbs: Modulation of estrogen action. Era of Hope Meeting for the Department of Defense Breast Cancer Research Program, Atlanta, GA, June 8–11, 2000.

178 *This herbal supplement has:* Belford-Courtney R (1993). Comparison of Chinese and western users of angelica sinensis. *Austr J Me Herbs,* 5(4)87–91; Fackelmann K (1998). Medicine for menopause. *Science News,* 153:392–393.

179 *However, like many other herbs:* Though not all studies agree on this herb's activity, many do believe that, similar to other phytoestrogens, dong quai competitively inhibits excess estrogen levels from binding to estrogen receptors in the brain and the body. Studies suggest it may also promote nerve growth and delay atrophy. Leung AY and Foster S (1996). *Encyclopedia of Common Natural Ingredients Used in Food, Drugs, and Cosmetics,* 2nd edition, New York, John Wiley; Hirata JD (1997). Does dong quai have estrogenic effects in post-menopausal women? *Fertil Steril,* 68:981–986; Schimizu M, et al (1991). Evaluation of angelica radix by the inhibitory effect on platelet aggregation. *Chem Pharm Bull,* 39:2046–2048.

179 *red clover may block the proliferation:* Soffa VM (1996). Alternatives to hormone replacement for menopause. *Alternative Therapies,* 2(2):34–39.

179 *Since it can enhance or block:* LeBail JC, et al (2000). Effects of phytoestrogens on aromatase, 3-beta, and 17-beta hydroxysteroid dehydrogenase activities and human breast cancer cells. *Life Sci,* 66:1281–1291; Kurzer, MS and Xu X (1997). Dietary phytoestrogens. *Ann Rev Nutr,* 17:353–381.

179 *this whole food:* Lock M (1991). Contested meaning of menopause. *Lancet,* 337:1270–1272. For a more complete discussion of the benefits and risks of soy, please read *The Wisdom of Menopause,* by Dr. Christiane Northrup (New York, Bantam 2001, pp. 180–186, 548–549).

180 *Low magnesium levels:* Facchinitti F, et al (1991). Oral magnesium successfully relieves premenstrual mood changes. *Obstet Gynecol,* 78:177–181; Hull RCW and Joffee JR (1990). Hypomagnesemia: Physical and psychiatric symptoms. *JAMA,* 224:1749–1751.

180 *Magnesium deficiency may in fact increase:* Britton J, et al (1994). Dietary magnesium, lung function, wheezing and airway hyper-reactivity in a random adult population sample. *Lancet,* 334:357–362; deLourdes, Lima M, et al (1998). The effect of magnesium supplementation in increasing doses in the control of type 2 diabetes. *Diabetes Care,* 21:682–686; Sojka JE (1995). Magnesium supplementation and osteoporosis. *Nutr Rev,* 53:71–80.

180 *Low calcium levels:* Linder J, et al (1989). Calcium and magnesium concentrations in affective disorder. *Acta Psychiatr Scand,* 80:527–537; Bowden CL, et al (1988). Calcium function in affective disorders and healthy controls. *Biol Psychiatry,* 23(4):367–376.

180 *Taking calcium buffered with citrate and carbonate:* Thys-Jacobs S, et al (1998). Calcium carbonate and PMS: Effects on premenstrual menstrual symptoms. *Am J Obstet Gynecol,* 179:444–452.

181 *Even though one approach:* Harte JL, et al (1995). The effects of running and meditation on beta-endorphin corticotrophin-releasing hormone and cortisol in plasma and on mood. *Biol Psychology,* 40:251–265.

183 *People who are able to laugh:* Martin RA and Lefcourt HM (1983). Sense of humor as a moderator of the relation between stressors and moods. *J of Personality and Social Psychology,* 45:1313–1324; LaRoche L (1998). *Relax—You May Only Have a Few Minutes Left: Using the Power of Humor to Overcome Stress in Your Life and Work,* New York, Villard.

183 *Patients who saw a funny film:* Richman L (2001). *I'd Rather Laugh: How to Be Happy Even When Life Has Other Plans for You,* New York, Warner Books (quote is on jacket); Berk L (1989). Neuroendocrine and stress hormone changes during mirthful laughter. *Am J Med Sci,* 298(6):390; Cogan R, et al (1987). Effects of laughter and relaxation on discomfort levels. *J of Behav Med,* 10:139–144; Cousins

N (1991). *Anatomy of an Illness: As Perceived by the Patient,* New York, Bantam; Hafen BQ, et al (1996). Mind body health: the effects of attitudes, emotions, and relationships. Ch. 27, *The Healing Power of Humor and Laughter,* pp. 541–561, Boston, Allyn and Bacon; LaRoche L (1997). Living with the heart and soul of humor. In: *The Psychology of Health, Immunity, and Disease,* 9th International Conference. Hilton Head Island, South Carolina, December 12–13, 1997, pp. 105–117.

183   *Aerobic exercise for at least twenty minutes:* Krucoff C and Krucoff M (2001). Ch. 3: Mental health conditions, pp. 89–98, in: *Healing Moves: How to Cure, Relieve, and Prevent Common Ailments with Exercise,* New York, Three Rivers Press.

183   *Even if you exercise:* Camacho TC, et al (1991). Physical activity and depression. *Am J Epidemiol,* 134:220–231; Farmer ME, et al (1998). Physical activity and depressive symptoms. *Am J Epidemiol,* 128:1340–1351.

183   *Regular, challenging exercise:* Hughes JR (1984). Psychological effects of habitual aerobic exercise: A critical review. *Prev Med,* 13:33–78; Byrne A and Byrne DG (1993). The effect of exercise on depression, anxiety and other mood states. *J Psychosom Research,* 37:565–574; Martinsen EW (1990). Benefits of exercise for the treatment of depression. *Sports Med,* 9:380–389.

184   *Regular exercise improves many health conditions:* Hollenbach CB, et al (1985). Effect of habitual activity on the regulation of insulin. *J Amer Gerontol Soc,* 33:273–277.

184   *exercising to exhaustion:* King AC and Brassington G (1997). Enhancing physical and psychological function in older family caregivers: The role of regular physical activity. *Ann Behav Med,* 19:91–100; Esterling BA, et al (1990). Emotional expression, emotional repression, stress disclosure responses, and Epstein Barr virus viral capsid antigen titers. *Psychosom Med,* 52:397–410; Keast D (1996). Immune responses to overtraining and fatigue. In: L Hoffman-Goetz, ed., *Exercise and Immune Function,* pp. 121–141, Boca Raton, FL: CRC Press.

184   *after twelve to sixteen weeks of aerobic exercise:* Folks C and Simes W (1981). Physical fitness and mental health. *Am Psychol* 36(4):373–389; Hatfield BD, et al (1987). Serum ß-endorphin and affective responses to graded exercises in young and elderly men. *J Gerontology,* 42(4):429–431; Hoffman-Goetz L, et al (1986). Chronic exercise stress in mice depresses splenic T-lymphocyte mitogenesis in vitro. *Clin Exper Immunol,* 65:551–559; Plante T and Rodin J (1990). Physical fitness and enhanced psychological health. *Curr Psychol Res Rev,* 9:3–24.

184   *Physical inactivity in older adults:* Simmisick EM, et al (1993). Risk due to inactivity in physically capable older adults. *Am J Pub Health,* 83:1443–1450.

185   *Massage has been shown:* Field TF, et al (1997). Massage therapy effects on depression and somatic symptoms in chronic fatigue syndrome. *J of Chronic Fatigue Syndrome,* 3:43–61; Field T, et al (1996). Massage and relaxation therapies: Effects on depressed adolescent mothers. *Adolescence,* 31:903–911; Field T, et al (1997). Massage therapy lowers blood glucose levels in children with diabetes. *Diabetes Spectrum,* 10:237–239; Sunshine W, et al (1996). Massage therapy and transcutaneous electrical stimulation effects in fibromyalgia. *J of Clin Rheumatol,* 2:18–22; Irmson G, et al (1996). Massage therapy is associated with enhancement of the immune system's cytotoxic capacity. *Int J of Neurosci,* 84:205–218; Field T, et al (1997). Juvenile rheumatoid arthritis: Benefits from massage therapy. *J Ped Psychol,* 22(5):607–617.

185   *by releasing endorphins:* Calenda E and Weinstein E (2001). Ch. 3, Therapeutic Massage. In: M Weintraub, ed. *Alternative and Complementary Treatment in Neurologic*

Illness, New York, Churchill Livingstone, p. 27; Puustjarvi K, et al (1990). Effects of massage in patients with chronic tension headache. *Acupunct Electrother Res,* 15(2):159–162; Lipton SA (1986). Prevention of classic migraine headache by Digra massage of superficial temporal arteries during visual aura. *Ann Neurol,* 19(5):515–516; Kaada B and Tosteinbo O (1989). Increase of plasma and beta-endorphin in massage. *Gen Pharmacol,* 20(4):487–489; Day JA, et al (1987). Effect of massage on serum levels of ß-endorphin and ß-lipoprotein in healthy adults. *Phys Therapy,* 67:926–930; Field T, et al (1992). Massage reduces anxiety in child and adolescent pediatric psychiatric patients. *J Am Acad Child Adolesc Psychiatry,* 31:12; Field T (1995). Massage therapy for infants and children. *Dev Behav Pediatri,* 16:105–111; Ferrell-Torry AJ and Glick OJ (1993). The use of therapeutic massage as a nursing intervention to modify anxiety and the perception of cancer. *Cancer Nursing,* 16:93–101.

185 *Meditation and prayer and other intentional practices:* Kabat-Zinn J (1982). An outpatient program in behavioral medicine for chronic pain patients based on a practice of mindfulness meditation. *Gen Hosp Psychiat,* 4:33–47.

185 *Meditation may also stimulate:* Blauke O, et al (2002). Stimulating illusory own body perceptions. *Nature,* 419:269.

185 *because blood cells have many:* Dossey L (1993). Ch. 11: Prayer and healing: Reviewing the research. In: *Healing Words,* pp. 177–178, New York, HarperCollins.

185 *has helped to bolster red blood cells:* Dr. Larry Dossey has written a well-respected, scholarly book on the therapeutic effects of prayer called *Healing Words* (HarperCollins, 1993). Brand WG (1990). Distant mental influence of rate of hemolysis of human red blood cells. *J of Am Soc Psychatr Res,* 84(1):1–24; Byrd RC (1988). Positive therapeutic effects of intercessing prayer in a coronary care unit. *S Med J,* 81(7):826–829.

185 *Prayer is recognized as a complementary therapy:* Krebs K (2000). Stress management: CAM approach. In: *Encyclopedia of Stress,* vol. 3, p. 533, New York, Academic Press.

186 *Yoga has successfully treated:* Murthy PJ (1998). P300 amplitude and antidepression response to Sudarshan Kriya yoga (SKY). *J Affect Disorders,* 30:45–48.

186 *It can also improve:* Jedrezik, et al (1995). The TM-Sidh program pure consciousness, creativity, and intelligence. *J Creativity and Behav,* 19:270–275; Gackenbach J (1992). Interhemispheric EEG coherence in REM sleep and meditation. In: J Antrobus, ed. *The Neuropsychology of Sleep and Dreaming,* Hillsdale, NJ, Erlbaum; Gellhorn F and Kiely W (1972). Mystical states of consciousness: Neurophysiology and clinical aspects. *J Nerv Ment Dis,* 154:399–405.

186 *Daily bright light exposure alone:* Yamada N, et al (1995). Clinical and chronological effects of light therapy on nonseasonal affective disorders. *Biol Psychiatry,* 37:866–873; Kripke DF (1998). Light treatment for nonseasonal depression: Speed, efficacy, and combined treatment. *J Affect Disord,* 49:109–117; Corral M, et al (2000). Light therapy's effect on post-partum depression (letter). *Am J Psychiatry,* 157:303–304.

186 *You sit at a distance of 33 centimeters:* Oren DA, et al (2002). Open trial of morning light therapy for treatment of depression. *Am J Psychiatry,* 159:666–669.

Chapter Six

190 *the amygdala and the bed nucleus:* Del Abril A, et al (1987). The bed nucleus of the stria terminalis in the rat: Regional stress differences controlled by gonadal steroids

early after birth. *Dev Brain Res,* 32:295–300; Mizukami S, et al (1983). Sexual differences in nuclear volume and its autogeny in the rat amygdala.

190   *Changes in estrogen and progesterone:* Gray JA (1982). *The Neuropsychology of Anxiety,* Oxford, UK, Oxford University Press; LeDoux, JE (1996). *The Essential Brain,* New York, Simon & Schuster.

191   *signs of the brain's fear circuits firing away:* Wittstein IS, et al (2005). Neurohormonal features of myocardial stunning due to sudden emotional stress. *NEJM,* 352(6):539–548.

192   *They may come from her:* Sackhorn H, et al (1982). Hemisphere asymmetry in the expression of positive and negative emotions. *Archiv Neurol,* 39:210–218; Mendez MF, et al (1989). Neurobehavioral changes associated with caudate lesions. *Neurology,* 39:349–354; Starkstein SE, et al (1987). Comparison of cortical and subcortical lesions in the production of post-stroke mood disorders. *Brain,* 220:1045–1059; Altemus M, et al (1989). Neuropsychological correlates of menstrual mood changes. *Psychosom Med,* 51:329–336.

193   *People with this personality style:* Polowsky I (1973). Hypertension and personality. *Psychosom Med,* 35(1):50–56; Van Egeron LF (1974). Social interactions, communications, and coronary-prone behavior patterns. *Psychosom Med,* 44(1):2–18; Lane RD and Schwartz GE (1987). Induction of lateralized sympathetic output to the heart by the central nervous system during emotional arousal: A possible neurophysiological trigger of sudden cardiac death. *Psychosom Med,* 49:274–284; Smith WK (1945). The functional emotional significance of the rostral cingulate as revealed by its responses to electrical stimulation. *J Neurophysiol,* 8:241–255.

197   *Being in a threatening situation:* Bremner JD, et al (1993). Neurobiology of PTSD. In: *Ann Rev Psychiatry,* Washington, DC, APA Press; McFarlane AC (1984). Life events, disasters, and psychological distress. *Mental Health in Australia,* 1(13):4–6.

199   *In effect, with PTRD:* Van der Kolk BA (1989). The compulsion to repeat trauma, revictimization, attachment, and masochism. *Psychiatric Clinics of NA,* 12:389–411; Van der Kolk BA, et al (1985). Inescapable shock, neurotransmitters, and addition to trauma: Toward a psychobiology of post-traumatic stress. *Biol Psychiatry,* 20:314–325.

200   *In response to even the slightest changes in her environment:* Kraemer GW (1985). Effects of differences in early social experiences in primate neurobiological behavioral development. In: M. Reite and TM Fields, eds., *The Psychology of Attachment and Separation,* Orlando, FL, Academic Press, pp. 125–161; LeDoux JE, et al (1991). Indelibility of subcortical emotional memories. *J Cognitive Neuroscience,* 2:238–243; Pitman RK, et al (1993). Once bitten, twice shy. Beyond the conditioning model of PTSD. *Biol Psychiatry,* 33:145–148.

200   *Women who have experienced physical abuse:* Van der Kolk BA (1989). The compulsion to repeat trauma, revictimization, attachment, and masochism. *Psychiatric Clinics of NA,* 12:389–411; Freud S (1920). Beyond the pleasure principle. In: J Strachey, ed. translated, *The Standard Edition of the Complete Psychological Works of Sigmund Freud,* 18:3–64, London, Howarth Press; Finkelhor D and Brown A (1984). The traumatic impact of child sexual abuse. *Am J Orthopsychiatry,* 55:530–541.

201   *Previous traumatic experience:* Pitman RK, et al (1993). Once bitten, twice shy. Beyond the conditioning model of PTSD. *Biol Psychiatry,* 33:145–148; LeDoux JE (1990). Information flow from sensation to emotion: Plasticity of the neutral

computation of stimulus value. In: M Gabriel and J Moore, eds. *Learning Computational Neuroscience*, Cambridge, MA, MIT Press.

201 *Despite the genetic differences:* Mitchell D, et al (1985). Habituation under stress: Shocked mice show non-associative learning in T-maze. *Behav and Neurol Biol*, 43:212–217.

202 *The nicer, normal men and women don't seem:* Van der Kolk B (1989). The compulsion to repeat trauma: Revictimization, attachment, and masochism. *Psychiatric Clinics of NA*, 12:389–411.

202 *The PSA morphine pump:* Ademac RE (1991). Normal and abnormal limbic mechanism of emotive biasing. In: KE Livingston and O. Hornykiewicz, eds. *Limbic Mechanisms*, New York: Plenum Press; Squire LR and Zola Morgan S (1991). The medial temporal lobe memory system. *Science*, 153:2380–2386; Ademac RE (1991). Partial kindling of the ventral hippocampus: Identification of changes in limbic physiology which accompany changes in feline aggression and defense. *Physiol and Behav*, 49:443–454.

202 *Yet the fear circuits:* Axelrod J and Reisine TD (1984). Stress hormones: Their interaction and regulation. *Science*, 224:452–459; Yehuda R, et al (1990). Interaction of the HPA Axis and catecholaminergic system of stress disorder. In: EB Griller, ed. *Biological Assessment of PTSD*, Washington, DC, APA Press; Reita M and Field JM (1985). *The Psychobiology of Attachment and Separation*, Orlando, FL, Academic Press; Dorn LD, et al (1996). Responses to CRH in depressed and non-depressed adolescents: Does gender make a difference? *J Am Acad Child Adolesc Psychiatry*, 35:764–773.

203 *Yet ironically, a woman may have an enhanced intuitive capacity:* Kulka RA, et al (1990). *Trauma and the Vietnam War Generation: Report of Finding from National Vietnam Veteran Readjustment Study*, New York, Brunner/Mazel; Squire L (1987). *Memory and the Brain*, New York: Oxford University Press; Reiker PP and Carmen EH (1986). The victim-patient process: The disinformation and transformation of abuse. *Am J Orthopsychiatry*, 56:360–370; Burgess AW and Holstrom E (1979). Adaptive strategies in recovery from rape. *Am J Psychiatry*, 136:1278–1282; Van der Kolk BA and Eisler R (1994). Childhood abuse and neglect and loss of self-regulation. *Bull Menninger Clinic*, 58:145–168; Kraemer GW (1985). Effects of difference in early social experiences on primates' neurobiological/behavioral development. In: M Reite and TM Fields, eds. *The Psychobiology of Attachment and Separation*, pp. 135–161, Orlando, FL, Academic Press; Simpson CA and Porter GL (1981). Self-mutilation in children and adolescents. *Bull Menninger Clinic*, 45:428–438; Gardner DL and Cowdry RW (1985). Suicidal and parasuicidal behavior in borderline personality disorder. *Psychiatric Clinics of NA*, 8:389–403; Stone MH (1987). A psychodramatic approach: Some thoughts on the dynamics and therapy of self-mutilation in borderline personality disorder. *J Personality Disorder*, 1:347–349; Hernandez JT and Clemente RS (1992). Emotional and behavioral correlates of sex abuse among adolescents. *J Adolesc Health*, 13:658–662; Herzog DB, et al (1993). Childhood sex abuse in anorexia nervosa and bulimia nervosa. *J Amer Acad Child Adolesc Psychiatry*, 32:962–966.

211 *What are my thoughts telling me:* Vermitten E, et al (2002). Anxiety. In: VS Ramachradran, ed. *Encyclopedia of the Human Brain*, Vol. 1, p. 161, New York, Elsevier Science; Linehan M (1993). *Skills Training for Borderline Personality Disorder*, pp. 148–149, New York, Guilford Press; Jeffers S (1987). *Feel the Fear and Do It Anyway*, p. 13, New York, Harcourt-Brace Jovanovich.

Chapter Seven

221 *These activities numb your brain's anxiety circuits:* Gold M, et al (1997). Eating disorder.
     In: JH Lowinson, et al, eds. *Substance Abuse: A Comprehensive Textbook,* 3rd edition.
     Baltimore, Williams and Wilkins, pp. 319–330; Koob GF and Nestler EJ (1997).
     Neurobiology of drug addictions. *J Neuropsychiatry Clin Neurosciences,*
     9(3):482–497.

221 *Most of your brain circuits will have been altered neurochemically:* Snyder FR, et al
     (1989). The tobacco withdrawal syndrome: Performance decrement assessed on a
     computerized test battery. *Drug Alcohol Dependency,* 23(3):259–266; Steward SH, et
     al (1997). Anxiety sensitivity and self-reported reasons for drug use. *J Subst Abuse,*
     9:223–240; Gilbert DG, et al (1989). Effects of smoking and nicotine on anxiety.
     Psychophysiology, 26(3):311–320; McGehee DS, et al (1995). Nicotine
     enhancement of fast excitatory synaptic transmission in the CNS. *Science,*
     269:1692–1696; Hall SM, et al (1993). Nicotine, negative affect, and depression. *J
     Consult Clin Psychol,* 61(5):761–767; Balfour DJ (1994). Sensitization to
     mesoaccumbens dopamine response to nicotine. *Pharmacol Biochem Behav,*
     59(4):1021–1030; Koob CF, et al (1994). Alcohol, the reward system, and
     dependence. In: E Jansson, et al, eds. *Toward a Molecular Basis for Alcohol Use and
     Abuse,* Boston: Birkhuser-Verlag, pp. 103–114; Gold MS, et al (1997). Eating
     disorder. In: JH Lowinson, et al, eds. *Substance Abuse: A Comprehensive Textbook,* 3rd
     edition. Baltimore: Williams and Wilkins, pp. 319–330; Aceto MD, et al (1996).
     Dependence in 9THC. *J Pharmacol Experimental Therapeutic,* 278:1290–1295;
     Ditoro R, et al (1998). Regulation of delta-opoid receptors by tetra-hydro-
     cannabinol in NG108-15 hybrid cell. *Life Sciences,* 63:197–204; Jentsch JD, et al
     (1998). Repeated exposure to delta-9 tetra-hydrocannabinol to prefrontal cortex
     dopamine metabolism in the rat. *Neurosci Lett,* 246:169–172; Compton DR, et al
     (1990). Cannabis dependence and tolerance production. *Adv in Alcohol and Sub
     Abuse,* 9:129–147; Goritti MA, et al (1999). Chronic 9THC treatment induces
     sensitization to the psychomotor effects of amphetamines in rats. *Eur J Pharmacol,*
     365:133–142; Navarro M, et al (1998). CB_1 receptor cannabinoid receptor
     antagonist receptor antagonist-induced opiate withdrawal in morphine-dependent
     rats. *Neuroreport,* 9:3397–3402.

223 *Scientists have discovered that a tendency to anxiety:* Solvason HB, et al (2003).
     Predictors of response in anxiety disorders. *Psychiatr Clin NA,* 26:411–433;
     Hettema JM, et al (2001). A review and meta-analysis of the genetic epidemiology
     of anxiety disorders. *Am J Psychiatry,* 158:1568–1578.

223 *The medicines or other solutions that successfully treat:* Noyes R (2001). Generalized
     anxiety disorder: Co-morbidity in generalized anxiety disorder. *Psychiatr Clin NA,*
     24:41–55.

223 *People with untreated or poorly treated anxiety disorders:* Noyes R (2001). Generalized
     anxiety disorder: Co-morbidity in generalized anxiety disorder. *Psychiatr Clin NA,*
     24:41–55.

228 *If your parents had an addiction to alcohol:* Ciraulo DA, et al (1989). Parental
     alcoholism as a risk factor in benzodiazepine abuse. *Am J Psychiatry,* 146:1333.

231 *By relaxing muscles that go into spasm:* Spinella M (2001). Ch. 6, Herbal sedatives and
     anxiolytics. In: M. Spinella, *The Psychopharmacology of Herbal Medicines,* Cambridge,
     MA, MIT Press, p. 205; Gruenwald J, et al (1988). *PDR of Herbal Medicines,* 1st
     edition. Montvale, NJ, Medical Economics.

231 *Valerian increases GABA activity in the brain:* Upton R, ed. (1999). Valerian root: Analytical, quality control, and therapeutic monograph. Santa Cruz, CA, *American Herbal Pharmacopeia,* 1–25; Klepser TB and Klepser ME (1999). Unsafe and potentially safe herbal therapies. *Am J Health Syst Pharm,* 56:125–138.

231 *valerian is used in combination:* Schulz H, et al (1994). The effect of Valerian extract on sleep polygraphy in poor sleepers: a pilot study. *Pharmacopsychiat,* 27(4):147–151; Leathwood PD, et al (1982). Agneus extract of Valerian root (Valeriana officinalis L.) improves sleep quality in men. *Pharmacol Biochem Behav,* 17(1):65–71.

231 *It is not a safe, long-term solution:* Murray MT and Pizzorno JE (1999). Piper methysticum (kava). In: JE Pizzorno and MT Murray, eds. *Textbook of Natural Medicine,* 2nd edition, Edinburgh, Churchill Livingstone, pp. 887–92; Mathews JD, et al (1998). Effects of heavy usage of kava in physical health. *Med J Aust,* 148:548–555.

231 *Like valerian, kava kava may work:* Brinker F (1998). *Herb Contraindications and Drug Interactions,* 2nd edition, Sandy, OR, Eclectic Medical Publications.

232 *Antianxiety Medicinal and Herbal Primer:* Singh YN & Blumenthal M (1996). Kava: an overview. *Herbalgram,* 39:33–55; Lindenberg D and Pitule-Schodel HD. (1990). D.L. Kavain in comparison with oxazepam and anxiety disorder. *Fortsch Med,* 108:49–50; Almeida JC and Grimsley EW (1996). Coma from the health food store: Interaction between Kava and alprazolam. *Ann Int Med,* 125:940–941; Volz HP and Keizer M (1997). Kava-Kava extract WS 1490 vs. placebo in anxiety disorders. *Pharmacopsychotherapy,* 30:1–5; Jussofie A, et al (1994). Kavapyrone-enriched extract from piper methysticum as modulator of the GABA binding site in different regions of the rat brain. *Psychopharmacology,* 116(4):469–474.

233 *It prevents the histamine release:* Safayhi H, et al (1994). Chamazulene: An antioxidant-type inhibitor of leukotriene-B₄ formation. *Planta Med,* 60(5):410; Miller TH, et al (1996). Effects of some components of the essential oil of chamomile on histamine release from mast cells. *Planta Med,* 62(1):60–61; Viola H, et al (1995). Apigenin, a component of Matricaria recutita flowers, is a central benzodiazepine receptor–ligand with anxiolytic effects. *Planta Med,* 61(3):213–216.

233 *Some susceptible individuals:* Newall CA, et al (1996). *Herbal Medicines: A Guide for Healthcare Professionals.* London, The Pharmaceutical Press; Bradley PR (1992). *British Herbal Compendium,* Vol. 1, Bournemouth, British Herbal Medicine Association; Wichtl M and Bisset NG, eds. (1994). *Herbal Drugs and Phytopharmaceuticals.* Stuttgart: Medpharm Scientific Publishers; Bourin M, et al (1997). A combination of plant extracts in the treatment of outpatients with adjustment disorder with anxious mood: Controlled study vs. placebo. *Fundam Clin Pharmacol,* 11:127–132; Yoshioka T, et al (1998). Anti-inflammatory potency of dehydrocardione, a zedoary-derived sesquiterpine. *Inflamm Res,* 47(12):476–481.

233 *Ultimately, your health and longevity depend:* Hyytia P and Koub GF (1999). GABA receptor agonist in the extended amygdala decreases alcohol self-administration in rats. *Eru J Pharmacology,* 283:151–159; Koob CF, et al (1994). Alcohol, the reward system, and dependence. In: B Jansson et al, eds. *Toward a Molecular Basis for Alcohol Use and Abuse,* Boston, Birkhauser-Verlag, pp. 103–114; Richards S, et al (1991). Benzodiazepine receptors: New vistas. *Sem in the Neurosciences,* 3:191–203.

234 *It also helps some women with other chronic viral or bacterial syndromes:* Cohen RA, et al (1964). Anti-viral activity of Melissa officinalis (lemon balm) extract. *Proc Soc Exp Biol Med,* 117:431–434; Herman ES and Kucera LS (1967). Antiviral substances in

plants of the mint family (labiatae). II. Nontanninia polypherols of Melissa officinalis. *Proc Soc Exp Biol Med,* 124:869.

235 *You do, however, have to be careful:* Brinker F (1997). Contraindications and drug interactions. Sandy, OR, Eclectic Medical Publications; Blumenthal M, ed. (2000). *Herbal Medicine: Expanded Commission E Monographs,* Newton, MA, Integrative Medicine Connections, pp. 230–231.

235 *Herbal combinations of hops and valerian root:* Schmitz M and Jackel M (1998). Comparative study for assessing quality of life of patients with exogenous sleep disorders (temporary sleep onset and sleep interruption syndromes) with a hops-valerian preparation and a benzodiazepine drug. *Wien Med Wochenscle,* 148(13):291–298.

235 *Gingko biloba improves attention:* Sasaki K, et al (1999). Effects of bilobolide on GABA levels and glutamic acid decarboxylase in mouse brain. *Eur J Pharmacol,* 367(2–3):165–173.

235 *Ginseng is used by many people:* Bhattocharga SK and Mitten SK (1991). Anxiolytic activity of Panax ginseng roots: An experimental study. *J Ethnopharmacol,* 34(1):87–92.

236 *Ginseng also treats insomnia:* Nguyen TT, et al (1997) Majonoside-R_2 reverses social isolation stress-induced decrease in pentobarbital sleep in mice: Possible involvement of neuroactive steroids. *Life Sciences,* 61(4):395–402.

236 *Similar to benzodiazepine medications:* Nguyen TT, et al (1997). Majonoside-R_2 reverses social isolation stress-induced decrease in pentobarbital sleep in mice: Possible involvement of neuroactive steroids. *Life Sciences,* 61(4):395–402; Zhang JT, et al (1990). Preliminary study of antiamnestic mechanism of ginsenoside. *Chin Med J Engl,* 932–838; Tachikawa E, et al (1999). Effects of ginseng seponins on responses induced by various receptor stimuli. *Eur J Pharmacol,* 369(1):23–32.

238 *Several Chinese herbs treat:* Watanabe K (1975). Studies of the active principle of magnolia bark. Centrally acting muscle relaxant activity of magnolia and honokoil. *Jpn J Pharmacol,* 25:605–607; Naeser MA (1990). *Outline Guide to Chinese Herbal Medicines in Pill Form,* Boston: Boston Chinese Medicine; Xhu XZ (1990). Development of natural products as drugs acting on the CNS. *Mem Inst Oswaldo Cruz,* 86(supp. II):173–175.

238 *Like any medicine, herbs can have complex side effects:* Bensky D and Barolet R (1990). *Chinese Herbal Medicine Formulas and Strategies,* Seattle: Eastland Press.

239 *It lowers panic:* Baulieu EE (1997). Neurosteroids of the nervous system, by the nervous system, and for the nervous system. *Recent Progress in Hormone Research,* 52:1–32.

240 *If you have severe anxiety, panic, and fatigue:* Compagnone NA and Mellon SH (2000). Neurosteroids: Biosynthesis and function of these novel neuromodulation. *Frontiers Neuroendocrinol,* 21:1–56; Bayart F, et al (1989). The role of gender and hormonal state in aggressions during encounters between residential and intruder mice. *Med Sci Res,* 17:517–519; Majewska MD, et al (1987). Pregnenolone sulfate: An endogenous antagonist of the GABA receptor complex in the brain. *Brain Res,* 404:355–360; Simon NG (2002). Chapter 5, Hormonal process in aggressive behavior. In: *Hormones, Brain, Behavior,* Vol. 1, New York, Elsevier Science, p. 373.

240 *However, when the individuals took medicines:* Baxter LR, et al (1992). Caudate glucose metabolic rate changes with both drug and behavior therapy for obsessive compulsive disorder. *Arch Gen Psychiatry,* 48:681–689.

242   *It helps regulate anxiety and panic:* Linehan M (1993). *Skills Training Manual for Treating Borderline Personality Disorder,* New York: Guilford Press.

244   *Regular exercise of all kinds:* Krucoff C and Krucoff M (2001). *Healing Moves: How to Cure, Relieve, and Prevent Common Ailments with Exercise,* New York: Three Rivers Press, pp. 89–98.

244   *However, if you have a history of posttraumatic stress disorder:* Kaadu B, et al (1989). Increase in plasma endorphins in connective tissue massage. *Gen Pharmacol,* 20(4):487–489; Day JA, et al (1987). Effect of massage on serum level of beta endorphins and beta lipoprotein in healthy adults. *Phys Therapy,* 67(67):926–930.

245   *In fact, one type of CBT:* Fenwick P (1987). *Meditation and the EEG: The Psychiatry of Meditation.* Oxford, England: Clarendon Publishers, pp. 104–117; Mandall A (1979). Psychiatric aspects of sports. *Psychiatric Annals,* 9:154–160.

245   *Some authorities have documented:* Becker I (2000). Ch. 3. Uses of yoga in psychiatry and medicine. In: *Complementary and Alternative Medicine and Psychiatry,* PR Muskin, ed. Washington, APA Press; Shannah FF, et al (1996). Clinical case report: Efficacy of yoga techniques in the treatment of obsessive compulsive disorder. *Int J Neuroscience,* 85:1–17; Woods CJ (1993). Mood changes and perception of vitality: A comparison of the effects of relaxation, visualization, and yoga. *J Royal Soc. Med,* 86:254–258; Vahaia NS, et al (1966). Some ancient Indian concepts in the treatment of psychiatric disorders. *Br J Psychiatry,* 112:1089–1096; Miller JJ, et al (1995). 3 year follow-up and clinical implications of mindfulness-based stress-reduction intervention in the treatment of anxiety disorders. *Gen Hospital Psychiatry,* 17:192–200; Sundar S (1984). Role of yoga in the management of essential hypertension. *Acta Cardiol,* 39:203–208; Nagendra HR and Nagaranthna R (1986). An integrated approach of yoga therapy for bronchial asthma. *J Asthma,* 23:123–127; Schmidt T, et al (1997). Changes in cardiovascular risk factors and hormones during 3 months of Kriya yoga training and vegetarian nutrition. *Acta Physiol Scand,* supp 640:158–162; Ornish DM, et al (1979). Effects of vegetarian diet and selected yoga techniques in the treatment of coronary heart disease. *Clin Res,* 27:720A; Shaffer HJ, et al (1997). Comparing hatha yoga with dynamic group therapy for enhancing methadone maintenance treatment. *Altern Ther Health Med,* 3:57–66.

Chapter Eight

257   *it suppresses the immune system:* Cohen S, et al (1993). Negative life events, perceived stress, negative effect and susceptibility to the common cold. *J of Personal and Social Psychol,* 64:131–140; Rector N and Roger D (1997). The stress buffering effects of self-esteem. *Personal and Individ. Differences,* 23:799–808.

258   *Having good self-esteem about the quality:* Cobb S (1976). Social support as a moderator of life stress. *Psychsom Med,* 38:300–314; Sarason IG, et al (1985). Events, social support and illness. *Psychsom Med,* 47(2):156–163; Hofer MA (1984). Relationships as regulators: A psychobiologic perspective on bereavement. *Psychosom Med,* 46(3):196–195; Schulz ML (1998). *Awakening Intuition,* Ch 6, Blood and bones: Helplessness and hopelessness, pp. 139–166. New York: Crown Publishing.

259   *Having good self-esteem about your relationships:* Holmes TH and Wolff HG (1952). Life situations, emotions and backache. *Psychom Med,* 14:18; Kasl S, et al 1975). The experience of losing a job: Reported changes in health, symptoms, and illness behavior. *Psychosom Med,* 37:106–122; Saarijarn S, et al (1992). Couple therapy

improves mental well-being in lower back pain patients. *J Psychosom Res,* 36(7):651–626; Tarlau M and Smalheiser I (1951). Personality patterns in patients with malignant tumors of the breast and cervix. *Psychosom Med,* 13:117; Antoni MH and Goodkin K (1988). Host moderator variables in the promotion of cervical neoplasm: I. Personality facets. *J Psychosom Res,* 32(3):327–338; Bachman GL, et al (1988). Childhood sexual abuse and consequences in adult women. *Obstet Gynecol,* 71(4):631–640; Schulz ML (1998). *Awakening Intuition,* Ch. 7, Sex Organs and the Lower Back, pp. 167–196. New York: Crown Publishing.

259   *Or to be happy, do you continuously have to carry burden:* Bradley AJ, et al (1980). Stress and mortality in the small marsupial (antechinus stuartii). *Gen and Comp Endocrinol,* 40:188–200; Hencke PG (1992). Stomach pathology and the amygdala. In: *The Amygdala: Neurobiological Aspects of Emotion, Memory, and Mental Dysfunction,* pp. 323–328; New York: Williams and Wilkins, Sen RN and Anand BK (1967). Effect of electrical stimulation of the limbic system of the brain (visceral brain) on gastric secretory activity and ulceration. *Ind J Med Res,* 45:515–521; Glavin GB (1980). Restraint ulcer: History of current research and future implications. *Brain Res Bull,* 5(sup 1):51–55; Green JJ and Van der Valk JM (1966). Psychosomatic aspects of ulcerative colitis. *Gastroenterology,* 86:519; Bogdonoff MD, et al (1959). Acute effect of psychologic stimuli upon plasma non-esterified fatty acid level. *Proc Soc Exp Biol Med,* 100:503; Meyer A, et al (1945). Correlation between emotions and carbohydrate metabolism in 2 cases of diabetes mellitus. *Psychosom Med,* 7:335–341; Rosen H and Lidz T (1949). Emotional factors in precipitation of recurrent diabetic acidosis. *Psychosom Med,* 11:211–215.

259   *In addition, the health of the organs in your chest region:* Theorell T and Rabe RH (1971). Psychosocial factors and myocardial infarction. *J Psychosom Res,* 15:25; Parkes CM, et al (1969). Broken heart: A statistical study of increased mortality among widowers. *Brit Med J,* 1:740; Clayton PJ (1974). Mortality and morbidity after the first year of widowhood. *Arch Gen Psychiatry,* 30:747–750; Razavi D, et al (1990). Psychosocial correlates of estrogen and progesterone receptors in breast cancer. *Lancet,* 335:931–933; Levy SM, et al (1987). Correlation of stress factors with sustained depression of natural killer cell activity and predicted prognosis in patients with breast cancer. *J Clin Oncol,* 5(3):348–353; Dembroski TM, et al (1989). Components of hostility as predictors of sudden death and MI. *Psychosom Med,* 51:514–522; Van Egeron LF (1979). Social interactions, communications, and coronary-prone behavior pattern. *Psychosom Med,* 41(1):2–18; Lane RD and Schwartz GE (1987). Induction of lateralized sympathetic input to the heart by the central nervous system during emotional arousal. *Psychosom Med,* 49:274–284.

259   *The health of the thyroid, throat, and neck area:* Sonino N, et al (1993). Life events in the pathogenesis of Graves' disease: A controlled study. *Acta Endocrinologica,* 128:293–296; Voth HM, et al (1970). Thyroid hot spots in relationship to life stress. *Psychosom Med,* 32(6):561–568; Johansson G, et al (1987). Examination stress affects plasma levels of TSH and thyroid hormones differently in women and men. *Psychosom Med,* 49:390–396.

259   *If you do not have good self-esteem about your unique intuitive and intellectual gifts:* Barber HO, et al (1970). Psychosomatic disorders of the ear, nose, and throat. *Postgrad Med,* May 1970:156–159; Van Egeron LF (1979). Social interactions, communications, and coronary-prone behavior. *Psychsom Med,* 41(1):2–18; Martin C, et al (1991). Ménière's disease: A psychosomatic disease. *Rev Laryngol Otol Rhinol,*

112(2):109–111; Paulson GW and Dadmehr N (1991). Is there a premorbid personality typical for Parkinson's disease? *Arch Neurol,* 41(2):73–76; Cloninger RC (1991). Brain network underlying personality development. In: BJ Carroll and JE Barrett, eds. *Psychopathology and the Brain,* New York, Raven.

260 *The inability to feel good about your purpose in life:* Schulz ML (1998). *Awakening Intuition: Using Your Mind-Body Network for Insight and Healing* New York, Crown; MacDonald ER, et al (1994). Survival in amyotrophic lateral sclerosis: The role of psychological factors. *Arch Neurol,* 51:17–23; Philippoulos GS, et al (1958). The etiologic significance of emotional factors in onset and exacerbation of multiple sclerosis. *Psychosom Med,* 20:458–474.

263 *And once you get insight into how your mood circuits are wired:* Kosslyn SM, et al (2001). Neural foundations of imagery. *Nature Reviews,* 2:625–664.

263 *The treatment gave patients a sense of well-being:* Hull RS, et al (1991). Psychosocial intervention and immunity. In: R Adler, et al, eds. *Psychoneuroimmunology,* 2nd edition, pp. 1068–1072, New York, Academic Press; Achterberg J (1984). Imagery and medicine: Psychophysiological speculations. *J of Mental Imagery,* 8:1–4; Achterberg J and Lawlis GF (1979). The relationship between blood chemistries and psychological variables in cancer patients. *Multivariate Exp Res,* 41:1–10; Simonton C, et al (1978). *Getting Well Again,* Los Angeles, T. Archer; Gruber BL, et al (1989). Immune system and psychological changes in metastatic cancer patients while using revitalized relaxation and guided imagery. *Scand J of Behav Ther,* 17:25–46; Langer ES and Rodin J (1976). The effects of choice and enhanced personal responsibility for the aged. *J of Personal and Soc Psychol,* 34:191–198; Linehan MM (1993). *Skills Training Manual for Treating Borderline Personality Disorder,* New York, Guilford Press, p. 63.

264 *Using a psychological and behavioral version of Zen:* Linehan MM (1993). *Skills Training Manual for Treating Borderline Personality Disorder,* New York, Guilford Press, p. 63.

264 *You can also imagine "hurtful emotions":* Linehan MM (1993). *Skills Training Manual for Treating Borderline Personality Disorder,* New York, Guilford Press, p. 168.

264 *Affirmations are like mental aspirin:* Hay LL (1984). *Heal Your Body,* Carson, CA, Hay House; Hay LL (1984). *You Can Heal Your Life,* Santa Monica, CA, Hay House; For a discussion of how I used Louise Hay's affirmations to put my life-threatening sleep disorder in remission, please see the introduction of Schulz ML (1989). *Awakening Intuition: Using your Mind-Body for Insight and Healing.* New York, Crown.

265 *Suppose that you've figured out the intuitive message:* Linehan M (1993). Distress tolerance handout 5: Basic principles of accepting reality, p. 176. In: *Skills Training for Treating Borderline Personality Disorder,* New York, Guilford Press.

267 *Faith becomes a way of life:* Rosenblatt N and Horowitz J (1996). *Wrestling with the Angels: What Genesis Teaches Us About Our Spiritual Identity, Sexuality, and Personal Relationships,* New York: Delta, p. xvi; Kuscher HS (1983). *Why Bad Things Happen to Good People,* New York: Avon.

Chapter Nine

284 *The feminine brain structure tends to prevent:* Skuse DH, et al (1977). Evidence for Turner's syndrome of an impaired X-linked focus affecting cognitive function. *Nature,* 387:705–708, June 1993.

284 *but it is not clear if:* Brown, ET, et al (1989). ADHD gender differences in a clinically

referred sample. Paper presented at the Annual Meeting of the American Academy of Child and Adolescent Psychiatry. New York, October 1989.

287   *He was easily distracted and his impulsive:* Speck O, et al (2000). Gender differences in functional organization of the brain for working memory. *Neuroreport,* 11(11):2581–2585.

287   *Women who developed in utero in an androgen-excess:* Shaywitz BA, et al (1994). A conceptual framework for learning disabilities and ADHD. *Canad J Sp Ed,* 9:1–32, 1994; Berry CA, et al. Girls with ADD: A silent majority. *Pediatrics,* 76:801–809.

287   *Even though she was postmenopausal:* Quinn PO and K Nadeau (2000). Ch. 11. *Gender Hyperactivity in Children and Adults,* pp. 215–226, New York, Marcel Dekker; Brown, RT, et al, 1989. ADHD gender differences in a clinical referred sample. Paper presented at the Annual Meeting of the American Academy of Child and Adolescent Psychiatry, New York, October 1989.

287   *Girls with ADD may have increasingly severe problems:* Huessey HR (1990). The pharmacotherapy of personality disorders in women. Annual Meeting of the American Psychiatric Association, New York, 1990; Zametkin AS, et al (1990). Cerebral Glucose Metabolism in Adults with Hyperactivity of Childhood Onset. *New Eng J Med,* 232:1361–1366; Arpels, JC (1966). The female brain hyperestrogenic continuum from PMS to menopause. *J Reprod Med,* 41:633–939; Fink G, et al (1996). Estrogen control of central neurotransmission: Effect on mood, mental state, and memory. *Cell Molec,* 16:325–344.

288   *Thyroid disorders:* Weiss RE and MA Stern (2000). Ch. 25, Thyroid function and ADHD, pp. 414–429. In: *Attention Deficits and Hyperactivity in Children and Adults,* New York, Marcel Dekker.

288   *Suzanne's son got older, his attention style:* Barkley RA, et al (1991). ADD With and without hyperactivity. *Pediatrics,* 87:519–531; Weiss G and Hechtman LT (1993). *Hyperactive Children Grown Up.* New York, Guilford; Hart EL, et al (1995). Developmental change in ADHD in boys. *J Ab Child Psych,* 23:729–749.

289   *In fact she was inhibited:* Brann RT, et al (1989). ADHD gender differences in a clinical referral sample. Paper presented at the Annual Meeting of the American Academy of Child and Adolescent Psychiatry, New York, October 1989; Wheeler J and Carlson CL (1994). The social functioning of children with ADD with and without hyperactivity. *J Emot. Behav Dis,* 21:2–12.

296   *suspended the use of British-made Adderall:* G Harris and B Carey (Feb. 11, 2005). Senator says FDA asked Canada not to suspend drug. *New York Times.* www.nytimes.com/2005/02/11/politics/11drug.html.

296   *They can be abused and addictive:* Powers, CA (2000). The pharmacology of drugs used for the treatment of ADHD. In: PJ Accardo, et al, eds. *Attention Deficits and Hyperactivity in Children and Adults,* New York, Marcel Dekker.

298   *Ginkgo biloba prevents or inhibits blood platelets:* Spinella M (2001). Ch 5, Cognitive enhancers. In: *The Psychopharmacology of Herbal Medicine,* Cambridge, MA, MIT Press, p. 148; Krieglstein, J et al, (1986). Influence of an Extract of Ginkgo Biloba in Cerebral Blood Flow and Metabolism. *Life Sci,* 39(24):2327–34; Kim, YS, et al (1988). Antiplatelet and Antithrombotic Effects of a Combination of Ticlopidine and Ginkgo Biloba Extract (EGB 761). *Thromb Res,* 91(1)33–38.

298   *If you are concerned about bleeding:* Newall, CA, et al (1996). *Herbal Medicine: A Guide for Healthcare Professionals.* London, Pharmaceutical Press; Brinker, F. (1998). *Herb*

Contraindications and Drug Interactions, 2nd edition. Sandy, OR, Eclectic Medical Publishers.

299 *If you are concerned about your fertility:* Ondrisek, RR, et al (1999). Inhibition of human sperm motility by specific herbs used in alternative medicine. *J Assist Reprod,* 16:87–91; Ondrisek, RR et al (1999). An alternative medicine study of herbal effects on the penetration of zona-free hamster oocytes and the integrity of sperm DNA. *Fert Ster,* 171:517–22.

299 *Ultimately, if the brain cells don't have the proper amount:* Stevens, LJ, et al (1995). Essential fatty acid metabolism in boys of ADHD. *Am J Clin Nutr,* 62:761–768.

300 *There are no available studies examining SAMe's effect on the female brain:* Shekim, WD, et al (1990). SAMe in adults with ADHD: preliminary results from an open trial. *Psychopharm Bull,* 26:249–253.

300 *SAMe has been shown to help fibromyalgia:* Benedetto P, et al (1993). Clinical evaluation of SAMe versus TENS in primary fibromyalgia. *Curr Therap Research Clin Experimental,* 53:222–229; Grassetto M and Varotto A (1994). Primary Fibromyalgia Is Responsive to SAMe. *Curr Therap Research Clin Experimental,* 55:797–806; Barcelo HA, et al (1984). Effect of SAMe on experimental osteoarthritis in rabbits. *Am J Med,* 83(SA):55–59.

301 *Dosages of Siberian ginseng vary:* Blumenthal M, et al (1998). *The Complete German Commission E Monographs:Therapeutic Guide to Herbal Medicines.* Trans. S Klein, Boston American Botanical Council; Robbers JE, et al (1996). *Pharmacognosy and Pharmacobiotechnology,* Baltimore, Williams and Wilkins; Voylor, BK, et al (1999). The efficacy of ginseng: A systemic review of randomized clinical trials, *Eur J Clin Pharmacol,* 55:567–575; Persson J, et al (2004). The memory-enhancing effects of ginseng and gingko biloba in healthy volunteers. *Psychopharmacology,* 172:430–434; Tode T, et al (1999). Effect of Korean red ginseng on psychological functions in patients with severe climacteric syndromes. *Int J Gynecology Obstetrics,* 67:169–174.

301 *Avoid gotu kola:* Tyler VE, et al (1981). *Pharmacognosy.* Philadelphia, Lea and Febiger.

301 *Low levels of caffeine added to Ritalin:* Garfinkel, et al (1981). Response to methylphenidate and varied doses of caffeine in children with ADD. *Canad J Psychiatry,* 26(6)395–401.

301 *It makes me fall asleep:* Fenwick P (1987). In: M West, ed. *Meditation and the EEG: The Psychiatry of Meditation.* Oxford, England, Clarendon Press, pp. 104–117.

Chapter Ten

310 *Your choice of mates, your likes and dislikes:* Tulving E and Markonitsch HJ (1998). Episodic and declarative memory: Role of the hippocampus. *Hippocampus,* 8:198–204; Wise SP (1996). The role of the basal ganglia in procedural memory. *Semin-Neurosci,* 8:39–46.

311 *Women's two brains communicate more:* Allen LS and Gorskin RA (2002). "Sex differences in the human brain," in Vol. 4, *Encyclopedia of the Brain,* New York, Elsevier, pp 287–308; Allen LS, et al (1991). Sex differences in the corpus callosum in the living human being. *J Neuroscience,* 11(9):933.

311 *However, high doses of stress push the cells:* Diamond DM, et al (1996). Psychological stress impairs spatial working memory. *Behav Neuroscience,* 110:661–672; McEwen BS (1997). Possible mechanism for atrophy of the human hippocampus. *Mol Psychology,* 2:255–262.

312 *Severe maternal stress increases a child's chance:* Vallee M, et al (1997). Prenatal stress induces high anxiety and postnatal handling induces low anxiety in adult offspring,

J Neuroscience, 17:2626–2636; McEwen BS, et al (1968). Selective retention of corticosterone by limbic structures in the rat brain. *Nature,* 220:911–912.

312   *Premenopausally, the feminine brain has some protection:* Wolf OT, et al (2001). The relationship between stress-induced cortisol levels and memory differs between men and women. *Pseudoneuroendocrinology,* 26(7):711–720.

312   *Their brains' chronic, elevated levels of cortisol:* Dellu F, et al (1996). Reactivity to novelty during youth as a predictor of cognitive impairment in the elderly. *Psychoneuroendocrinology,* 21(5):441–453; DeRoche V, et al (1993). Individual differences in the psychomotor effects of morphine are predicted by reactivity to novelty and influenced by corticosterone secretion. *Brain Research,* 623:341–344; Meaney M, et al (1994). Early environmental programming of hypothalamus, pituitary, and adrenal responses to stress. *Seminars Neurosci,* 6:247–259.

313   *Ultimately, however, many of these factors:* Mesulan, MM (2002). Ch. 10. Aging, Alzheimer's disease, and dementia: Clinical and neurobiological perspectives. In: *Principles of Behavioral and Cognitive Neurology,* New York, Oxford Press, p. 441; Launer LJ, et al (1995). Medial temporal lobe atrophy in an open population of very old persons: Cognitive, brain atrophy, and sociomedical correlates. *Neurology,* 45:747–752.

313   *the cellular and anatomic changes:* Barnes CA and McNaughton BL (1980). Physiologic compensation for loss of afferent synapses in rat hippocampal granule cells during senescence. *J Physiol,* 309:473–485; Peters A, et al (1998). Are neurons lost from the primate cerebral cortex during aging. *Cerebral Cortex,* 8:295–300.

313   *Normal aging does not necessarily mean:* Peters A, et al (1998). Are neurons lost from the primate cerebral cortex during aging. *Cerebral Cortex,* 8:295–300.

313   *In normal aging, there is a cumulative* increase: Buell SJ and Coleman PD (1979). Dendritic growth in the aged human brain and failure of growth in senile dementia. *Science,* 206:854–856; Berwitz LI, et al (1989). Localization of the growth associated phosphoprotein GAP43 (B-SO, F') in the human cerebral cortex. *J Neurosci,* 9:990–995.

313   *By continuously putting yourself in novel environments:* Diamond M, et al (1985). Plasticity in the 904 day male rat cerebral cortex. *Exper Neurol,* 87:309–317; Connor JR, et al (1980). Aging and environmental influences on 2 types of dendritic spines in the rat occipital cortex. *Exptl Neurology,* 70:371–379.

314   *Wear and tear vs. Use it or lose it:* Rosenweig M and Bennett E (1996). Psychobiology of plasticity effects of training and experience in brain behavior. *Behav Brain Res,* 78:57–65; Ryff C and Singer B (1998). The contours of positive human health. *Psychol Inquiry,* 9:1–28; Weisel T and Hubal D (1965). Comparison of effects of unilateral and bilateral eye closure on cortical unit response in kittens. *J Neurophysiol,* 28:1029–1040.

314   *Adults like Felice who continue learning:* Shimamura A, et al (1995). Memory and cognitive abilities in university professors: Evidence of successful aging. *Psychol Science,* 6:271–277.

314   *The longer we hold emotional beliefs:* Alwin DF, et al (1991). *Political Attitudes Over the Life Span. The Bennington Women over 50 years,* Madison, University of Wisconsin Press.

315   *Normal aging may slow us down so we can think things through:* Mesulan MM (1989). Involutional and developmental implication of age-related neural changes in search of an engram of wisdom. *Neurobiol Aging,* 8:581–583.

316   *Immune cells become activated:* Rogers J (1993). Clinical trial of indomethacin in Alzheimer's patients. *Neurology,* 43:1609–1611.

317   *In the later stages of the illness:* Mesulan MM (2000). Ch. 10. Alzheimer's disease and dementia. In: *Principles of Behavioral and Cognitive Neurology,* New York: Oxford University Press, pp. 444–445.

318   *She may have had a mild forgetfulness for years:* Fox NC, et al (1998). Presymptomatic cognitive deficits in individuals at risk of familial Alzheimer's disease. *Brain,* 121:1631–1639.

318   *ApoE₄ in women seems to have a worse effect:* Hardy J (1997). Amyloid: the presenilins and Alzheimer's disease. *Trends Neurosci,* 20:154–157; Levy-Lahad E and Bird JD (1996). Genetic factors and Alzheimer's disease. *Ann Neurol,* 40:829–840.

319   *But if you keep your cholesterol levels low:* Simmons M, et al (1998). Cholesterol depletion inhibits generation of ß-amyloid in hippocampal neurons. *Proc Natl Acad Sci USA,* 95:6460–6464; Raber J, et al (2002). Androgens protect against apolipoprotein E₄-induced cognitive deficits. *J Neuroscience,* 22(12):5204–5209; Bartres D, et al (2002). Apo-lipoprotein E gender effects on cognitive performance in age-associated memory impairment. *J Neuropsychiatry Clin Neurosc,* 14(1):80–83.

319   *Brain-irritating amyloid plaques:* Bondareff W, et al (1989). Neurofibrillary degeneration and neuronal loss in Alzheimer's disease. *Neurobiol Age,* 10:709–715.

319   *Tangles also spread to areas in the brain:* Convit A, et al (1997). Specific hippocampal volume reduction in individuals at risk for Alzheimer's disease. *Neurobiol Age,* 18:131–138; Geula C and Mesulan MM (1994). Cholinergic systems and related neuropathological predictive patterns in Alzheimer's disease. Terry RD, et al, eds. *Alzheimer's Disease,* New York, Raven Press, pp 263–294.

321   *In women, significant atrophy is found at average by age fifty:* Hogervorst E, et al (2001). Serum total testosterone is lower in men with Alzheimer's disease. *Neuroendocrino Lett,* 11(3):163–168; Gibbs RB (1998). Impairment of basal forebrain cholinergic neurons associated with aging and long term loss of ovarian function. *Exp Neurol,* 151:289–302.

321   *Unresolved grief could turn into a major depression:* Berman KF, et al (1997). Modulation of cognition specific cortical atrophy by gonadal steroids: A PET study of women. *Proc Natl Acad Sci USA,* 94:8836–8841.

323   *They can't freely recall information:* Cummings JL (1990). Introduction. In: JL Cummings, ed. *Subcortical Dementia,* New York, Oxford University Press, pp. 3–16; Butter N, et al (1986). An assessment of verbal recall, recognition, and verbal abilities in patients with Huntington's Disease. *Cortex,* 22:11–32.

324   *Too little or too much thyroid hormone:* Arem R (1999). *The Thyroid Solution,* New York, Ballantine Books, Ch. 16: Curing the lingering effects of thyroid imbalances, p. 347.

325   *In fact, major depression occurs in between 1 and 15 percent:* Meyers CA (2002). Cancer patient's cognitive function. In: *Encyclopedia of the Human Brain,* New York, Elsevier Science, p. 592.

325   *taking bioidentical estrogen:* Arpels JAC (1996). The female brain: Hypoestrogenic continuum from PMS to menopause. *J Reprod Med,* 41:633–639.

326   *To age gracefully, you have to exercise every area:* Cotman CW and Niclo-Sanpedro M (1984). Cell biology of synaptic plasticity. *Science,* 225:1287–1294; Neill D (1995). Alzheimer's disease, maladaptive synaptoplasticity hypothesis. *Neurodegeneration,* 4:217–232; Verghese J, et al (2003). Leisure activities and the risk of dementia in the elderly. *New Eng J Med,* 348:2508–2516; Snowden A, et al (1996). Linguistic

ability in early life and cognitive function and Alzheimer's in late life. *JAMA*, 274(7):528–532; Wilson RS, et al (2002). Participation in cognitively stimulating activities and risk of incident Alzheimer's disease. *JAMA*, 287(6):742–748; Bell M, et al (2001). Neurocognitive enhancement therapy with work therapy. *Arch Gen Psychiatry*, 58:763–768; Hausdorff JM, et al (1999). The power of ageism on physical function of older persons: Reversibility of age-related gait. *J Am Geriatric Soc*, 47:1346–1349; Friedland RP (1993). Epidemiology, education, and the ecology of Alzheimer's disease. *Neurology*, 43:246–249; Katzman R (1993). Education and the prevalence of dementia and Alzheimer's disease. *Neurology*, 43:13–20; Mortimer JA (1997). Brain reserve and the clinical expression of Alzheimer's disease. *Geriatrics*, 52(supp 2):S50–S53.

327 *The more you learn, the more "connections" you build in your brain:* Zhang M, et al (1990). The prevalence of dementia and Alzheimer's disease in Shanghai, China: Impact of age, gender, and education. *Ann Neurol*, 27:428–437; Fratiglioni L, et al (1991). Prevalence of Alzheimer's disease and other dementias in an elderly population: Relationship with age, sex, and education. *Neurology*, 41:1886–1892; Mortimer JA (1993). Education and other socioeconomic determinants of dementia and Alzheimer's disease. *Neurology*, 43:539–544; Roth M (1986). The association of clinical and neuropsychological findings and its bearing on the classification and etiology of Alzheimer's disease. *Br Med Bulletin*, 42:42–50; Mortimer JA (1989). Do psychosocial risk factors contribute to Alzheimer's disease? In: AS Henderson and JH Henderson, eds., *Etiology of Dementia of the Alzheimer's Type,* Chichester, England, John Wiley and Sons, pp. 39–53; Kemper S, et al (1990). Telling stories: The structure and adult narratives. *Eur J Cognitive Psych*, 2:205–228; Ohm J, et al (1995). Close-meshed prevalence rates of different stages as a tool to uncover the rate of Alzheimer's disease-related neurofibrillary changes. *Neuroscience*, 64:209–217.

328 *Frequently participating in these relatively simple activities:* Fabrigoule C, et al (1995). Social and leisure activities and risk of dementia: A prospective, longitudinal study. *J Am Geriatr Soc*, 43:485–490.

329 *Usually, it's just associated with inactivity:* Alexander NB (1996). Gait disorders in older adults. *J Am Geriatr Soc*, 44:434–451; Chandler JM and Hadley EC (1996). Exercise to improve physiologic and functional performance in old age. *Clin Geriatr Med*, 12:761–784; Judge JO, et al (1996). Effects of age on the biomechanics and physiology of gait. *Clin Geriatr Med*, 12:659–678; Guralnik JM, et al (1995). Lower-extremity function in persons over the age of 70 years as a predictor of subsequent disability. *New Eng J Med*, 332:556–561; Sudarsky L (1990). Gait disorders in the elderly. *New Eng J Med*, 20:1441–1446; Oberg T, et al (1993). Basic gait parameters: Reference data for normal subjects, 10–79 years of age. *J Rehabil Res Dev*, 30:210–223; Guralnik JM, et al (1994). A short physical performance battery assessing lower extremity function: Association with self-reported disability and prediction of mortality and nursing home admission. *J Gerontol*, 49:M85–M94.

329 *The authors of the study concluded:* Cotman CW and Niclo-Sanpedro M (1984). Cell biology of synaptic plasticity. *Science*, 225:1287–1294.

329 *Many of the risk factors:* McGeer PL and Rogers J (1992). Anti-inflammatory agents as a therapeutic approach to Alzheimer's disease. *Neurology*, 42:447–449; McGeer PL, et al (1996). Arthritis and anti-inflammatory agents as a negative risk factor for Alzheimer's disease. *Neurology*, 47:425–432; McGeer EG and McGeer PL (1999). Chapter 26, Role of inflammatory processes and microglial

activation in Alzheimer's disease. In: RD Terry, et al, eds. *Alzheimer's Disease,* 2nd edition. Philadelphia, Lippincott, Williams, and Wilkins; Hull M, et al (1996). The participation of IL_6, a stress-inducible cytokine, in the pathogenesis of Alzheimer's disease. *Behav Brain Res,* 78:37–41; Walker DG et al (1997). Involvement of inflammation and complement in Alzheimer's disease. In: Antel J and Hartung HP, eds. *Clinical Neuroimmunology,* Oxford, Blackwell Science, pp 172–188; Fukumoto H, et al (1996). Association of a beta 40-positive senile plaques with microglial cells in the brains of patients with Alzheimer's disease and in non-demented aged individuals. *Neurodegeneration,* 5:13–17; DiPatre PL and Gelman BB (1997). Microglial cell activation in aging and Alzheimer's disease: Partial linkage with neurofibrillary tangle burden in hippocampus. *J Neuropathol Exp Neurol,* 56:143–149; Uchihara T, et al (1997). Activated microglial cells are co-localized with perivascular deposits of amyloid-beta protein in Alzheimer's disease brain. *Stroke,* 28:1948–1950; Sheng JG, et al (1997). Glia-neuronal interactions in Alzheimer's disease: Progressive association of IL-1 alpha + microglia and S100 beta + astrocytes with neurofibrillary tangle stages. *J Neuropath Exp Neurol,* 56:285–290; Klegeris A and McGeer PL (1997). b-amyloid protein enhances macrophage production of oxygen free radicals and glutamate. *J Neurosci Res,* 49:229–235; McGeer EG and McGeer PL (1997). Inflammatory cytokines in the CNS. *CNS Drugs,* 7:214–228; Shen Y, et al (1996). Characterization of neuronal cell death induced by complement activation. *Brain Res Protocols,* 1:186–194; Hull M et al (1996). Interleukin-6 associated inflammatory processes in Alzheimer's disease: New therapeutic options. *Neurobiol Aging,* 17:795–800; Fiebich BL, et al (1996). Effects of NSAID's on IL-1 beta-induced IL-6 mRNA and protein synthesis in human astrocytoma cells. *Neuroreport,* 7:1209–1213.

329 *So many of the anti-inflammatory treatment approaches:* Meziane H, et al (1998). Memory enhancing effects of secreted forms of ß-amyloid precursor protein in normal and amnesic mice. *Proc Natl Acad Sci,* 95:12683–12688; Roch JM, et al (1994). Increase of synaptic density and memory retention by a peptide representing the trophic domain of the amyloid $ß/A_4$ protein precursor. *Proc Natl Acad Sci (USA),* 9:7450–7454; Cotman CW and Nielo-Sampedroy M (1984). Cell biology of synaptic plasticity. *Science,* 225:1287–1294.

330 *However, frailty is not caused simply by advanced age:* Buchnes DM and Wagner EH (1992). Preventing frail health. *Clin Geriatri,* 8:1–17; Fried LP (1993). The epidemiology of frailty: The scope of the problem. In: HM Perry, et al, eds. *Aging Musculoskeletal Disorders and Care of the Frail Elderly,* New York, Springer, pp. 3–16; Fried LP, et al (2001). Frailty in older adults: Evidence of a phenotype. *J Gerontol,* 56A:M1–M11; Fried LP, et al (1998). Risk factors for 5 year mortality in older adults. *JAMA,* 279:585–592; Jarrett PG, et al (1995). Illness prevention in elderly patients. *Arch Int Med,* 155:1060–1064; Rockwood K, et al (2000). Conceptualization and measurement of frailty in elderly people. *Drugs Aging,* 17:295–302; Roubenoff R and Rall LC (1993). Humoral mediation of changing body composition during aging and chronic inflammation. *Nutr Rev,* 51:1–11; Fried LP and Walston J (1998). Frailty and failure to thrive. In: W Hazzard, ed. *Principles of Geriatric Medicine and Gerontology,* Columbus, OH, McGraw-Hill.

330 *Vitamin E (2000 iu/day):* Dickson DW (1997) The pathogenesis of senile plaques. *J Neuropath Exp Neurol,* 56:321–339; Rogers J, et al (1997) Inflammatory Mediators in Alzheimer's Disease. In: W Wasco and RE Tanzi, eds. *Molecular Mechanism of*

Dementia, Totowa, NJ, Humana Press, pp. 177–198; Steward WF, et al (1995). Risk of Alzheimer's disease and duration of NSAID use. *Neurology,* 50:1541–1545; Karpus TM and Saag KG (1998). NSAIDs and cognitive function: Do they have beneficial and deleterious effects? *Drug Safety,* 19(6):427–433; Luterman JO, et al (2000). Cytokine gene expression as a function of the clinical progression of Alzheimer's disease dementia. *Arch Neurology,* 57:1153–1160; Rogers J (1993). Clinical trial of indomethacin in Alzheimer's disease. *Neurology,* 43:1609–1611; Perry VH, et al (1996). Microglia activation and inflammation in the CNS. *J Neurochem,* 66:sup 70–sup 72.

330   *Its mechanism is similar to aspirin's:* Ladislav V (1990). Involvement of free radicals. *Neurobiol of Aging,* 11:567–571; Jeandel C, et al (1989). Lipid peroxidation, free radical scavenges in Alzheimer's disease. *Gerontology,* 35:272–282.

330   *High levels of antioxidants correlate:* Perrig WJ, et al (1997). The relationship between antioxidants and memory performance in the old and very old. *J Am Geriatr Soc,* 45:718–724; Yamada K, et al (1999). Protective effect of Idebeane and ∂-tocopherol in ß-amyloid 1-42 induced learning and memory deficits in rates: Implication of oxidative stress in ß-amyloid-induced neurotoxicity *in vivo, Eur J Neurosc,* 11(1):83–90.

331   *Zinc also bolsters immunity:* Cuajungco MP and Lees GJ (1977). Zinc metabolism in the brain: Relevance to human neurodegenerative disorders. *Neurobiol Dis,* 4:137–169; Duchateau J, et al (1981). Beneficial effects of oral zinc duration on the immune response of old people. *Am J Med,* 70:1001–1004; Fabris N and Mocchegiani E (1995). Zinc, human disease and aging. *Aging Clin Exp Res,* 7:77–93; Mares–Perlman JA, et al (1996). Association of zinc and antioxidant nutrients with age-related maculopathy. *Arch Opthalmol,* 114:991–997 Sandstead HH, et al (2000). History of zinc as related to brain function. *J Nutr,* 130:496s–502s.

331   *Selenium functions with d-alpha-tocopherol:* Berry MJ, et al (1991). Type I iodothyronine deiodinase is a selenocysteine-containing enzyme. *Nature,* 349:438–440; *Dietary Reference Intakes for Vitamin C, Vitamin E, Selenium, and Carotenoids.* Washington, DC, National Academy Press, 2000; Kohrle J (1996). Thyroid hormone deiodinases—a selenoenzyme family acting as gatekeepers to thyroid hormone action. *Acta Med Austrialia,* 23:17–30.

332   *In fact, some researchers have suggested that tocotrienols:* Elson CE (1995). Suppression of mevalenate pathway activities by dietary isoprenoids: Protective roles and cardiovascular disease. *J Nutr,* 125 (6 suppl):16665–16725; Kamat JP and Devasagayam TP (1995). Tocotrienols from palm oil as inhibitors of lipid peroxidation and protein oxidation in rat brain mitochondria. *Neurosci Letter,* 195:179–182; McIntyre BS, et al (2000). Antiproliferative and apopotic effects of tocopherols and tocotrienols on normal mouse mammary epithelial cells. *Lipids,* 35:171–180; Nesaretnam K, et al (1995). Effects of tocotrienols in the growth of human breast cancer cell line in culture. *Lipids,* 30:1139–1143; Nesaretnam K, et al (1998). Tocotrienols inhibit the growth of human breast cancer cells irrespective of estrogen receptor status. *Lipids,* 33:461–469; Parker RA, et al (1993). Tocotrienols regulate cholesterol production in mammalian cells by post-transcriptional suppression of 3-hydroxy-3-methylglutasyl coenzyme A reductase. *J Biol Chem,* 268:11230–11238; Pearce BC, et al (1994). Inhibitors of cholesterol biosynthesis; 2. Hypocholesterolemic and antioxidant activities of benzopyran and tertrahydronaphthalene analogue of the tocotrienols. *J Med Chem,* 37:526–514;

Tomeo AC, et al (1995). Antioxidant effects of tocotrienols in patients with hyperlipidemia and carotid stenosis. *Lipids*, 30:1179–1183.

332 *Long-term treatment with these drugs may prevent:* Shepherd J, et al (1995). Prevention of coronary artery disease with Pravastatin in men with hypercholesterolemia. *New Engl J Med*, 333:1301–1307; Donns JR, et al (1998). Primary prevention of acute coronary events with Lovastatin in men and women with average cholesterol levels. *JAMA*, 279:1615–1622.

332 *In addition to lowering the risk of osteoporosis:* Wolozin B, et al (2000). Decreased prevalence of Alzheimer's disease associated with 3-hydroxy-3-methylglutaryl Coenzyme A reductase inhibitors. *Arch Neurol*, 57:1439–1443.

332 *Coenzyme Q_{10} (200 mg/day) also seems to lower inflammation:* Rosenfeld FL, et al (1999). Coenzyme Q_{10} improves the tolerance of senescent myocardium to aerobic and ischemic stress: Studies in rat and in human atrial tissues. *Biofactors*, 9(2–4):291–299; Bergossi AM, et al (1994). Exogenous CoQ_{10} supplementation prevents plasma Vbiquione reduction induced by HMG-CoA reductase inhibitors. *Mol Aspects Med*, 15(suppl):187–193; Blznakov EM and Wilkins DJ (1998). Biochemical and clinical consequences of inhibiting Coenzyme Q_{10} biosynthesis by lipid lowering HMG-CaA reductase inhibitors (statins). *Advanc Therapy*, 15:218–228; Folkers K, et al (1990). Lovastatin decreases Coenzyme Q_{10} levels in humans. *Proc Natl Acad Sci USA*, 87:8931–8934; Lass A and Sohal RS (2000). Effect of Coenzyme Q_{10} and a-tocopherol content of mitochondria on the production of superoxide anion radicals. *FASEB J*, 14:87–94; Matthews RJ, et al (1998). Coenzyme Q_{10} administration increases mitochondrial concentrations and exerts neuroprotective effects. *Proc Natl Acad Sci USA*, 95:8892–8897.

333 *Acetyl-L-carnitine may improve levels:* Calvani M, et al (1992). Action of acetyl-L-carnitine in neurodegeneration and Alzheimer's disease. *Ann NY Acad Sci*, 663:483–486; DiDonato S, et al (1986). Systemic carnitine deficiency secondary to lack of electron transfer flavoprotein Vbiquione oxidoreductase. *Neurology*, 36:957–963; Arrigo A, et al (1990). Effects of acetyl-L-carnitine on reaction times and cerebrovascular insufficiency. *Int J Clin Pharmacol Res*, 10:133–137.

333 *Most supplements and medicine treatments:* Geula C and Mesulan MM (1994). Cholinergic systems and related neuropathological predilection patterns in Alzheimer's disease. In: RD Terry et al, eds. *Alzheimer's Disease*, New York, Raven Press, pp. 263–294.

334 *no major side effects have been associated:* Little A, et al (1985). A double blind placebo controlled trial of high dose lecithin in Alzheimer's disease. *J Neuro Neurosurg Psych*, 48:736–742; Wurtman RJ, et al (1981). Precursor cause of neurotransmitter synthesis. *Pharmac Rev*, 32:315–335; Rathman KL and Conner CS (1984). Alzheimer's disease: Clinical features, pathogenesis, and treatment. *Drug Intelligence and Clinical Pharmacology*, 18:684–691.

334 *Side effects of high doses include:* Spiers PA, et al (1996). Citicholine improves verbal memory in aging. *Arch Neurol*, 53:441–448; Babb SM, et al (1996). Different effect of CDP-choline on brain cytosolic choline levels in younger and older subjects as measured by proton magnetic resonance spectroscopy. *Psychopharmacol*, 127:88–94; Galletti P, et al (1991). Biochemical rationale for the use of CDP-choline in traumatic brain injury: Pharmacokinetics of the orally administered drug. *J Neurol Sci*, 130 suppl:S19–S25.

334 *Acetyl-L-carnitine:* Provesan P, et al (1995). Acetyl-L-carnitine restores choline acetyl transferase activity in the hippocampus of rats with partial unilateral fimbria-fornix

transection. *Int J Dev Neuroscience,* 13:13–19; White HL and Scates PW (1990). Acetyl-L-carnitine as a precursor of acetylcholine. *Neurochem Res,* 15:597–601; Livingston GA, et al (1991). Acetyl-L-carnitine in dementia. *Int J Geriatr Psychiatry,* 6:853–860; Sano M, et al (1992). Double-blind parallel design pilot study of acetyl-levo-carnitine in patients with Alzheimer's disease. *Arch Neurology,* 49:1137–1141.

334 *Combining lecithin/phosphatidylcholine with tacrine:* Eagger SA, et al (1991). Tacrine in Alzheimer's disease. *Lancet,* 337:989–992.

335 *Only 20 to 30 percent of patients have a positive response:* Wilcock G, et al (1993). An evaluation of the efficacy and safety of PTHA (tacrine) without lecithin in the treatment of Alzheimer's disease. 22:316–324; Nordbery A, et al (1997). Imaging of nicotinic and muscarinic receptors in Alzheimer's disease: Effect of tacrine treatment. *Dement Geriatri Cogn Disord,* 8(2):78–84.

335 *Tacrine also seems to decrease levels:* Lahiri DK, et al (1998). The secretion of amyloid b peptide is inhibited by tacrine. *Brain Res Mil Brain Res,* 62(2):131–40; Qizilbash N, et al (1998). Cholinesterase inhibitors of Alzheimer's disease: Metanalysis of tacrine trials. *JAMA,* 280(20):1777–182; Hake Am (2001). Use of cholinesterase inhibitors for treatment of Alzheimer's disease. *Cleveland Clinic J Med,* 68(7):608–615; Knapp MJ, et al (1994). A 30 week randomized controlled trial of high dose tacrine in patients with Alzheimer's disease. *JAMA,* 271:985–991; Rogers SL (1998). A 24 week double-blind placebo controlled trial of donepazol in patients with Alzheimer's disease. *Neurology,* 50:136–145.

335 *There are a few very rare individuals:* Krasowski MD, et al (1997). Natural inhibitors of cholinesterase: Implication for adverse drug reactions. *Can J Anaesthesiol,* 44(5):525–534.

336 *Siberian ginseng (625 mg 2/day) precipitates acetylcholine release:* Benishin CG (1992). Actions of ginsenoside Rb_1 on choline uptake in central cholinergic nerve endings. *Neurochem Int,* 21(1):1–5.

336 *and increases choline uptake:* Salim KM, et al (1997). Ginsenoside Rb_1 regulates ChAT NGF, and TrkA, mRNA expression in the rat brain. *Brain Res Mol Brain Res,* 47(1–2):177–182.

336 *This effect has been shown in diabetic patients:* Sotanicemi EA, et al (1995). Ginseng therapy in NIDDM, diabetic patients. *Diabetes Care,* 19:1373–1375.

336 *Ginseng is also an "adaptogen,":* Winther K, et al (1997). Russian root, Siberian ginseng improves cognitive function in middle-aged people whereas ginkgo biloba seems effective only in the elderly. XVI World Congress of Neurology, Buenos Aires, *J Neurol Sci,* 150 (suppl 90).

336 *Ginseng maintains and supports:* Salim KM, et al (1997). Ginsenoside Rb_1 regulates ChAT NGF, and TrkA, mRNA expression in the rat brain. *Brain Res Mol Brain Res,* 47(1–2):177–182; Liu M and Zhang JT (1996). Effect of ginsenoside Rb_1 on C-fos gene expression on cAMP levels in the rat hippocampus. *Chung Kao Yao C Hsudn Pao,* 17(2):171–174.

336 *It may facilitate behavioral adaptation to stress:* Raptin JR et al (1994). Demonstration of the anti-stress activity for the extract of ginkgo biloba using a discrimination learning task. *General Pharmacol,* 25:1009–1016; Oken BS, et al (1998). The efficacy of ginkgo biloba on cognitive function in Alzheimer's disease. *Arch Neurol,* 55:1409–1415; Kanowski S, et al (1996). Proof of efficacy of the ginkgo biloba special extract EGb761 in outpatients suffering from mild to moderate dementia. *Pharmacopsychiatry,* 29(2):47–56; Wettstein A (1999). Cholinesterase inhibitors and ginkgo extracts are comparable in the treatment of dementia. *Fortschr Med,*

117(5):48–49 (German); LeBars PL, et al (1997). A placebo-controlled, double-blind, randomized trial of an extract of ginkgo biloba of dementia. *JAMA*, 278(16):1327–1332; Itil JM, et al (1998). The pharmacological effects of ginkgo biloba in the brain of dementia patients. *Psychopharmacol Bull*, 34(3):391–397; Allain H, et al (1993). Effect of 2 doses of ginkgo biloba extract (EGb761) on the dual coding test in elderly patients. *Clin Ther*, 15(3):549–533; Hofferberth B (1994). The efficacy of EGb761 in patients with senile dementia of Alzheimer's type, a double-blind, placebo-controlled study of ginkgo biloba extract in elderly outpatients with mild to moderate memory impairment. *Curr Med Res Opin*, 12:350–355; Kristofikova Z, et al (1992). Change in high affinity choline uptake in the hippocampus of old rats after long term administration of two nootropic drugs (Tacrine and ginkgo biloba). *Dementia*, 3:304–307; Kleijnen J and Knipschold P (1992). Ginkgo biloba. *Lancet*, 340:1136–1139; Kleijnen J and Knipschold P (1992). Ginkgo biloba for cerebral insufficiency. *Br J Clin Pharmacol*, 34:352–358; Decker MW, et al (1988). Effect of training on a spatial memory task on high affinity choline uptake in hippocampus and cortex in young adults and aged rats. *J Neurosci*, 8(1):90–99; Taylor AE (1986). Frontal lobe dysfunction in Parkinson's disease: The cortical focus of neostriatal outflow. *Brain*, 105(pt 5): 845–883; Rogers SL, et al (1998). A 24 week double-blind, placebo-controlled trial of Donepezil in patients with Alzheimer's: Donepezil Study Group. *Neurology*, 50(1):136–148; Soholm B (1998). Clinical improvement of memory and other cognitive function by ginkgo biloba: A review of relevant literature. *Adv Ther*, 15(1):54–65; Hasse J, et al (1996). Effectiveness of brief infusion with ginkgo biloba special extract in dementia of vascular, Alzheimer's type. *J Gerontol Geriatr*, 29(4):302–309; Subhan Z and Hindmarch I (1984). The psychopharmacologic effects of ginkgo biloba extract in normal healthy volunteers. *In J PharmacolRes*, 4(2):89–93; Waret D, et al (1991). Comparative effects of ginkgo biloba extracts on psychomotor performance and memory in healthy subjects. *Therapie*, 46(1):33–36; Weather K, et al (1998). Effects of ginkgo biloba extract on cognitive function and blood pressure in elderly subjects. *Curr Therapeutic Res*, 59(12):881–888.

337 *Any vitamin E/alpha-tocopherol/alpha-tocotrienol supplement used with ginkgo:* Rosenblatt M, et al (1997) Spontaneous hyphema associated with ingestion of ginkgo biloba extract. *New Engl J Med*, 336:1108; Rowin J and Lewis SL (1996). Spontaneous bilateral subdural hematoma associated with chronic ginkgo biloba ingestion. *Neurology*, 46:1775–1776; Field B and Vadual R (1998). Ginkgo biloba and memory: An overview. *Nutr Neurosci*, 1:2565–2567.

337 *However, most people tolerate it very well:* Rosenblatt M, et al (1997). Spontaneous hyphema associated with ingestion of ginkgo biloba extract. *New Engl J Med*, 336:1108.

337 *However, huperzine A is supposed to be:* Cheng DH and Tang XC (1998). Comparative studies of Huperzine A, E_{2020}, and Tacrine on behavior and cholinesterase activities. *Pharmacol Biochem Behav*, 60(2):377–386.

337 *It has been used as a prescription drug:* Skolnick AA (1997). Old Chinese herbal medicine used for fever yields possible new Alzheimer's disease therapy. *JAMA*, 277(10):776; Cheng DH, et al (1996). Huperzine A: A novel and promising acetylcholinesterase inhibitor. *Neuro Report*, 8(1):97–101.

337 *One study showed that it prevented oxidative nerve cell death:* Ved HS, et al (1997). Huperzine A: A potential therapeutic agent for dementia reduces neuronal cell death caused by glutamate. *Neuro Report*, 8(4):963–968.

337   *Huperzine A hasn't been fully studied:* Tang XC, et al (1994). Comparison of the effects of natural and synthetic Huperzine A on rat brain cholinergic function *in vitro* and *in vivo. J Ethnopharmacol,* 44(3):147–155; Hanin I, et al (1993). Natural and synthetic Huperzine A: Effect on cholinergic function *in vitro* and *in vivo. Ann NY Acad Sci,* 695:304–306.

337   *people who smoke have been reported:* Van Duijn C and Hofman A (1991). Relation between nicotine intake and Alzheimer's disease. *BMJ,* 302:149–154; Warburton DM (1992). Nicotine as a cognitive enhancer. *Prog Neuropsychopharmacol Biol Psychiatry,* 16(2): 181–191; Sunderland T, et al (1985). Differential responsivity of mood, behavior, and cognition to cholinergic agents in elderly neuropsychiatric populations. *Brain Res,* 472(4):371–389.

338   *Since cyclic changes in serotonin levels:* LaDisich W (1994). Effect of progesterone on regional serotonin metabolism in the rat brain. *Neuropharmacology,* 13:877–883; Mendelson SD, et al (1993). Autoradiographic analysis of the effects of estradiol benzoate on ^{3}H-paroxetine binding on the cerebral cortex and dorsal hippocampus of gonadectomized male and female rats. *Brain Res,* 601:299–302.

338   *SAMe has been used for years:* Bell KM, et al (1998). S-adenosylmethionine treatment of depression: A controlled clinical trial. *Am J Psychiatry,* 145:1110–1114; Bottiglieri T, et al (1990). Cerebrospinal fluid SAMe in depression and dementia: Effects of treatment with parenteral and oral SAMe. *J Neuro Neurosurg Psych,* 53:1096–1098; Bottiglieri T and Hyland K (1994). SAMe levels in psychiatric and neurological disorders: A review. *Acta Neurol Scand,* 154:19–26; Morrison LD, et al (1996). Brain SAMe levels are severely decreased in Alzheimer's disease. *J Neurochem,* 67:1328–1331.

338   *In one study of 260 women and men:* Goodwin JS, et al (1983). Association between nutritional status and cognitive function in healthy elderly population. *JAMA,* 249:2917–2922.

338   *Everyone who has memory complaints:* Reynolds EH (1999). Interrelationships between the neurology of folate and B$_{12}$ deficiency. In: *Folic Acid in Neurology, Psychiatry, and Internal,* New York, Raven; Thornton NE and Thornton BP (1977). Geriatric mental function and serum folate. *South Med J,* 70:919–922.

338   *SAMe, B$_6$, B$_{12}$, folic acid, and L-carnitine:* Hutto BR (1997). Folate and cobalaminin in psychiatric illness. *Compr Psychiatry,* 38:305–314; Nilsson-Ehle H (1998). Age-related changes in cobalamin (vitamin B$_{12}$) handling: Implication for therapy. *Drugs Aging,* 12:277–292.

338   *Interestingly, high blood homocysteine levels:* Bots ML, et al (1997). Homocysteine, atherosclerosis, and prevalent cardiovascular disease in the elderly: The Rotterdam Study. *J Intern Med,* 242:339–347; Bostom AG, et al (1999). Non-fasting plasma total homocysteine levels and all-cause and cardiovascular disease mortality in elderly Framingham men and women. *Arch Intern Med,* 159:1077–1080; Bell IR, et al (1992). Plasma homocysteine in vascular disease, and in non-vascular demential of depressed elderly people. *Acta Psychiatr Scand,* 86:386–390; Riggs KM, et al (1996). Relations of vitamin B$_6$, vitamin B$_{12}$, folate, and homocysteine in cognitive performance in the normative aging study. *Am J Clin Nutr,* 63:306–314; Clarke R, et al (1998). Folate, vitamin B$_{12}$, and serum total homocysteine levels in confirmed Alzheimer's disease. *Arch Neurol,* 55:1449–1455; Beal MF (1995). Aging, energy, and oxidative stress in neurodegenerative diseases. *Ann Neurol,* 38:357–366; White AR, et al (2001). Homocysteine potentiates copper and amyloid beta peptide mediated toxicity in primary neural cultures: Possible risk factors in Alzheimer's

type neurodegenerative pathway. *J Neurochem,* 76:1509–1520; Homocysteine
Lowering Trialists Collaboration (1998). Lowering blood homocysteine with folic
acid based supplements: Meta-analysis of randomized trials. *BMJ,* 616:894–898.

338   *B$_6$, B$_{12}$, and folic acid:* Sheshadri S, et al (2002). Plasma homocysteine as a risk factor
for dementia and Alzheimer's disease. *New Eng J Med,* 346(7):476–483.

339   *Low levels of DHA (docosahexaenoic acid):* Kyle DJ, et al (1998). Low serum
docosahexaenoic acid (DHA) is a significant risk factor for Alzheimer's disease.
Presented at the 3rd Issfal Congress, Lyon, France, June 1–5, 1998; Niducker A
(1997). Probing genes, drugs, fatty acids in dementia. *Clinical Psychiatry News,*
December 1997, p. 4; Soderberg M, et al (1991). Fatty acid composition of brain
phospholipids in aging and in Alzheimer's Disease. *Lipids,* 26:421–425.

339   *Phosphatidyl Serine:* Pepeu G, et al (1996). A review of phosphatidyl serine
pharmacological and clinical effects. *Pharmacol Res,* 33(2):73–80; Crook JH, et al
(1991). Effects of phosphatidyl serine in age-associated memory impairment.
Neurology, 41:644–649.

339   *Phosphatidyl serine may make the membrane:* Crook JH, et al (1992). Effects of
phosphatidyl serine on Alzheimer's disease. *Psychopharmacol Bull,* 28:61–66.

339   *After the "mad cow" scare:* Cenacchi T, et al (1993). Cognitive decline in the elderly:
A double-blind, placebo-controlled, multi-center study of the efficacy of
phosphatidyl serine administration. *Aging (Milano),* 5(2): 123–133; Hibbeln JR and
Salem N (1995). Dietary polyunsaturated fatty acids and depression: When
cholesterol does not satisfy. *Am J Clin Nutrition,* 62:1–9.

339   *A woman's risk for getting Alzheimer's is reduced:* Kawas C, et al (1997). A prospective
study of estrogen replacement therapy and the risk of developing Alzheimer's
disease. *Neurology,* 48(6):1517–1521; Inestrosa NC, et al (1998). Cellular and
molecular basis for estrogen's neuroprotection: Potential relevance in Alzheimer's
disease. *Mol Neurobiol,* 17(1–3):73–86.

339   *A growing body of evidence suggests that long-term use:* Clen CL, et al (2002). Hormone
replacement therapy in relation to breast cancer. *JAMA,* 287(6):734–741.

340   *And it is very possible that the dosage of the neurosteroid:* Baulieu EE (1997).
Neurosteroids of the nervous system, by the nervous system, for the nervous
system. *Recent Progress in Hormonal Research,* 52:1–32.

341   *Excessive DHEA supplementation:* Brown RP, and Gerbary PL (1999). Chapter 1:
Integrative psychopharmacology. In: PR Muskin, ed. *Complementary and Alternative
Medicine and Psychiatry.* APA Press, Washington, DC, p. 44.

341   *Hormonal treatment improves reaction time:* Fedor-Freyburgh P (1977). The influence
of estrogen on well-being, and mental performance in climacteric and post-
menopausal women. *Acta Obstetrica Gynecologica,* Scandinavia, 64:5–6; Sherwin BB
(1988). Estrogen and/or androgen replacement treatment and cognitive
functioning in surgical menopausal women. *Psychoneuroendocrinology,* 13:345–357;
Luine VN (1985). Estradiol increases choline acetyl transferase activity in specific
basal forebrain nuclei and projection areas of female rats. *Experimental Neurol,*
89:484–490; Veliskova J, et al (1999). Estrogens have neuroprotective effects on
hippocampal cells in adult females following kainic acid–induced status epilepticus.
Epilepsia, 40(7):27; Henderson VW (1997). The epidemiology of estrogen
replacement therapy and Alzheimer's disease. *Neurol,* 48(suppl. 7):27–35; Sherwin
BB (1997). Estrogen effects on cognition in menopausal women. *Neurol,* 48(suppl.
7):21–26.

341   *Red wine has both a protective neuroeffect:* Gehn BD, et al (1997). Resveratol, a

polyphenolic compound found in grapes and wine, an agonist for the E_2 receptor. *Proc Natl Acad Sci USA*, 94:14138–14143.

342   *Your cognition and memory:* Hausdorff JM, et al (1999). The power of ageism on physical function of older persons: Reversibility of age-related gait changes. *J Am Geriatr Soc*, 47:1346–1349.

343   *Women who increase their level of baseline activity:* Jaffe K, et al (2000). Prospective study of physical activity and cognitive decline in elderly women. *Arch Intern Med*, 161:1703–1708.

344   *Studies indicate that learning new things:* Wilson RS, et al (2002). Participation in cognitively stimulating activities and the risk of Alzheimer's disease. *JAMA*, 287(6):742–747.

Acknowledgments

Charlie Brown had a whole gang of people who helped him play the game of life. I have been blessed with so many wonderful people who help me field balls, who pinch hit when I need it, and coach me into home plate.

The Coaches: I first thank God, who keeps me in the game and drafted me in the first place. I am grateful to Edith Kaplan, Marsel Mesulam, the work of the great Norman Geschwind, Deepak Pandya, and Marney Naeser, whose ideas and words have shaped what I know about the brain.

I am thankful to the staff of "P6," Dr. George McNeil, Dr. Gerry Robinson, Mary Romano-Liberty, Diane Boyce, the work of Marsha Linehan, Patrice Roy, and the MMC library, especially May Ann Lamont, for helping to teach me how to take what I know about the brain and ground it in psychiatry. I am grateful to Dr. Heather McClelland for great, honest, "plain English" phone conversations about neuropsychology and other things.

I am grateful to Dr. Satya Ambrose, Dr. Ted Kaptchuk, and Dr. Dan Bensky for teaching me so much about traditional Chinese medicine, acupuncture, and Chinese herbs.

I want to acknowledge the contributions of Edgar Cayce, Caroline Myss, Louise Hay, Winter Robinson, Teresa Moreira, the curandera, and others who helped shape the field of medical intuition and who all continue to inspire me every day.

The Team: I am grateful to Muriel Nellis, who helped me start this book in the first place. Thanks to Lisa Gorman, my "Jewish godmother," for teaching me how to fundraise and for giving me the Mont Blanc pen (among other things) with which I wrote this entire book on three-by-five-inch Post-it notes scotch-taped together. Thanks to Karen Kinne for taking my "chicken scratch" handwritten notes and translating them into a typed manuscript. You are one of Maine's great treasures. Thank you to Scott Leighton for expert graphic support. Then, of course, there is the greatest coach in the world, Leslie Meredith, senior editor at Free Press/Simon & Schuster, smart, quick, and open-minded. I am so thankful for being able to work with such a legend in publishing.

To the team at William Morris, including Cara Stein, Jennifer Rudolph-Walsh, and Joni Evans, for helping me to get in the left-hand lane. Thanks to Reid Tracy, Jill Kramer, and the staff at Hay House for supporting my work and for being a revolutionary in the publishing industry. Thank you to Naomi Judd for being a loving and supportive career coach and southern godmother who always is on hand with Kool-aid, Diet Rite, and great advice. You are truly an inspiration.

The Clubhouse: Thanks to Harraseeket Inn in Freeport, Maine, for the greatest five-star fast food. To Rhonda, the bartender, for serving up those "stiff Diet Cokes" daily, putting the TV on CNN, and understanding my peculiar affection for *The Boston Herald,* ketchup, chocolate ice cream, bananas, and peanut butter; Mary-Anne, Pierre, and all the other chefs; Peggy and Denise, the waitresses; Chip and Nancy Gray, the owners, all create a place where "everyone always knows your name." If it weren't for you, I'd be doing drive-thru.

Thanks to John Carpenter, for legal work when things are going well, and to Marshall Bellovin, Kate Debevoise, and Ben Campo at Drummond and Drummond, when they don't. In gratitude to Stacy, "your travel expert," for getting me bulkhead seats and understanding the frequent schedule changes; to Stacie, for the great cut, and Jen at Kiowa for the great color. Thank you to Ashley, who's brilliant, talented, and classy; your tireless work to improve yourself and the planet is an inspiration. To Joseph Saucier, at Escada, for rehabilitating my clothing personality, introducing me to sequins, and showing me the sales rack.

I am in deep gratitude to Laura Day ("The Real Thing") for being my NYC business yenta, intuitive colleague, confidant, and email "pen pal."

Why am I thankful for Wy and Roach? I treasure the long bus rides on the road, the antics in the hotel suites, and the general "ADHD" merriment we have. I love you guys! I am grateful to Bill Goddard for helping me with insurance and not yelling at me for totaling that rental car in the flash flood in Nashville. I also appreciate Jenny Adams, my southern Yoda. Thanks to Gil Levin, of the Cape Cod Institute, for inviting me to teach each summer, and giving me that great house on the ocean so I can spend a week with my friends, family, and a bunch of drag queens.

Thanks to the TV people: Thanks to Becker Entertainment and 480 Digital. Mikie, the casting person, you're a TV yenta. Thank you to Judge Judy and Judge Hatchett for being a daily, daytime TV inspiration and "keeping it real."

Thanks to Sue Abel, for keeping it clean; Mike Brewer, for keeping it mowed and plowed; and the two musketeers Pedro and Paulo for keeping it balanced. I am in gratitude to Paul Glazer, for putting up the steel girders in my spine; to Deb Merrill, for helping me walk upright; and to the great and powerful Fern Tsao, for rearranging my meridians. You help keep me in the game . . . if it weren't for you, I'd be out on waivers.

The Front Office: I am in gratitude to Noah Levy, a combination personal assistant, stylist, and all-around mensch. I can always depend on you for great food, company, advice, gossip, and getting front-row tickets to Joan Rivers. Thanks to Lizette, my Portuguese hair stylist and Feng Shui master, who's got a great big heart. I am grateful to Paulina for being a calming presence during my not-so-calm clinics. Thank you to Diane "What-A-Babe" Grover for lunches, scheduling, and occasional clandestine activities.

I am deeply grateful to Chris Northrup for being a wonderful mentor, colleague, friend, and angel. She pushes me when I need it and tolerates my unique driving habits. I cherish the lunches, the intellectual conversations, shopping expeditions, movies, and road trips (even the time the limo burned to the ground). I have laughed, cried, and learned so much. Thank you. Then there is Siggy, the receptionist, Dolly and Molly in the secretarial pool, Oscar, who does billing, and Francine and Buddy in the mail room. You make me human.

Index

About the Author

MONA LISA SCHULZ M.D., Ph.D., is a clinical assistant professor of psychiatry at the University of Vermont School of Medicine, Maine Medical Center, Portland, Maine. She holds a B.A. from Brown University, an M.D. from the Boston University of Science and Medicine, and a Ph.D. from their department of Behavioral Neurosciences. Dr. Schulz is also a practicing neuropsychiatrist specializing in head injury, dementia, stroke, Parkinson's disease, and the psychiatric aspects of medical conditions and a medical intuitive who does readings on individuals from all over the world, helping patients understand the connections between their health problems and their emotional states. She is the author of *Awakening Intuition: Using Your Mind-Body Network for Insight and Healing* and has been research partners with best-selling author Dr. Christiane Northrup since 1992. She is a frequent contributor to Dr. Northrup's popular monthly newsletter at Hay House as well as her monthly eletter at www.drnorthrup.com. She lives in Yarmouth, Maine, with her four cats, Miss Dolly, Miss Molly, Mr. Oscar, and the great Dr. Sigmund Feline. Visit the author's website at www.drmonalisa.com.